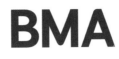

BMA

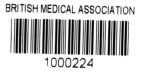

DRUG METABOLISM
IN DISEASES

DRUG METABOLISM IN DISEASES

Edited by

WEN XIE, MD, PhD

Professor of Pharmaceutical Sciences and Pharmacology,
The Joseph Koslow Endowed Chair in Pharmaceutical Sciences,
Director of the Center for Pharmacogenetics School of Pharmacy,
University of Pittsburgh, Pittsburgh, PA, United States

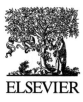

ELSEVIER

AMSTERDAM • BOSTON • HEIDELBERG • LONDON
NEW YORK • OXFORD • PARIS • SAN DIEGO
SAN FRANCISCO • SINGAPORE • SYDNEY • TOKYO
Academic Press is an imprint of Elsevier

Academic Press is an imprint of Elsevier
125 London Wall, London EC2Y 5AS, United Kingdom
525 B Street, Suite 1800, San Diego, CA 92101-4495, United States
50 Hampshire Street, 5th Floor, Cambridge, MA 02139, United States
The Boulevard, Langford Lane, Kidlington, Oxford OX5 1GB, United Kingdom

Library of Congress Cataloging-in-Publication Data
A catalog record for this book is available from the Library of Congress

British Library Cataloguing-in-Publication Data
A catalogue record for this book is available from the British Library

ISBN: 978-0-12-802949-7

For information on all Academic Press publications
visit our website at https://www.elsevier.com/

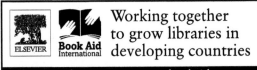

Working together
to grow libraries in
developing countries

www.elsevier.com • www.bookaid.org

Publisher: Mica Haley
Acquisition Editor: Kristine Jones
Editorial Project Manager: Molly McLaughlin
Production Project Manager: Edward Taylor
Designer: Mark Rogers

Typeset by TNQ Books and Journals

Contents

Contributors vii
Preface ix

1. Introduction of Drug Metabolism and Overview of Disease Effect on Drug Metabolism
R. SANE, M. SINZ

Introduction 2
Overview of Drug Metabolism 3
Disease Effects on Drug Metabolism 5
Disease Effects on Absorption Parameters 8
Changes in Blood Flow to Organs 10
Changes in Protein Binding 11
Disease Effects on Transporter Expression 13
Summary 14
References 16

2. Regulation of Drug-Metabolizing Enzymes and Drug Metabolism by Inflammatory Responses
E.T. MORGAN

Introduction 22
The Inflammatory Response 23
Regulation of DMEs by Inflammatory Mediators 28
Regulation of P450 Enzymes in Specific Disease States and Models 32
Disease-Dependent Drug–Drug Interactions 43
Mechanisms of Regulation 44
Conclusion 47
References 47

3. Regulation of Drug Transporters by Inflammation
D. KOJOVIC, M. PIQUETTE-MILLER

Introduction 59
Acute Inflammation 60
Models of Acute Inflammation 61

Effect of Acute Inflammation on Drug Transporters 62
Chronic Inflammation 75
Impact of Chronic Inflammation on Drug Transporters 75
Conclusion 80
References 80

4. Drug Metabolism in Kidney Disease
T.D. NOLIN

Conventional Drug-Dosing Paradigm in Kidney Disease 92
Nonrenal Clearance 93
Influence of Experimental Kidney Disease on Drug Metabolism 94
Influence of Kidney Disease on Drug Metabolism in Humans 99
Mechanisms of Altered Drug Metabolism in Kidney Disease 105
Summary 107
References 107

5. Drug and Fatty Acid Cytochrome P450 Metabolism in Critical Care
S.M. POLOYAC

Introduction 115
Stroke 118
Traumatic Brain Injury 123
Cardiac Arrest 127
Summary 133
References 133

6. Drug Metabolism in Cardiovascular Disease
J.C. COONS, P. EMPEY

Introduction 139
Cardiovascular Diseases 140
Cytochrome P-450 Expression in Cardiovascular Disease 147

Pharmacogenomics Related to Cardiovascular Drugs
    and Disease   148
Conclusion   153
References   153

7. Pharmacogenetic Factors That Affect Drug Metabolism and Efficacy in Type 2 Diabetes Mellitus
X. LI, Z.Q. LIU

Introduction   158
Sulfonylureas   158
Meglitinides   163
Metformin   166
Thiazolidinediones   169
α-Glucosidase Inhibitors   172
DPP-4 Inhibitors   173
Conclusion   173
References   173

8. Hepatic Drug Metabolism in Pediatric Patients
E.H.J. KREKELS, J.E. ROWER, J.E. CONSTANCE, C.A.J. KNIBBE, C.M.T. SHERWIN

Ontogeny of Hepatic Drug Metabolism   181
Ontogeny of Intrinsic Hepatic Clearance   184
Ontogeny of Hepatic Blood Flow   194
Ontogeny of Plasma Protein Binding   195
Ontogeny of Hepatic Drug Transporters   196
Conclusion   196
References   197

9. Drug Metabolism in Pregnancy
J.E. MOSCOVITZ, L. GORCZYCA, L.M. ALEKSUNES

Introduction   208
Physiological Adaptations During
    Pregnancy   208
Hepatic Phase I Enzymes   210
Hepatic Phase II Enzymes   215
Hepatic Transporters   218
Nuclear Receptors   220

Hormonal Regulation   221
Extrahepatic Regulation   230
Case Example: Bile Acid Metabolism and
    Transport   230
Conclusion and Future Directions   234
References   234

10. Estrogen-Metabolizing Enzymes in Systemic and Local Liver Injuries: A Case Study of Disease—Drug Interaction
X. CHAI, S. ZENG, W. XIE

Estrogen Sulfotransferase and Steroid Sulfatase in
    Estrogen Homeostasis: An
    Introduction   241
Estrogen Sulfotransferase and Its Regulation in Sepsis
    Response   243
Estrogen Sulfotransferase and Its Regulation in Liver
    Ischemia and Reperfusion Response   245
Steroid Sulfatase and Its Regulation in Estrogen
    Homeostasis and Inflammation in Chronic Liver
    Disease   248
Conclusions and Perspectives   251
Acknowledgment   251
References   252

11. Xenobiotic Receptors in the Crosstalk Between Drug Metabolism and Energy Metabolism
P. LU, W. XIE

Introduction   258
Xenobiotic Receptors as Master Regulators of Drug
    Metabolism   258
Drug Metabolism can be Affected by Energy
    Metabolism   260
Energy Metabolism can be Affected by Drug
    Metabolism and Xenobiotic Receptors   264
Conclusion and Perspectives   270
References   271

Index   279

Contributors

L.M. Aleksunes Rutgers University, Piscataway, NJ, United States

X. Chai University of Pittsburgh, Pittsburgh, PA, United States; Zhejiang University, Hangzhou, China

J.E. Constance University of Utah, Salt Lake City, UT, United States

J.C. Coons University of Pittsburgh, Pittsburgh, PA, United States

P. Empey University of Pittsburgh, Pittsburgh, PA, United States

L. Gorczyca Rutgers University, Piscataway, NJ, United States

C.A.J. Knibbe Leiden University, Leiden, The Netherlands; St. Antonius Hospital, Nieuwegein, The Netherlands

D. Kojovic University of Toronto, Toronto, ON, Canada

E.H.J. Krekels Leiden University, Leiden, The Netherlands

X. Li Xiangya Hospital Central South University, Changsha, China

Z.Q. Liu Xiangya Hospital Central South University, Changsha, China

P. Lu University of Pittsburgh, Pittsburgh, PA, United States

E.T. Morgan Emory University, Atlanta, GA, United States

J.E. Moscovitz Rutgers University, Piscataway, NJ, United States

T.D. Nolin University of Pittsburgh, Pittsburgh, PA, United States

M. Piquette-Miller University of Toronto, Toronto, ON, Canada

S.M. Poloyac University of Pittsburgh, Pittsburgh, PA, United States

J.E. Rower University of Utah, Salt Lake City, UT, United States

R. Sane Bristol Myers Squibb, Wallingford, CT, United States

C.M.T. Sherwin University of Utah, Salt Lake City, UT, United States

M. Sinz Bristol Myers Squibb, Wallingford, CT, United States

W. Xie University of Pittsburgh, Pittsburgh, PA, United States

S. Zeng Zhejiang University, Hangzhou, China

Preface

I am very happy to present you with this special topic book titled *Drug Metabolism in Diseases*.

Drug metabolism is essential for both drug therapy and drug safety. In addition to the genetic and environmental factors, diseases and physiological states of patients have profound effects on drug metabolism and disposition. Examples of diseases known to affect drug metabolism include liver and kidney diseases, inflammation and sepsis, cardiovascular diseases, and diabetes. Physiological conditions that can affect drug metabolism exist in pediatric and pregnant populations, and patients in critical care, among others. Understanding the pathophysiological effect on drug metabolism will help to guide better and safer use of clinical drugs. Armed with the knowledge of disease effects on drug metabolism, the use of drugs can be tailored to specific diseases or physiological conditions, which is highly relevant to personalized medicine and precision medicine. For these reasons, there is a great need for a book in this area. The topics mentioned earlier have been systemically covered in this book.

Another key feature of this book is the mechanistic insights by which diseases and physiological states affect drug metabolism. Examples of the mechanistic insights throughout the chapters include pharmacogenetics, xenobiotic receptors, nuclear receptors, transcriptional regulation of genes encoding drug metabolizing enzymes and transporters, crosstalk between xenobiotic metabolism and endobiotic metabolism, as well as the reciprocal effect of the expression and activity of drug-metabolizing enzymes and transporters on the clinical outcome of diseases. Understanding these mechanistic insights is paramount in harnessing the benefits of the knowledge communicated in this book and to improve the effective and safe use of drugs in the clinic.

I want to thank all of the contributing authors who are experts in the forefront of this emerging and exciting field of research. Special thanks go to Kristine Jones, Senior Acquisitions Editor at Elsevier, who initially approached me for a book project. I also want to thank Molly McLaughlin, Editorial Project Manager at Elsevier, who has been extremely helpful in all stages of the development of this book.

Wen Xie, MD, PhD
Professor of Pharmaceutical Sciences and
Pharmacology
The Joseph Koslow Endowed Chair in
Pharmaceutical Sciences
Director of the Center for Pharmacogenetics
School of Pharmacy
University of Pittsburgh, Pittsburgh, PA

CHAPTER

1

Introduction of Drug Metabolism and Overview of Disease Effect on Drug Metabolism

R. Sane, M. Sinz

Bristol Myers Squibb, Wallingford, CT, United States

OUTLINE

Introduction	2	*Changes in Gastric Emptying Time*	9
Overview of Drug Metabolism	3	**Changes in Blood Flow to Organs**	10
Disease Effects on Drug Metabolism	5	**Changes in Protein Binding**	11
Liver Disease	6	*Small Molecules*	12
Influence of Infection and Inflammation	6	*Protein Therapeutics*	12
Chronic Kidney Disease	7	**Disease Effects on Transporter Expression**	13
Disease Effects and Genetic Disorders	8		
Disease Effects on Absorption Parameters	8	**Summary**	14
Changes in Permeability	8	**References**	16
Changes in Gut and Lung Surface Area	9		

List of Abbreviations

AAG Alpha-1 acid glycoprotein
ADME Absorption, distribution, metabolism, and elimination
AUC Area under the curve
BCRP Breast cancer resistance protein
CHF Chronic heart failure
CL$_{int}$ Intrinsic clearance

COPD Chronic obstructive pulmonary disease
CYP Cytochrome P450
ER Extraction ratio
FcRn Neonatal Fc-receptor
GIT Gastrointestinal tract
IFN Interferon
IL Interleukin

Drug Metabolism in Diseases
http://dx.doi.org/10.1016/B978-0-12-802949-7.00001-8

MRP Multidrug resistance-associated protein
OATP Organic anion transporter protein
P-gp P-glycoprotein

TNF Tumor necrosis factor
UGT UDP-glucuronosyltransferase

INTRODUCTION

In today's contemporary medical arena, medical practitioners have at their disposal numerous drugs to treat acute and chronic diseases. Furthermore, many patients take multiple drugs daily to treat one or more illnesses, in particular, the increasing elderly population. This combination of events naturally leads to an increased number of drug–drug interactions. Although drug–drug interactions are becoming more predictable due to our understanding of the effect drugs can have on drug-metabolizing enzymes (expression and inhibition), our understanding of the effect of disease states on drug metabolism and disposition is less well comprehended. Many diseases are accompanied by one or more physiological and biochemical changes that affect the absorption, distribution, metabolism, and elimination (ADME) of drugs. These physiological/biochemical changes can lead to changes in the clearance, exposure, and distribution of drugs. There are often multiple changes that occur simultaneously during the course of a disease; therefore the overall effect of a disease on the pharmacokinetics of a drug can be complex. In addition, the degree of disease severity will also impact these changes, i.e., increasing severity of disease leading to increased physiological/biochemical changes.

The most significant organs related to absorption, drug metabolism, and elimination include the liver, intestine, and kidneys. Changes in the normal function of these organs due to disease will have the greatest impact on drug exposure and efficacy. For example, celiac disease and changes in drug absorption (Tran et al., 2013) or irregular drug absorption in Parkinson's disease (Nyholm and Lennernas, 2008). Liver disease has been shown to have an effect on the expression of drug-metabolizing enzymes and elimination of some drugs, as well as significant interindividual variations in drug elimination in the case of nonalcoholic fatty liver disease or cirrhosis (Merrell and Cherrington, 2011; Palatini et al., 2010). Lastly, kidney disease has been shown to have effects beyond the expected reduction in renal clearance with effects on drug-metabolizing enzymes and drug transporters in the kidney and liver (Nolin et al., 2003; Yeung et al., 2014).

In regards to drug interactions, the pharmaceutical industry has concentrated on the ability to predict and eliminate drug–drug interactions, but is less likely to incorporate the effects of various diseases on drug ADME disposition (drug–drug interactions) in the development process. This is particularly true during the drug discovery stage where the emphasis is bringing forward compounds that have appropriate potency to the target, reasonable overall ADME properties, and a satisfactory safety profile. It is not until clinical development that particular attention is given to how a drug may need to be tailored (changes in dose or dosing regimen) when administered while treating certain diseases or concomitant diseases associated with the primary disease.

This chapter begins with a survey of general drug metabolism principles, such as biotransformation reactions, major drug-metabolizing enzymes, drug absorption and elimination, and enzyme expression. For a more comprehensive review of drug metabolism principles, the reader is referred to Parkinson et al. (2013). The remainder of the chapter describes major physiological and biochemical changes that occur in various disease states and the impact they have on the ADME characteristics of drugs. These changes and their effects are illustrated throughout the chapter using pharmacokinetic principles and literature examples from animal and human studies. The majority of the chapter is devoted to drug metabolism and the effects that naturally occurring or inherited diseases can have on drug exposure. However, keeping in mind that metabolism is only one element that controls drug exposure, the remaining portion of the chapter describes how disease can affect the absorption and distribution of drugs, as well as physiological changes like blood flow, and how disease affects the expression of drug transporters.

OVERVIEW OF DRUG METABOLISM

Once administered, drugs can be eliminated from the body by one of three major pathways or routes. Polar drugs are often eliminated intact in urine via the kidneys, and both polar and nonpolar drugs can be eliminated directly through bile. Lastly, and most importantly, drugs are most often metabolized by endogenous enzymes and then eliminated in urine or bile. Drug metabolism or drug biotransformation is the process by which xenobiotics are enzymatically modified to make them more readily excretable and eliminate pharmacological activity. In most cases, this involves modifications to the parent drug or addition of functional groups that make the parent drug molecule more hydrophilic and more amenable to elimination. The liver is the major organ where drug metabolism occurs followed in significance by the intestine and kidneys and a variety of additional organs to a lesser degree (e.g., blood, skin, and brain).

Drug-metabolizing enzymes are generally categorized into two classes (phases 1 and 2) based on the type of biotransformation they perform. Phase 1 enzymes are considered oxidative or hydrolytic enzymes. They typically increase the polarity of molecules by the addition of a hydroxyl group (oxidative) or the unmasking of a more polar functionality (hydrolytic), such as the cleavage of an amide or ester bond to expose the free amine or carboxylic acid, respectively (both being more polar than the original amide or ester). Typical phase 1 oxidative enzymes include: cytochrome P450 (CYP) enzymes, flavin monoxidases, monoamine oxidases, alcohol/aldehyde oxidoreductases, and aldehyde/xanthine oxidases. Phase 1 hydrolytic enzymes include: epoxide hydrolases, esterases, and amidases. The CYP family of enzymes is by far the predominant biotransformation pathway or elimination process for the majority of marketed drugs. The second class of drug-metabolizing enzymes is called phase 2 conjugative enzymes. Phase 2 enzymes are responsible for conjugating parent drug molecules or metabolites derived from phase 1 metabolism by enzymatic addition of a polar group. Typical phase 2 enzymes and their conjugates include: UDP-glucuronosyltransferases (UGTs) that conjugate UDP-glucuronic acid, sulfotransferases that conjugate a sulfate group, glutathione S-transferases that conjugate the tripeptide glutathione, N-acyltransferases that conjugate an acetyl group to an amine, and methyltransferases (MTs) that conjugate a methyl group. All of these reactions create larger and more polar metabolites, making them easier for the body to eliminate in bile or urine. A notable exception is the MTs, which generally make the parent drug or metabolite less water soluble (less hydrophilic); fortunately MTs constitute a minor phase 2 pathway for drugs. Of all the phase 2 pathways, the UGT family of enzymes metabolizes the greatest number of drugs and metabolites.

The systemic exposure of the drug depends on its bioavailability. Following an oral dose, the drug moves through the lumen of the gastrointestinal tract (GIT) and is absorbed by the epithelial cells. The fraction that is absorbed from the lumen (f_a) can be metabolized by the enzymes in the gut wall. The fraction that escapes gut wall metabolism (f_g) then moves through the portal vein to the liver, where it undergoes first-pass metabolism. The bioavailability of a drug is the product of the fraction absorbed (f_a), the fraction that escapes gut wall metabolism (f_g), and the fraction that escapes hepatic clearance (f_h). Fig. 1.1 describes the processes a drug goes through before it reaches the systemic circulation (drug exposure). Disease states can influence one or more of these processes ultimately influencing the bioavailability of the drug and these will be discussed throughout the chapter.

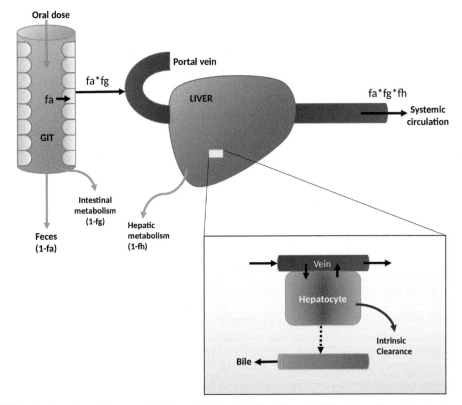

FIGURE 1.1 Overview of factors affecting oral bioavailability. Bioavailability depends on the fraction of dose absorbed (f_a), the fraction that escapes gut wall metabolism (f_g), and hepatic metabolism. The inset illustrates the route a drug may take once in the liver: from blood to hepatocyte, back to blood or into bile (either as parent drug or metabolite).

Changes to the expression (or activity) of these phase 1 and 2 enzymes, in particular the CYPs and UGTs, due to disease can have a significant impact on the rate of metabolism and systemic clearance of many drugs. Hepatic or liver clearance (CL_h) is related to liver blood flow (Q_h) and intrinsic clearance (CL_{int}) as shown in Eq. (1.1).

$$CL_h = Q_h \left(\frac{CL_{int}}{Q_h + CL_{int}} \right) \tag{1.1}$$

CL_{int} represents the ability of the liver to clear unbound drug from the blood when there is no flow limitation demonstrating the inherent enzyme activity of the drug-metabolizing enzyme. Any increase or decrease in the CL_{int} of an enzyme results in a commensurate change in the hepatic clearance of a drug that is significantly metabolized by that particular enzyme.

The regulation or expression of drug-metabolizing enzymes is controlled by two main mechanisms. The most common mechanism of enzyme expression is mediated by nuclear receptors or transcription factors, such as the aryl hydrocarbon receptor, pregnane X receptor, or constitutive androstane receptor (Xie, 2009). Combined, these three transcription factors control the normal expression of most drug-metabolizing enzymes and drug transporters. These receptors can be activated through binding of drugs to the receptor leading to an increase in the expression of drug-metabolizing enzymes (increased CL_{int} and CL_h). The second less common mechanism of enzyme regulation is stabilization of the mRNA or protein (Koop and Tierney, 1990). By decreasing the degradation of mRNA or protein (with no change in expression level), the pool of active enzyme accumulates and can be responsible for enhanced metabolism and greater elimination of drug.

Most often, diseases cause suppression of expression of drug-metabolizing enzymes (Gandhi et al., 2012; Shah and Smith, 2015). The suppression of CYPs is predominately attributed to decreases in transcription; however, it can also be due to decreased translation or posttranslational modification of CYPs (Riddick et al., 2004). This suppression leads to a reduction in enzyme expression and pool of active enzyme (decreased CL_{int} and CL_h), leading to decreases in drug elimination. Cytokines (small proteins associated with cell signaling) have been shown to suppress CYP expression and enzyme activity in human hepatocyte cultures, and the effect has been shown to be gene specific. For example, interleukin 1 (IL-1) has been shown to downregulate CYP2C8 and CYP3A4 mRNA expression by 75–95%, with no effect on CYP2C9 or CYP2C19 (Aitken and Morgan, 2007). Additional studies have shown that an increase in IL-6 concentration results in suppression of CYP3A4 in primary human hepatocytes (Dickmann et al., 2011).

DISEASE EFFECTS ON DRUG METABOLISM

Although aging is not considered a disease, studies on the liver changes that occur with age do provide insight into how diseases may affect the liver and its ability to metabolize drugs. As we age, our ability to metabolize drugs decreases; this is thought to be due to several physiological changes that occur in the liver, such as an ~40% decrease in liver volume, an ~40% decrease in liver blood flow, and a decline in the expression of CYP enzymes (Tajiri and Shimizu, 2013). Not surprisingly, acute or chronic diseases of the liver (e.g., cirrhosis or infection) that reduce the number of viable hepatocytes, alter blood flow, or reduce enzyme levels have an effect on drug clearance and exposure (Bruha et al., 2012).

Liver Disease

Liver cirrhosis is associated with several different effects that can influence drug exposure. A common phenomenon associated with liver cirrhosis is portal-systemic shunting, a physiological change that diverts blood drained from the intestine to the systemic circulation consequently bypassing its normal route to the liver. This shunting of blood away from the liver has the effect of increasing the bioavailability of orally administered drug as they do not enter the liver to be metabolized. In addition, a lack of oxygen (oxygen is an obligatory cofactor for all CYP enzymes) could lead to decreased enzyme function (Verbeeck, 2008). It has also been shown that CYP levels (reduced activity) in patients suffering from cirrhosis change with the severity of the disease. In the early stages of the disease, CYP3A4 and CYP2C19 are affected, whereas in the later stages of the disease CYPs 1A2, 2D6, and 2E1 are also affected (Verbeeck, 2008). The effects of liver cirrhosis appear to have a greater impact on the CYP enzymes than on phase 2 enzymes, such as glucuronidation, although in severe states of cirrhosis, glucuronidation is also affected.

Hypoxia is a deficiency in the amount of oxygen reaching tissues. Hypoxia due to cardio-respiratory disease has been shown to affect the metabolism and exposure of several drugs. The elimination of theophylline (CYP1A2 substrate) and tolbutamide (CYP2C substrate) was shown to change in patients with hypoxia. The elimination of theophylline was decreased, whereas the elimination of tolbutamide was increased (du Souich and Fradette, 2011). The clearance of both drugs is blood flow independent, so the changes in elimination are likely due to changes in mRNA expression or enzyme activity of CYP1A2 and CYP2C.

Influence of Infection and Inflammation

Infection and inflammation are known to have effects on the hepatic and extrahepatic metabolism of drugs, and many chronic diseases are often associated with inflammation (Gandhi et al., 2012; Morgan, 2001, 2009; Shah and Smith, 2015). Wooles and Borzelleca (1966) demonstrated that inflammation led to a decrease in drug metabolism activity in mice. After a decade, it was shown that infection along with inflammation led to an increase in quinine exposure (due to reduced metabolism) in patients suffering from malaria (Trenholme et al., 1976). Inflammation is the result of a tissue's attempt to adapt to cellular stress by releasing inflammatory cytokines IL-1β, IL-6, tumor necrosis factor alpha (TNF-α), and interferons (IFNs) α/γ, all of which are thought to affect (suppress) the expression of CYP enzymes (Feghali and Wright, 1997).

In patients with rheumatoid arthritis, chronic inflammation results in downregulation of CYP3A4 activity. In clinical studies with tocilizumab, an anti-IL-6 antibody approved for use in rheumatoid arthritis, an increase in the CYP3A4 function was observed by way of increased clearance of simvastatin, a substrate of CYP3A4 (Schmitt et al., 2011). Infusion with the anti-IL-6 antibody results in restoring the CYP3A4 levels to normal levels, leading to a significant decrease in simvastatin exposure [fourfold decrease in the area under the curve

(AUC), 1 week post dose] and a twofold increase in simvastatin clearance. Interestingly, there was no change in the pharmacokinetics of other concomitant medication, such as omeprazole (CYP2C19 substrate) or dextromethorphan (CYP2D6 substrate) (Evers et al., 2013).

Cancer is another disease associated with inflammation and inflammation-associated cytokines. Patients with cancer often exhibit higher levels of the cytokines IL-6 and TNF-α than normal healthy individuals (Filella et al., 1996). These elevated levels of cytokines are likely to downregulate the expression and enzyme activity of CYP3A4, which will affect the pharmacokinetics of many drugs, including anticancer drugs such as docetaxel, erlotinib, and vemurafenib.

Immunotherapy is a rapidly advancing field for the treatment of cancer. Ipilimumab is an anti-CTLA-4 (cytotoxic T-lymphocyte associated protein 4) antibody that has been approved for use in advanced melanoma. Inhibition of the CTLA-4 protein results in upregulation of T-cell activity and proliferation. Nivolumab is an anti-PD1 antibody, approved for use in non–small cell lung cancer and melanoma. PD1 is an immune checkpoint that dampens the immune response to prevent damage to tissues. Production of TNF-α, IL-6, and interferon γ is increased following anti-CTLA-4 and anti-PD-1 treatment (Curran et al., 2010; Dulos et al., 2012). In addition to the inflammation already inherent to cancer, these immunomodulators also have the potential to further impair CYP-mediated metabolism (Harvey and Morgan, 2014).

A study by Dostalek et al. found that the activity and expression level of CYP3A4 in patients with diabetes mellitus are significantly reduced. Human liver microsomes isolated from diabetic livers were shown to have decreased expression and activity of CYP3A4, which corresponds with observations from animal models of diabetes (Dostalek et al., 2011; Wang et al., 2007). The downregulation of CYP3A4 was attributed to elevated levels of IL-6 and TNF-α found in diabetic patients (Morgan, 1997).

Chronic Kidney Disease

The kidney contributes to the elimination and metabolism of a wide variety of drugs; it is highly distinct from other organs of metabolism since it has specific regions of cellular activity. The CYP enzymes are found in the renal tubular epithelial cells of the renal cortex. Studies in animal models of renal failure show a decrease in protein expression and activity of CYP2C11 and CYP3A2 (Leblond et al., 2002). Rat hepatocytes treated with uremic serum from patients with advanced chronic renal failure led to a 35% reduction in the protein and mRNA expression of CYP2C6, 2C11, 3A1, and 3A2, as well as a reduction in CYP enzyme activity (Dreisbach and Lertora, 2008). As in Eq. (1.1), hepatic clearance depends on intrinsic clearance, as well as drug-free fraction [Eq. (1.4)]. A decrease in CYP expression results in a decrease in intrinsic clearance, thus increasing the bioavailability. In renal failure, along with a decrease in enzyme expression, there is also a decrease in serum albumin levels, increasing the free fraction of the drug. The relative magnitude of changes in free fraction and intrinsic clearance will determine the net effect on the bioavailability. Moreover, phase 2 drug-metabolizing enzymes are also affected in patients with kidney disease as observed by the increase in morphine exposure (due to reduced glucuronidation of morphine) in patients as compared with control subjects (Osborne et al., 1993).

Disease Effects and Genetic Disorders

Some genetic disorders can lead to physiological/biochemical changes that may have profound effects on endogenous components, as well as drugs. Crigler—Najjar syndrome and Gilbert syndrome are disorders affecting the metabolism of bilirubin. In both Gilbert syndrome and Crigler—Najjar syndrome, activity of the phase 2 enzyme UGT1A1 is diminished or absent. Therefore drugs that are substrates of UGT1A1 cannot be metabolized/eliminated and can cause potential toxicity. A good example of this is irinotecan, an anticancer prodrug that is converted to its active form SN-38, which has a narrow therapeutic index. SN-38 is mainly inactivated by UGT1A1. The lack of the UGT1A1 enzyme leads to toxicity in oncology patients treated with irinotecan (Cecchin et al., 2009). Ethinylestradiol is also a substrate for UGT1A1 (Ebner et al., 1993). Therefore women using ethinylestradiol as a component of an oral contraceptive and who have Gilbert or Crigler—Najjar syndrome are at increased risk for hyperbilirubinemia and/or estrogen-related adverse effects. Glucuronidation and the impact of these genetic disorders have been reviewed in detail by Strassburg (2010) and de Wildt et al. (1999).

DISEASE EFFECTS ON ABSORPTION PARAMETERS

Absorption of drugs takes place by passive diffusion, paracellular transport, or carrier-mediated transport. Paracellular transport (i.e., movement of compounds through fenestrations in the membrane) depends on the size of the molecule (<500 g/mole) and largely occurs with water-soluble compounds that cannot move through cells. Active transport (carrier-mediated transport) is carried out by transporters that may exist on the luminal or abluminal side of cell membranes. Additional discussion of drug transporters and disease effects are described later in the chapter.

Changes in Permeability

A major mechanism of drug absorption through the GIT as well as transport through membranes is by passive diffusion. The rate of diffusion/transport in turn depends on the concentration gradient of the solute across the membrane, the surface area available for absorption, and the permeability of the compound as described by Eq. (1.2).

$$\text{Rate of transport} = \text{Permeability} \times \text{Surface area} \times \text{Concentration gradient} \qquad (1.2)$$

The permeability of a drug depends on its intrinsic properties such as size, lipophilicity, and charge. Small, lipophilic, and unionized molecules are able to cross membranes more easily than larger hydrophilic molecules, such as peptides and proteins. Permeability also depends on the thickness of the membrane. Patients with irritable bowel syndrome typically have damaged, thinner intestinal mucosa, leading to increased gut permeability (Spiller et al., 2000). In addition to changes in permeability, delayed gastric emptying observed in patients with irritable bowel syndrome is likely to change the rate and extent of absorption of drugs.

The distribution of compounds can also be influenced by permeability into tissues. The blood—brain barrier is vital in protecting the brain from xenobiotics. The endothelial cells in the brain capillaries have tight junctions as well as glial processes that limit the permeability of most polar drugs. In addition, a range of efflux transporters are expressed on the luminal side of brain capillaries and actively pump compounds out of the brain. Growth of certain brain tumors can cause changes in the vasculature of tumor microvessels leading to development of fenestrations in the endothelial layer (Loscher and Potschka, 2005). Preclinical tumor models have demonstrated that the permeability of certain drugs such as methotrexate is enhanced when tumors are present, allowing more drugs to reach the brain (Groothuis, 2000).

Changes in Gut and Lung Surface Area

Patients with celiac disease show atrophy of the villi in the small intestine, decreasing the surface area available for absorption. A study in patients with hypothyroidism showed that patients with celiac disease required higher doses of levothyroxine than patients without celiac disease (Tran et al., 2013). Interestingly, patients who were treated for celiac disease, who would presumably have repaired/improved small intestines over time, required lower doses of levothyroxine, supporting the hypothesis that the small intestine atrophy limited the absorption of levothyroxine.

The pulmonary route of administration is useful because absorption through the lungs can bypass first-pass metabolism in the liver. In addition, the lungs are highly vascularized and have a high surface area, allowing for efficient absorption. Several anesthetics and other drugs, such as nicotine, antibiotics, and protein therapeutics are administered via the lungs, resulting in good systemic exposure. Pulmonary disorders that result in airflow obstruction or airway inflammation due to asthma or chronic obstructive pulmonary disease (COPD) could potentially alter the extent of systemic absorption. However, in the case of inhaled corticosteroids, such as fluticasone, it has been shown that lowered systemic absorption of the steroids in patients with COPD and asthma actually reduces undesired suppression of the adrenal and pituitary glands as compared with healthy volunteers (Singh et al., 2003). In this situation, the limited systemic absorption is beneficial as it decreases drug exposure to the adrenal and pituitary glands thereby decreasing the undesired side effects.

Changes in Gastric Emptying Time

Gastric emptying and intestinal transit time determine the available time that a drug is in contact with the absorptive surfaces in the GIT. According to the pH-partition hypothesis, only unionized drugs can cross cellular membranes. Even weakly acidic drugs, more likely to be unionized in the stomach, are mostly absorbed from the small intestine due to its larger surface area. For example, for a weakly acidic drug such as paracetamol, the rate of absorption is directly related to the rate of gastric emptying; faster absorption is observed in subjects with faster gastric emptying (Prescott, 1974). On the other hand, the absorption of drugs that have slow dissolution characteristics could be enhanced by a decrease in gastric motility and increased intestinal transit time. The following examples help illustrate how these changes affect the absorption of drugs.

The treatment of Parkinson's disease depends on oral administration of the dopamine precursor levodopa. Levodopa is primarily absorbed from the small intestine; therefore gastric emptying is the rate-limiting step for onset of activity. Irregular gastric emptying time is common in patients with Parkinson's disease. Delays in gastric emptying cause the levodopa to be metabolized by amino acid decarboxylase enzyme in the gastric mucosa, decreasing the fraction absorbed by the gut (F_g), thus decreasing the bioavailability and limiting efficacy (Nyholm and Lennernas, 2008). Patients with celiac disease often exhibit faster gastric emptying than normal subjects. Using aspirin as a test substrate, Parsons et al. (1977) found that the time to reach maximal plasma concentration (T_{max}) is shorter in patients with celiac disease than in normal subjects.

Absorption of drugs also depends on their dissolution profile. Ketoconazole is an antifungal agent administered orally for the treatment of oral thrush. The oral absorption of ketoconazole is decreased in patients with AIDS, who exhibit achlorhydria, or decreased secretion of gastric acid (Chin et al., 1995). Ketoconazole is practically insoluble in water, except at a pH below 3. The decrease in gastric secretions due to achlorhydria or ingestion of food results in a stomach pH greater than 3, limiting the solubility of ketoconazole, resulting in incomplete absorption (Mannisto et al., 1982).

CHANGES IN BLOOD FLOW TO ORGANS

In all tissues perfused with blood, the vascular system acts as a transportation system delivering and removing substances. If the movement of a drug through a membrane (permeability) occurs readily, then the perfusion of the tissue is the rate-limiting step for drug distribution. The net rate of movement of drug in tissue (extravasation) is the difference between the rate of entry and the rate of exit of the drug and can be described by Eq. (1.3).

$$\text{Rate of extravasation} = Q \times (C_A - C_v) \tag{1.3}$$

where Q is the blood flow, C_A is the arterial blood concentration, and C_V is the concentration in venous blood. Therefore the rate of blood flow can determine the extent to which a drug can distribute into tissues and decrease systemic exposure.

Perfusion of metabolizing organs, like the liver, also drives the clearance of a drug, as described by the well-stirred model of hepatic metabolism, Eq. (1.4).

$$CL_h = Q_h \times ER = Q_h \times \left(\frac{f_u \times CL_{int}}{Q_h + f_u \times CL_{int}} \right) \tag{1.4}$$

where Q_h is the hepatic blood flow and CL_{int} is the intrinsic clearance. Therefore hepatic clearance/elimination depends on several factors, such as blood flow (Q_h), enzyme activity (CL_{int}), and protein binding (f_u). ER is the hepatic extraction ratio, a measure of the organ's relative efficiency in eliminating drug from blood. For example, an ER of 0.8 would be considered high as 80% of the drug is cleared from the blood as it passes through the liver.

Chronic heart failure (CHF) is associated with hypoperfusion (decreased Q_h) to the sites of drug clearance leading to decreased clearance of drugs. Decreased perfusion of tissues can also lead to a decrease in volume of distribution. This decrease in volume of distribution can be up to 40% of normal values, necessitating a decrease in loading doses (Woosley et al., 1986). In this situation, the half-life of a drug remains nearly unchanged due to the simultaneous decreases in volume and clearance. As described in Eq. (1.5), the half-life ($t_{1/2}$) of a drug is directly proportional to the volume of distribution (V) and inversely proportional to its clearance (CL).

$$t_{1/2} = \frac{0.693 \times V}{CL} \tag{1.5}$$

Therefore a simultaneous decrease in both the volume of distribution and clearance will minimize any changes in half-life.

Stenson et al. reported that patients with low cardiac output and therefore low hepatic blood flow exhibited higher exposures of lidocaine. They also observed that patients with CHF were more likely to have incidences of lidocaine toxicity and recommended that doses could be lowered while still maintaining therapeutic concentrations (Stenson et al., 1971). Quinidine, an antiarrhythmic, is another drug that shows altered kinetics in patients with CHF. The decreased perfusion of blood limits the absorption of quinidine, when administered orally, possibly due to the decreased blood flow to the intestine. The volume of distribution and the clearance of quinidine are also decreased, leading to no change in the elimination half-life (Crouthamel, 1975). Thus diminished blood perfusion to absorption sites, such as the GIT and muscle (intramuscular route of administration), can result in altered absorption of drugs.

As described previously, in liver cirrhosis, a fraction of the blood in the portal vein does not come in contact with the hepatocytes, thus decreasing the hepatic blood flow. This shunting of liver blood flow decreases the hepatic blood flow by 20—40% of normal (Moreno et al., 1967). As seen in Eq. (1.4), the hepatic clearance of a drug is directly proportional to the blood flow to the liver as well as intrinsic clearance. For a drug with high ER, a decrease in blood flow can decrease hepatic clearance, thus improving bioavailability. On the other hand, for drugs with low ERs, the clearance depends more on the intrinsic clearance (CL_{int}) and free fraction (f_u), than on blood flow. Therefore a change in blood flow should not greatly affect the hepatic clearance of low-ER drugs. However, in liver disease, both blood flow to the liver and enzyme activity are decreased, and it is not possible to distinguish between the influences of these two physiological changes, highlighting the complexity of effects that can occur even within a single disease.

CHANGES IN PROTEIN BINDING

The distribution of drugs within the body depends on its reversible binding to blood cells, plasma proteins, and tissues. The fraction of drug not bound to plasma proteins is available to distribute to tissues or sites of action. The protein—drug complex acts as a transport system to carry drugs to their site of action. This form of transport is particularly important for drugs with poor solubility. Protein-bound drug is also unavailable for clearance by hepatic/renal metabolism as only the free (unbound) drug is available for clearance. Therefore protein binding is an important factor that influences the distribution and clearance of drugs.

Small Molecules

The majority of small-molecule drugs bind to serum albumin, alpha-1 acid glycoprotein (AAG), lipoproteins, or erythrocytes. Albumin is the most abundant protein in human serum with a concentration of 35–50 g/L and a long half-life of about 20 days. Albumin binds to acidic drugs as well as endogenous compounds such as bile acids. AAG is another plasma protein that is present in the plasma but at much lower concentrations than albumin. Due to its acidic nature, AAG is much more likely to bind to basic drugs. The concentration of AAG in plasma is highly variable in healthy as well as diseased individuals. Increases in AAG concentration can result from chronic renal failure, inflammatory diseases, trauma, cancer, and acute myocardial infarction, but reduced in liver cirrhosis (Edwards et al., 1982; Paxton and Briant, 1984).

A decrease in plasma binding could result in an increase in the volume of distribution of certain drugs. In patients with cirrhosis of the liver, serum albumin concentrations are lowered; this can potentially increase the free fraction of drugs. Unbound drug is available to cross into tissues; therefore an increase in free fraction will increase the tissue distribution of a drug. Increased tissue distribution will in turn result in lower plasma concentrations, leading to a higher apparent volume of distribution. For example, the apparent volume of distribution for cefodizime is three times larger in patients with cirrhosis than in healthy individuals (el Touny et al., 1992). Also, patients with ascites (accumulation of fluid in the peritoneal cavity) have a significant increase in volume of distribution of some drugs due to the additional fluid possibly requiring the use of larger loading doses (Verbeeck, 2008).

A good example of the influence of protein binding on clearance is naproxen. Naproxen is a low-ER drug with high plasma binding, and thus has a very small volume of distribution (0.15 L/kg). The plasma binding of naproxen is decreased in patients with alcoholic cirrhosis, resulting in unbound free fractions that are two- to fourfold higher than in healthy subjects (Williams et al., 1984). However, there is no large change in the volume of distribution. This is because for drugs with a small volume of distribution, a large change in the unbound fraction will not result in major changes in the volume of distribution. Williams et al. (1984) did not find a difference in the total clearance of naproxen; however, the clearance of unbound drug ($CL \times f_u$) was decreased by about 60% in patients with cirrhosis.

Hypoalbuminemia can result from burns, malnutrition, or cirrhosis of the liver and patients with chronic kidney disease show decreased serum albumin levels (Liumbruno et al., 2009; Klammt et al., 2012). In patients with renal failure, the unbound fraction of cerivastatin is increased but the total exposure is more than doubled due to the decrease in hepatic uptake of the statin by organic anion transporter proteins (OATPs) (Vormfelde et al., 1999). This example once again illustrates the complex nature (i.e., multiple simultaneous changes) of pharmacokinetic modifications that occur in disease states sometimes leading to unpredictable changes.

Protein Therapeutics

Therapeutic proteins are extensively used in the treatment of cancer, HIV, and other diseases. Monoclonal antibodies, IFNs, and cytokines are examples of some of the macromolecular therapeutic proteins. Proteins are not good substrates for CYP enzymes and are generally cleared by renal filtration or degraded to smaller peptides or amino acids in several tissues by circulating phagocytic cells or by their target antigen-containing cells (Keizer et al., 2010). In addition, antibodies and endogenous immunoglobulins can sometimes be protected from degradation by binding to protective receptors [the neonatal Fc-receptor (FcRn)], which explains their long elimination half-lives (up to 4 weeks).

FcRn recycles both albumin and IgG thereby circumventing each from being degraded and extending their half-life (Sand et al., 2014). The fusion of a therapeutic protein with albumin enhances the half-life of the therapeutic protein by taking advantage of the recycling of human albumin by FcRn receptors. A deficiency in FcRn receptors due to a mutation (β2-microglobulin gene) can result in decreased plasma concentrations of IgG and albumin (Wani et al., 2006). This disorder is known as familial hypercatabolic hypoproteinemia, and the hypercatabolism (high clearance) of IgG and albumin can result in lower concentrations of albumin fusion proteins or therapeutic antibodies (Kim et al., 2007). Disorders such as this are likely to influence the pharmacokinetics of therapeutic antibodies and albumin-fused therapeutic proteins.

DISEASE EFFECTS ON TRANSPORTER EXPRESSION

ATP-binding cassette transporters (ABC transporters) play a major role in the maintenance of nutrient uptake and elimination of waste products, energy generation, and cell signaling. The normal function of some human ABC transporters is to secrete cytotoxic compounds (dietary cytotoxics and therapeutic drugs) from cells. These transporters [P-glycoprotein (P-gp), breast cancer resistance protein (BCRP), and multidrug resistance-associated protein (MRP) 1] are highly expressed in the gut, liver, and kidneys, where they restrict the bioavailability of administered drugs. P-gp and BCRP in particular are also expressed in the epithelia of sensitive tissues (e.g., the brain and placenta) and in stem cells, where they perform a barrier function.

The transporters in the kidney are located in the plasma membranes of epithelial cells of the proximal tubules and actively facilitate the movement of drug into the cells from the plasma against the membrane negative charge. The drug transporters are broadly divided into organic anion transporters, organic cation transporters, and ATP-dependent active transporters, e.g., P-gp. The renal and nonrenal clearances of many drugs are significantly reduced in patients with chronic renal failure. Animal models of chronic renal failure indicate that renal failure modulates the efflux transporter, Mrp2 in the liver and kidneys with an increase of 70−200% in protein and mRNA expression (Laouari et al., 2001). In contrast, a decrease in the expression and function of intestinal P-gp was found in a rat model of renal failure (Veau et al., 2001).

Inflammation modulates both the activity and expression of the CYP isozymes and transporters. For example, cytokines have been shown to decrease the mRNA expression of CYP 3A4 and increase the expression of MDR1A1 in a Caco2 cell model (Bertilsson et al., 2001). In a study by Ufer et al., P-gp mRNA and protein expression was decreased in patients with ulcerative colitis as compared with healthy volunteers. Expression of BCRP and P-gp in the intestinal tissue is reduced in patients with ulcerative colitis (Ufer et al., 2009). The effect of inflammatory mediators on expression of P-gp is not entirely understood and results from different studies seem to vary. In a study by Bauer et al. (2007), a time-dependent change in P-gp activity postexposure to TNF-α was observed in capillary preparations from rat brain. They observed a transient reduction in activity, followed by a sustained increase. A similar observation was made by Seelbach et al. (2007) using a carrageenan-induced inflammatory pain model in rats. In a rat model of lipopolysaccharide-induced inflammation, the authors found that the expression of Mdr1a mRNA in the brain and liver was decreased. In addition to this, the authors also found a loss of CYP3A and Oatp2 mRNA in the liver (Goralski et al., 2003). Downregulation of P-gp and BCRP in the intestinal tissue may increase the exposure of orally administered substrates of P-gp and BCRP. Decreased expression of these transporters in the brain may increase the distribution of transporter substrates across the blood–brain barrier leading to higher CNS exposures. However, there have been no reports that directly connect the change in transporter function in disease states with changes in the pharmacokinetics of drugs. Dubin–Johnson and Rotor syndromes are two genetic disorders that cause an increase in conjugated bilirubin. Dubin–Johnson syndrome is caused by a defect in the multiple drug-resistance protein 2 gene (ABCC2/MRP2), whereas Rotor syndrome is due to mutations in *SLCO1B1* (OATP1B1) and *SLCO1B3* (OATP1B3) transporters (Strassburg, 2010). OATP1B1 and OATP1B3 are localized on the basolateral membrane of hepatocytes and mediate the uptake of drugs from the portal vein into hepatocytes. Deletion or decreased expression of ABC transporters and OATPs may affect distribution of substrates into various tissues and lead to increased GaN toxicity. Individuals with mutations in these genes could be more susceptible to toxicity of drugs and metabolites. For example, patients with a mutation in the *SLCO1B1* gene exhibited higher concentrations (increased AUC) of repaglinide than those with the wild-type genotype (Kalliokoski et al., 2008).

SUMMARY

Table 1.1 provides an overview of the possible changes to pharmacokinetic parameters when changes in physiology, absorption, protein binding, or enzyme activity occur. As the table shows, a change in the extent of absorption should not influence the clearance and volume of distribution of a drug. However, the overall exposure of the drug could be affected. The clearance of a drug depends on the blood flow to the metabolizing organ (Q), intrinsic clearance (Cl_{int}), and drug free fraction (f_u) [Eq. (1.4)]. Therefore a change in blood flow or free fraction can affect drugs with high ER differently than drugs with low ER. The clearance of high-ER drugs is perfusion (blood flow) limited. A reduction in blood flow to organs of metabolism can affect drugs with a high ER by decreasing the clearance and extending the half-life, whereas the clearance of low-extraction drugs may not be affected. An increase in the free fraction of a drug can result in a higher volume of distribution and an increased half-life for high-ER drugs. For low-ER drugs, the increase in free fraction may increase both the clearance and the volume of distribution, minimizing any change in the half-life. Finally, changes in the level of enzymatic activity are more likely to influence the clearance of low-ER drugs compared with high-ER drugs.

As this chapter outlines, there are many physiological changes that take place in various disease states. Therefore the prediction of altered pharmacokinetics in the patient population

TABLE 1.1   Effect on Pharmacokinetic Parameters of Drugs due to Possible Changes in Physiology in Disease State for Drugs Eliminated by the Liver Administered Intravenously

Pharmacokinetic Changes	ER Status	Clearance	Volume of Distribution	Half-Life	Area Under the Curve
Decreased absorption		↔	↔	↔	↓
Increased absorption		↔	↔	↔	↑
Decreased blood flow to liver	High ER	↓	↔	↑	↑
	Low ER	↔	↔	↔	↔
Increased fraction unbound in blood	High ER	↔	↑	↑	↔
	Low ER	↑	↑	↔	↓
Decreased enzyme activity	High ER	↔	↔	↔	↔
	Low ER	↓	↔	↑	↑
Increased enzyme activity	High ER	↔	↔	↔	↔
	Low ER	↑	↔	↓	↓

↓, decreased; ↑, increased; ↔, little or no change; *ER*, extraction ratio.

is not a trivial task. Fig. 1.2 outlines and illustrates the many ways in which different diseases can influence the pharmacokinetics of drugs.

A significant challenge in predicting appropriate dose adjustments due to physiological/biochemical changes are the multiple stages or degrees of severity a disease may have over the time course of disease progression or between patients. The time-dependent changes and spectrum of severity that occur within a disease state make it challenging to anticipate dose adjustments for an entire patient population. There are, however, tools that the pharmaceutical scientist can utilize to predict the pharmacokinetics of drugs in the clinic. First and foremost, one should understand the route of metabolism, route of elimination, protein binding, and physicochemical properties of the drug in the preclinical and clinical settings. Physiologically based pharmacokinetic (PBPK) models can then be built and the parameters that are altered in the diseased population (e.g., blood flow or enzyme activity) can be entered into the PBPK model to predict changes that may occur in the diseased state. Simcyp (Certara, Princeton, NJ, USA) is one such modeling software that can allow the user to predict pharmacokinetic profiles of drugs in the diseased state.

Although the pharmaceutical industry has not specifically focused on the effects of disease states on the metabolism and disposition of developing drugs until clinical development, this approach is changing. An earlier awareness of how disease can affect drug disposition is now recognized as a key to faster and more successful development of safe and efficacious drugs. As such, the physiological and biochemical changes that occur with major diseases are being evaluated in greater depth to bring about a better understanding of how these changes can ultimately affect drug metabolism and disposition.

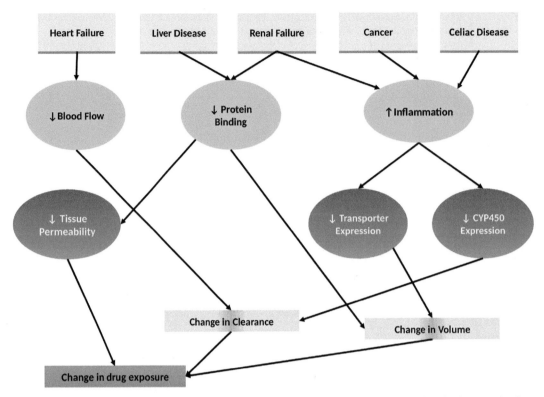

FIGURE 1.2   Change in pharmacokinetic parameters in disease states is complicated and often results from multiple mechanisms common to several diseases.

References

Aitken, A.E., Morgan, E.T., 2007. Gene-specific effects of inflammatory cytokines on cytochrome P450 2C, 2B6 and 3A4 mRNA levels in human hepatocytes. Drug Metab. Dispos. 35 (9), 1687—1693.

Bauer, B., Hartz, A.M., Miller, D.S., 2007. Tumor necrosis factor alpha and endothelin-1 increase P-glycoprotein expression and transport activity at the blood—brain barrier. Mol. Pharmacol. 71 (3), 667—675.

Bertilsson, P.M., Olsson, P., Magnusson, K.E., 2001. Cytokines influence mRNA expression of cytochrome P450 3A4 and MDR1 in intestinal cells. J. Pharm. Sci. 90 (5), 638—646.

Bruha, R., Dvorak, K., Petrtyl, J., 2012. Alcoholic liver disease. World J. Hepatol. 4 (3), 81—90.

Cecchin, E., Innocenti, F., D'Andrea, M., Corona, G., De Mattia, E., Biason, P., Toffoli, G., 2009. Predictive role of the UGT1A1, UGT1A7, and UGT1A9 genetic variants and their haplotypes on the outcome of metastatic colorectal cancer patients treated with fluorouracil, leucovorin, and irinotecan. J. Clin. Oncol. 27 (15), 2457—2465.

Chin, T.W., Loeb, M., Fong, I.W., 1995. Effects of an acidic beverage (Coca-cola) on absorption of ketoconazole. Antimicrob. Agents Chemother. 39 (8), 1671—1675.

Crouthamel, W.G., 1975. The effect of congestive heart failure on quinidine pharmacokinetics. Am. Heart J. 90 (3), 335—339.

Curran, M.A., Montalvo, W., Yagita, H., Allison, J.P., 2010. Pd-1 and CTLA-4 combination blockade expands infiltrating T cells and reduces regulatory T and myeloid cells within B16 melanoma tumors. Proc. Natl. Acad. Sci. USA 107 (9), 4275—4280.

de Wildt, S.N., Kearns, G.L., Leeder, J.S., van den Anker, J.N., 1999. Glucuronidation in humans. Pharmacogenetic and developmental aspects. Clin. Pharmacokinet. 36 (6), 439—452.

Dickmann, L.J., Patel, S.K., Rock, D.A., Wienkers, L.C., Slatter, J.G., 2011. Effects of interleukin-6 (IL-6) and an anti-IL-6 monoclonal antibody on drug-metabolizing enzymes in human hepatocyte culture. Drug Metab. Dispos. 39 (8), 1415—1422.

Dostalek, M., Court, M.H., Yan, B., Akhlaghi, F., 2011. Significantly reduced cytochrome P450 3A4 expression and activity in liver from humans with diabetes mellitus. Br. J. Pharmacol. 163 (5), 937—947.

Dreisbach, A.W., Lertora, J.J., 2008. The effect of chronic renal failure on drug metabolism and transport. Expert Opin. Drug Metab. Toxicol. 4 (8), 1065—1074.

du Souich, P., Fradette, C., 2011. The effect and clinical consequences of hypoxia on cytochrome P450, membrane carrier proteins activity and expression. Expert Opin. Drug Metab. Toxicol. 7 (9), 1083—1100.

Dulos, J., Carven, G.J., van Boxtel, S.J., Evers, S., Driessen-Engels, L.J., Hobo, W., Boots, A.M., 2012. PD-1 blockade augments TH1 and TH17 and suppresses TH2 responses in peripheral blood from patients with prostate and advanced melanoma cancer. J. Immunother. 35 (2), 169—178.

Ebner, T., Remmel, R.P., Burchell, B., 1993. Human bilirubin UDP-glucuronosyltransferase catalyzes the glucuronidation of ethinylestradiol. Mol. Pharmacol. 43 (4), 649—654.

Edwards, D.J., Lalka, D., Cerra, F., Slaughter, R.L., 1982. Alpha1-acid glycoprotein concentration and protein binding in trauma. Clin. Pharmacol. Ther. 31 (1), 62—67.

el Touny, M., el Guinaidy, M., Abdel Bary, M., Osman, L., Sabbour, M.S., 1992. Pharmacokinetics of cefodizime in patients with liver cirrhosis and ascites. Chemotherapy 38 (4), 201—205.

Evers, R., Dallas, S., Dickmann, L.J., Fahmi, O.A., Kenny, J.R., Kraynov, E., Zhang, L., 2013. Critical review of preclinical approaches to investigate cytochrome P450-mediated therapeutic protein drug-drug interactions and recommendations for best practices: a white paper. Drug Metab. Dispos. 41 (9), 1598—1609.

Feghali, C.A., Wright, T.M., 1997. Cytokines in acute and chronic inflammation. Front. Biosci. 2, d12—26.

Filella, X., Blade, J., Guillermo, A.L., Molina, R., Rozman, C., Ballesta, A.M., 1996. Cytokines (IL-6, TNF-alpha, IL-1alpha) and soluble interleukin-2 receptor as serum tumor markers in multiple myeloma. Cancer Detect. Prev. 20 (1), 52—56.

Gandhi, A., Moorthy, B., Ghose, R., 2012. Drug disposition in pathophysiological conditions. Curr. Drug Metab. 13 (9), 1327—1344.

Goralski, K.B., Hartmann, G., Piquette-Miller, M., Renton, K.W., 2003. Downregulation of MDR1a expression in the brain and liver during CNS inflammation alters the in vivo disposition of digoxin. Br. J. Pharmacol. 139 (1), 35—48.

Groothuis, D.R., 2000. The blood—brain and blood-tumor barriers: a review of strategies for increasing drug delivery. Neuro Oncol. 2 (1), 45—59.

Harvey, R.D., Morgan, E.T., 2014. Cancer, inflammation, and therapy: effects on cytochrome P450-mediated drug metabolism and implications for novel immunotherapeutic agents. Clin. Pharmacol. Ther. 96 (4), 449—457.

Kalliokoski, A., Neuvonen, M., Neuvonen, P.J., Niemi, M., 2008. The effect of SLCO1B1 polymorphism on repaglinide pharmacokinetics persists over a wide dose range. Br. J. Clin. Pharmacol. 66 (6), 818—825.

Keizer, R.J., Huitema, A.D., Schellens, J.H., Beijnen, J.H., 2010. Clinical pharmacokinetics of therapeutic monoclonal antibodies. Clin. Pharmacokinet. 49 (8), 493—507.

Kim, J., Hayton, W.L., Robinson, J.M., Anderson, C.L., 2007. Kinetics of FcRn-mediated recycling of IgG and albumin in human: pathophysiology and therapeutic implications using a simplified mechanism-based model. Clin. Immunol. 122 (2), 146—155.

Klammt, S., Wojak, H.J., Mitzner, A., Koball, S., Rychly, J., Reisinger, E.C., Mitzner, S., 2012. Albumin-binding capacity (ABIC) is reduced in patients with chronic kidney disease along with an accumulation of protein-bound uraemic toxins. Nephrol. Dial Transplant. 27 (6), 2377—2383.

Koop, D.R., Tierney, D.J., 1990. Multiple mechanisms in the regulation of ethanol-inducible cytochrome P450IIE1. Bioessays 12 (9), 429—435.

Laouari, D., Yang, R., Veau, C., Blanke, I., Friedlander, G., 2001. Two apical multidrug transporters, P-gp and MRP2, are differently altered in chronic renal failure. Am. J. Physiol. Ren. Physiol. 280 (4), F636—F645.

Leblond, F.A., Petrucci, M., Dube, P., Bernier, G., Bonnardeaux, A., Pichette, V., 2002. Downregulation of intestinal cytochrome P450 in chronic renal failure. J. Am. Soc. Nephrol. 13 (6), 1579—1585.

Liumbruno, G.M., Bennardello, F., Lattanzio, A., Piccoli, P., Rossettias, G., Italian Society of Transfusion Medicine and Immunohaematology (SIMTI) Working Party, 2009. Recommendations for the use of albumin and immuno-globulins. Blood Transfus. 7 (3), 216–234.

Loscher, W., Potschka, H., 2005. Role of drug efflux transporters in the brain for drug disposition and treatment of brain diseases. Prog. Neurobiol. 76 (1), 22–76.

Mannisto, P.T., Mantyla, R., Nykanen, S., Lamminsivu, U., Ottoila, P., 1982. Impairing effect of food on ketoconazole absorption. Antimicrob. Agents Chemother. 21 (5), 730–733.

Merrell, M.D., Cherrington, N.J., 2011. Drug metabolism alterations in nonalcoholic fatty liver disease. Drug Metab. Rev. 43 (3), 317–334.

Moreno, A.H., Burchell, A.R., Rousselot, L.M., Panke, W.F., Slafsky, F., Burke, J.H., 1967. Portal blood flow in cirrhosis of the liver. J. Clin. Invest. 46 (3), 436–445.

Morgan, E.T., 1997. Regulation of cytochromes P450 during inflammation and infection. Drug Metab. Rev. 29 (4), 1129–1188.

Morgan, E.T., 2001. Regulation of cytochrome P450 by inflammatory mediators: why and how? Drug Metab. Dispos. 29 (3), 207–212.

Morgan, E.T., 2009. Impact of infectious and inflammatory disease on cytochrome P450-mediated drug metabolism and pharmacokinetics. Clin. Pharmacol. Ther. 85 (4), 434–438.

Nolin, T.D., Frye, R.F., Matzke, G.R., 2003. Hepatic drug metabolism and transport in patients with kidney disease. Am. J. Kidney Dis. 42 (5), 906–925.

Nyholm, D., Lennernas, H., 2008. Irregular gastrointestinal drug absorption in Parkinson's disease. Expert Opin. Drug Metab. Toxicol. 4 (2), 193–203.

Osborne, R., Joel, S., Grebenik, K., Trew, D., Slevin, M., 1993. The pharmacokinetics of morphine and morphine glu-curonides in kidney failure. Clin. Pharmacol. Ther. 54 (2), 158–167.

Palatini, P., Orlando, R., De Martin, S., 2010. The effect of liver disease on inhibitory and plasma protein-binding displacement interactions: an update. Expert Opin. Drug Metab. Toxicol. 6 (10), 1215–1230.

Parkinson, A., Ogilvie, B., Buckley, D.K.,F., Czerwinski, M., Parkinson, O., 2013. Chapter 6: Biotransformation of xe-nobiotics. In: Klaassen CD (Klaassen CD.), Casarett and Odoull's Toxicology: The Basic Science of Poisons, eighth ed. McGraw-Hill Education.

Parsons, R.L., Kaye, C.M., Raymond, K., 1977. Pharmacokinetics of salicylate and indomethacin in coeliac disease. Eur. J. Clin. Pharmacol. 11 (6), 473–477.

Paxton, J.W., Briant, R.H., 1984. Alpha 1-acid glycoprotein concentrations and propranolol binding in elderly patients with acute illness. Br. J. Clin. Pharmacol. 18 (5), 806–810.

Prescott, L.F., 1974. Gastric emptying and drug absorption. Br. J. Clin. Pharmacol. 1 (3), 189–190.

Riddick, D.S., Lee, C., Bhathena, A., Timsit, Y.E., Cheng, P.Y., Morgan, E.T., Chiang, J.Y., 2004. Transcriptional sup-pression of cytochrome P450 genes by endogenous and exogenous chemicals. Drug Metab. Dispos. 32 (4), 367–375.

Sand, K.M., Bern, M., Nilsen, J., Noordzij, H.T., Sandlie, I., Andersen, J.T., 2014. Unraveling the interaction between FcRn and albumin: opportunities for design of albumin-based therapeutics. Front. Immunol. 5, 682.

Schmitt, C., Kuhn, B., Zhang, X., Kivitz, A.J., Grange, S., 2011. Disease-drug-drug interaction involving tocilizumab and simvastatin in patients with rheumatoid arthritis. Clin. Pharmacol. Ther. 89 (5), 735–740.

Seelbach, M.J., Brooks, T.A., Egleton, R.D., Davis, T.P., 2007. Peripheral inflammatory hyperalgesia modulates morphine delivery to the brain: a role for p-glycoprotein. J. Neurochem. 102 (5), 1677–1690.

Shah, R.R., Smith, R.L., 2015. Inflammation-induced phenoconversion of polymorphic drug metabolizing enzymes: hypothesis with implications for personalized medicine. Drug Metab. Dispos. 43 (3), 400–410.

Singh, S.D., Whale, C., Houghton, N., Daley-Yates, P., Kirby, S.M., Woodcock, A.A., 2003. Pharmacokinetics and sys-temic effects of inhaled fluticasone propionate in chronic obstructive pulmonary disease. Br. J. Clin. Pharmacol. 55 (4), 375–381.

Spiller, R.C., Jenkins, D., Thornley, J.P., Hebden, J.M., Wright, T., Skinner, M., Neal, K.R., 2000. Increased rectal mucosal enteroendocrine cells, T lymphocytes, and increased gut permeability following acute campylobacter en-teritis and in post-dysenteric irritable bowel syndrome. Gut 47 (6), 804–811.

Stenson, R.E., Constantino, R.T., Harrison, D.C., 1971. Interrelationships of hepatic blood flow, cardiac output, and blood levels of lidocaine in man. Circulation 43 (2), 205–211.

Strassburg, C.P., 2010. Hyperbilirubinemia syndromes (Gilbert-Meulengracht, Crigler-Najjar, Dubin-Johnson, and Rotor syndrome). Best Pract. Res. Clin. Gastroenterol. 24 (5), 555–571.

Tajiri, K., Shimizu, Y., 2013. Liver physiology and liver diseases in the elderly. World J. Gastroenterol. 19 (46), 8459–8467.

Tran, T.H., Smith, C., Mangione, R.A., 2013. Drug absorption in celiac disease. Am. J. Health Syst. Pharm. 70 (24), 2199–2206.

Trenholme, G.M., Williams, R.L., Rieckmann, K.H., Frischer, H., Carson, P.E., 1976. Quinine disposition during malaria and during induced fever. Clin. Pharmacol. Ther. 19 (4), 459–467.

Ufer, M., Hasler, R., Jacobs, G., Haenisch, S., Lachelt, S., Faltraco, F., Cascorbi, I., 2009. Decreased sigmoidal ABCB1 (p-glycoprotein) expression in ulcerative colitis is associated with disease activity. Pharmacogenomics 10 (12), 1941–1953.

Veau, C., Leroy, C., Banide, H., Auchere, D., Tardivel, S., Farinotti, R., Lacour, B., 2001. Effect of chronic renal failure on the expression and function of rat intestinal p-glycoprotein in drug excretion. Nephrol. Dial. Transplant. 16 (8), 1607–1614.

Verbeeck, R.K., 2008. Pharmacokinetics and dosage adjustment in patients with hepatic dysfunction. Eur. J. Clin. Pharmacol. 64 (12), 1147–1161.

Vormfelde, S.V., Muck, W., Freudenthaler, S.M., Heyen, P., Schmage, N., Kuhlmann, J., Gleiter, C.H., 1999. Pharmacokinetics of cerivastatin in renal impairment are predicted by low serum albumin concentration rather than by low creatinine clearance. J. Clin. Pharmacol. 39 (2), 147–154.

Wang, T., Shankar, K., Ronis, M.J., Mehendale, H.M., 2007. Mechanisms and outcomes of drug- and toxicant-induced liver toxicity in diabetes. Crit. Rev. Toxicol. 37 (5), 413–459.

Wani, M.A., Haynes, L.D., Kim, J., Bronson, C.L., Chaudhury, C., Mohanty, S., Anderson, C.L., 2006. Familial hypercatabolic hypoproteinemia caused by deficiency of the neonatal Fc receptor, FcRn, due to a mutant beta2-microglobulin gene. Proc. Natl. Acad. Sci. USA 103 (13), 5084–5089.

Williams, R.L., Upton, R.A., Cello, J.P., Jones, R.M., Blitstein, M., Kelly, J., Nierenburg, D., 1984. Naproxen disposition in patients with alcoholic cirrhosis. Eur. J. Clin. Pharmacol. 27 (3), 291–296.

Wooles, W.R., Borzelleca, J.F., 1966. Prolongation of barbiturate sleeping time in mice by stimulation of the reticuloendothelial system (RES). J. Reticuloendothel Soc. 3 (1), 41–47.

Woosley, R.L., Echt, D.S., Roden, D.M., 1986. Effects of congestive heart failure on the pharmacokinetics and pharmacodynamics of antiarrhythmic agents. Am. J. Cardiol. 57 (3), 25B–33B.

Xie, W., 2009. In: Xie, W. (Ed.), Nuclear Receptors in Drug Metabolism. John Wiley and Sons, Hoboken, NJ.

Yeung, C.K., Shen, D.D., Thummel, K.E., Himmelfarb, J., 2014. Effects of chronic kidney disease and uremia on hepatic drug metabolism and transport. Kidney Int. 85 (3), 522–528.

2

Regulation of Drug-Metabolizing Enzymes and Drug Metabolism by Inflammatory Responses

E.T. Morgan

Emory University, Atlanta, GA, United States

OUTLINE

Introduction   22

The Inflammatory Response   23
   Initiation of an Inflammatory Response   23
   Propagation of the Inflammatory Signal   24
   Cytokines and Acute Phase Proteins   25
     Cytokine Regulation of APP Genes   25
     Interleukin-6   25
     Interleukin-1   26
   Innate Immune Response in the Liver   27

Regulation of DMEs by Inflammatory Mediators   28
   TLR Ligands   28
     Toll-Like Receptor 4   28
     Toll-Like Receptor 2   28
     Toll-Like Receptor 3   28
   Proinflammatory Cytokines   29
     Caveats to Primary Hepatocyte Work   29
     Participation of Cytokines in DME
     Regulation In Vivo   30
   Other Cytokines   31

Regulation of P450 Enzymes in Specific Disease States and Models   32
   Liver Disease   32
   Viral Infections   33
     Influenza   33
     Human Immunodeficiency Virus   33
     Hepatitis C Virus   33
     Hepatitis B Virus   34
     Hepatitis A Virus   35
   Bacterial Infections   35
     Sepsis   35
     Helicobacter pylori   35
   Parasitic Infections   35
     Malaria   35
     Schistosomiasis   36
     Leishmaniasis   37
     Liver Flukes   37
     Amebiasis   37
   Sterile Inflammation   37
     Vaccination   37
     Arthritis   38

Drug Metabolism in Diseases
http://dx.doi.org/10.1016/B978-0-12-802949-7.00002-X

21

Cancer	39	Downregulation of Positive	
Lupus Erythematosus	42	Transcription Factors	45
Behçet Disease	42	Inhibitory Binding to Positive	
Critical Illness	43	Transcription Factors	45
Congestive Heart Failure	43	Induction Mechanisms	45
Bone Marrow Transplantation	43	Epigenetic Mechanisms	46
		Posttranscriptional Mechanisms	46
Disease-Dependent Drug—Drug		Nitric Oxide	46
Interactions	43	MicroRNAs	47
Mechanisms of Regulation	44		
Transcriptional Mechanisms	44	**Conclusion**	47
Direct Repression via Negative		**References**	47
Response Elements	44		

INTRODUCTION

The majority of drug-metabolizing enzymes (DMEs) are downregulated during an inflammatory response, resulting in reduced drug clearance. For drugs or toxicants that are inactivated by metabolism, this can lead to elevated parent drug levels and increased toxicity if exposure (dosage) is not changed. This was first illustrated by the reduced clearance and increased toxicity of theophylline during influenza infection in children (Chang et al., 1978; Kraemer et al., 1982). Reduced metabolism of a prodrug could lead to therapeutic inefficacy, although there are no good examples. Reduced bioactivation of drugs to toxic metabolites can be protective, as demonstrated for acetaminophen toxicity in rats pretreated with bacterial lipopolysaccharide (LPS) (Liu et al., 2000). Inflammatory regulation should also be considered in pharmacogenetic analyses, where the downregulation of a polymorphic P450 enzyme by inflammation can result in phenotype—genotype discordance, i.e., phenoconversion (Williams et al., 2000; Shah and Smith, 2015). Induction of DMEs, especially cytochrome P450 (P450) enzymes, is less common during inflammation but induction would result in the opposite consequences to those caused by downregulation. An example of an enzyme induced during certain inflammatory conditions is CYP2A6 (Su and Ding, 2004).

We will concentrate on infectious and inflammatory diseases that have been studied in humans, with insights from animal and cell culture studies that support the clinical data and shed light on the mechanisms and specificities of the effects. The reader is referred to review articles (Renton, 2005; Aitken et al., 2006; Gandhi et al., 2012; Morgan et al., 2012) for a more comprehensive coverage of animal experiments.

Inflammation is a component of almost all human chronic diseases, and so it is likely to be a contributing factor to the modulation of drug metabolism that will be discussed in subsequent chapters. Indeed, several systems biology studies have identified correlations of inflammatory pathways in human liver samples with expression of DMEs (Klein et al., 2010;

Yang et al., 2010b; Rieger et al., 2013; Schroder et al., 2013). Here, we will concentrate on basic principles and diseases not dealt with in later chapters, and we will focus on DMEs in the liver.

THE INFLAMMATORY RESPONSE

Inflammation was defined by Celsus as characterized by swelling, redness, heat, and pain (Celsus, c.100 BC). These responses reflect a complex cascade of cellular and molecular events. Many different factors can initiate inflammation at different anatomic sites, and as a result inflammatory responses are heterogeneous (Salazar-Mather and Hokeness, 2003). Molecular and cellular responses characteristic of inflammation, with important consequences for cell, tissue, and organ function, can occur in the absence of classical symptoms. Here, as in the modern literature, we will consider one or more of these characteristics to be indicatory of an inflammatory response, although inflammation per se may or may not occur.

Initiation of an Inflammatory Response

Inflammatory responses provide defense against invading pathogens, stimulate repair mechanisms in response to tissue damage, and protect against harmful chemicals. They are a function of the innate immune system and triggered by exposure of monocytes, macrophages, and dendritic cells to molecular signals associated with pathogens (pathogen-associated molecular patterns, PAMPs) and tissue damage products (damage-associated molecular patterns, DAMPs) (Medzhitov, 2008; Takeuchi and Akira, 2010). In turn, the proteins on host cells that recognize PAMPs and DAMPs are called pattern recognition receptors (PRRs).

Toll-like receptors (TLRs) are the most important PRRs involved in the initiation of inflammatory responses. TLRs are transmembrane proteins that, in response to PAMP or DAMP binding, activate cellular kinases to initialize signaling pathways that ultimately result in the activation of transcription factors controlling synthesis and release of cytokines such as interferons (IFNs), interleukin (IL)-1β, IL-6, and tumor necrosis factor (TNF) alpha. Humans have 10 distinct TLRs, which are localized in the plasma membrane, in endolysosomal membranes, or, in the sole case of TLR4 (Fig. 2.1), in both (De Nardo, 2015). TLRs are expressed on macrophages, monocytes, and other cells of the innate immune system, including Kupffer cells (KCs), stellate cells, and endothelial cells in the liver. TLRs 2, 3, 4, and 7 have also been detected in hepatocytes (Morgan et al., 2012).

The signaling pathways used by TLR4 are depicted in Fig. 2.1. TLR4 is the receptor for bacterial LPS, thus acting as the main sensor for gram-negative bacterial infection. Only TLR4 signals through both pathways. All other TLRs except TLR3 signal through the myeloid differentiation response gene 8 (MyD88)-dependent pathway, which as shown ultimately results in the activation of nuclear factor kappa-light-chain-enhancer of activated B cells (NF-κB), stimulating the production of IL-1β, IL-6, and TNFα, and thus initiating an inflammatory response (De Nardo, 2015). This arm of the pathway also involves other transcription factors via activation of mitogen-activated protein kinases (MAPKs), which contribute to the inflammatory response. The second signaling pathway of TLR4 involves the adaptor protein

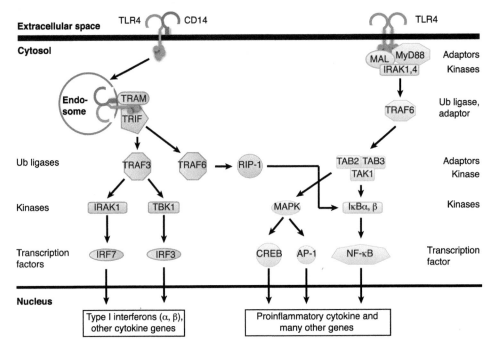

FIGURE 2.1   **Toll-like receptor (TLR) signaling.** For simplicity, the soluble protein MD-2, which associates with the extracellular domain of TLR4 and functions in ligand recognition, is not shown. CD14 also functions to deliver lipopolysaccharide (LPS) to the TLR4 complex at low LPS concentrations and thus is also required for MyD88 signaling under these conditions. MyD88 adapter-like (MAL) protein is also known as Toll interleukin 1 receptor domain containing protein (TIRAP). *AP*, activator protein; *CREB*, cAMP response element–binding protein; *IκB*, inhibitor of NF-κB; *IKK*, IκB kinase; *IRAK*, interleukin 1 receptor–associated kinase; *IRF*, interferon regulatory factor; *RIP*, receptor interacting protein; *TRAF*, TNF receptor-associated factor; *TAB*, transforming growth factor β-activated kinase binding protein; *TAK*, transforming growth factor β-activated kinase; *TBK*, TANK-binding kinase; *TRAM*, TRIF-related adaptor molecule; *STAT*, signal transducer and activator of transcription.

TIR-domain-containing adaptor-inducing IFNβ (TRIF) (De Nardo, 2015). CD14, which serves with TLR4 as an LPS coreceptor, is required for trafficking of TLR4 to the endosomes where it can bind TRIF via the bridging adaptor TRIF-related adaptor molecule (TRAM) (De Nardo, 2015). Ultimately, the kinase cascade initiated by TRIF binding results in the induction of a primarily IFN-based response. TLR3, a receptor for double-stranded DNA, is the only other TLR that signals via TRIF (De Nardo, 2015).

Other PRRs include the cytosolic Nod-like receptor, and retinoic acid–inducible gene 1 families, which are present in the cytoplasm of the cell. Their roles, if any, in regulation of DMEs are poorly understood.

Propagation of the Inflammatory Signal

The acute-phase response (APR) is the cumulative response to injury or infection, comprising the early inflammatory response and reactions that immediately follow it (Baumann and Gauldie, 1994). Activation of NF-κB in macrophages or other cell types via

TLRs results in the increased transcription of IL-1 and TNFα. These early response cytokines activate stromal cells and leukocytes to release cytokines and chemokines such as IL-6, IL-8, and monocyte chemoattractant protein-1, resulting in recruitment of neutrophils to the site of inflammation. These cells in turn release their own complement of cytokines, prostaglandins, and other inflammatory mediators that contribute to the APR (Baumann and Gauldie, 1994).

Cytokines and Acute Phase Proteins

Acute phase proteins (APPs) are a large set of proteins whose synthesis and secretion by the liver are stimulated in the early response to inflammation, comprising proteins such as C-reactive protein (CRP), serum amyloid A (SAA), and α1-acid glycoprotein (AAG) (Baumann and Gauldie, 1994). APP induction in humans ranges from a 50% increase in the case of ceruloplasmin, to three orders of magnitude for SAA and CRP. Negative APPs are downregulated by inflammation (e.g., albumin).

Cytokine Regulation of APP Genes

IL-1β, TNFα, and IL-6 have pivotal roles in the induction of APPs during inflammation (Baumann and Gauldie, 1994). The cellular signaling pathways involved are shown in Fig. 2.2. IL-6 is the most important cytokine for induction of APPs, which may be divided into two main classes (Baumann and Gauldie, 1994). Type 2 APPs such as haptoglobin and α-, β-, and γ-fibrinogen are formed in response to IL-6. Type 1 APPs such as CRP, SAA, and AAG are regulated synergistically by both IL-6- and IL-1-type cytokines (including TNFα) (Baumann and Gauldie, 1994). APP expression and regulation are species dependent: e.g., haptoglobin is a type 1 APP in rat and type 2 in humans, and CRP is a major APP in humans but a minor one in mice.

Interleukin-6

The IL-6 receptor (IL-6Rα) signals via two major arms (Fig. 2.2) (Heinrich et al., 2003; Xu et al., 2015), requiring its association with glycoprotein-130 (gp130). A family of IL-6-like cytokines have many commonalities with IL-6 in the effects they produce (Heinrich et al., 2003). The signal transducer and activator of transcription (STAT) protein-3 undergoes Janus kinase (JAK)-dependent phosphorylation, dimerization, and translocation to the nucleus where it binds to response elements on APP genes. Alternatively, activation of RAS and a MAPK cascade ultimately results in the phosphorylation and activation of CCAAT enhancer–binding protein (C/EBP)β (also called NFIL-6) to form an active transcription factor. C/EBPβ is rapidly induced in leukocytes, liver, and many other tissues in response to IL-1, IL-6, or LPS and plays a central role in the APR as it activates IL-6 transcription as well as that of many APPs (Akira et al., 1990). The human CRP gene has two synergistic IL-6/C/EBPβ response elements in its proximal promoter. The human SAA gene likewise has a C/EBP element that mediates induction by IL-6 (Betts et al., 1993).

The CRP gene contains a binding site for STAT3 that is required for optimal activation by IL-6 (Zhang et al., 1996). Although the SAA gene does not have a consensus STAT3 site, binding of activated STAT3 to NF-κB and subsequently to sequences adjacent to the NF-κB-binding site is essential for synergistic induction by IL-1 and IL-6 (Hagihara et al., 2005).

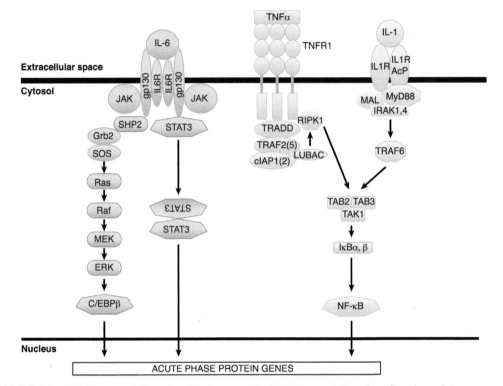

FIGURE 2.2   **Cytokine regulation of acute phase protein (APP) transcription.** Signaling through tumor necrosis factor α receptor 2 (TNFR2) is not shown, as this receptor is restricted mainly to immune cells and endothelial cells. *SHP2*, src homology protein 2; *SOS*, son of sevenless; *ERK*, extracellular signal–regulated kinase; *cIAP*, cellular inhibitor of apoptosis; *LUBAC*, linear ubiquitin chain assembly complex; *TRADD*, TNFR1-associated death domain protein; *RIPK*, receptor interacting protein kinase; *JAK*, Janus kinase; *C/EBP*, CCAAT enhancer–binding protein; *MEK*, mitogen-extracellular signaling-regulated kinase.

Soluble forms of both IL-6Rα and gp130, formed by alternative translation or limited proteolysis, are present in human serum. sIL-6Rα binding to membrane-bound gp130 confers agonist activity, whereas its binding to sgp130 enhances the antagonistic activity of the latter (Heinrich et al., 2003).

Interleukin-1

The IL-1 receptor 1(IL-1R1) is related to the TLRs and must dimerize with its signaling subunit IL-1RAcP to initiate signaling (Tsutsui et al., 2015), using the MyD88-dependent pathway to stimulate NF-κB activation (Fig. 2.2) and APP transcription (Fig. 2.2). NF-κB is a family of proteins including p50, p65, and RelA, that form homo- and heterodimers to bind to enhancer elements on responsive genes that usually stimulate (but sometimes inhibit) gene transcription. The canonical form is a p50–p65 dimer, in which the p65 subunit possesses a highly active transcription activation domain (Weber et al., 2010). IL-1 itself does not induce the transcription of CRP, but potentiates the effect of IL-6 (Zhang et al., 1995). It does so via a binding site for p50–p60 heterodimers that displace the repressive factor octamer-1 (Voleti and Agrawal, 2005). In contrast to CRP, the human SAA gene can be activated by IL-1 alone, and this is mediated via NF-κB binding to a site that synergizes with a C/EBP site to produce cooperative induction by IL-6 and IL-1 (Betts et al., 1993).

At least part of the effect of IL-1 in primary hepatocytes on CRP and SAA expression is due to stimulation of IL-6 formation (Moshage et al., 1988). The activity of IL-1β is controlled in part by the competitive IL-1 receptor antagonist (IL-1ra), which itself is an APP. Other members of the IL-1 family include IL-18 and IL-13, which have different receptors but ultimately regulate the same signaling pathways (Weber et al., 2010). IL-17 is a product of T helper-17 cells, and IL-17 receptors are expressed in the liver. It was shown to induce CRP in both primary hepatocytes and hepatoma cells, in an IL-1- and IL-6-independent manner (Patel et al., 2007; Eklund, 2009). This is perhaps not surprising since IL-17 activates both the NF-κB and C/EBPβ pathways (Onishi and Gaffen, 2010; Gaffen et al., 2014)

TUMOR NECROSIS FACTOR α

TNFα exists in both membrane-bound and soluble forms. There are two TNFα receptors (TNFR1 and 2), both of which exist as trimers on the cell surface (Fig. 2.2). TNFR1 is the most relevant for hepatic APP and DME regulation, as it is the form expressed in hepatocytes (Brenner et al., 2015). Like IL-1/IL-1R, TNFα binding to TNFR1 ultimately results in the activation of NF-κB transcriptional activity.

Although IL-6- and IL-1-type cytokines dominate the regulation of all of the APPs, the mechanisms and transcription factors involved are different for each. The earlier discussion highlights how the modes of action of C/EBP, STAT3, and NF-κB, and their interactions, are different for CRP and SAA. This is also true for other APPs, and together with differences in cytokine patterns and tissue and cell differences in response (Eklund, 2009), explains why the APPs are not coordinately expressed and differ according to disease state and severity.

Innate Immune Response in the Liver

The KCs are macrophages that are resident in the hepatic sinusoids. They are the first hepatic cells to come in contact with pathogens and their associated toxins, and they function to sense and phagocytize these agents (Bilzer et al., 2006). To do so, they express a full complement of TLRs (Wu et al., 2010; Morgan et al., 2012). TLR activation of KCs results in the synthesis and release of TNFα, IL-1β, and IL-6; induction of nitric oxidase synthase (NOS) 2 and activation of NADPH oxidase resulting in massive synthesis and release of NO and superoxide, respectively; and induction of cyclooxygenase-2 with resultant production of prostaglandins and thromboxanes (Bilzer et al., 2006; Woolbright and Jaeschke, 2015). The role of KC in inflammatory regulation of hepatic DMEs has been demonstrated in animals by the attenuation of enzyme downregulation when KCs are inactivated, in models of TLR4-dependent gram-negative (Xu et al., 2004; Kim et al., 2011) and TLR2-dependent gram-positive (Ghose et al., 2009) sepsis, whereas downregulation in a model of gastrointestinal bacterial infection did not require KCs (Kinloch et al., 2011).

REGULATION OF DMEs BY INFLAMMATORY MEDIATORS

TLR Ligands

Toll-Like Receptor 4

The prototypic TLR4 ligand LPS has been studied intensively as a model of bacterial sepsis, and much has been learned about inflammatory regulation of DMEs in this model. Very low doses of LPS administered to healthy human volunteers 24 and 0.5 h before a drug cocktail caused significant reductions of antipyrine, hexobarbital, and theophylline clearance in both men and women (Shedlofsky et al., 1994, 1997). Changes were on the order of 15—40%, and importantly the reductions in antipyrine clearance were negatively correlated with levels of IL-6 and TNFα in the plasma.

In rats, the major P450 mRNAs CYP2C11 and CYP3A2 are rapidly downregulated to 10—20% of control after LPS injection, and reduced P450 gene transcription can be observed within 1 h (Aitken et al., 2006). Other enzymes downregulated in rats include UGT1A1, 1A6, 2B1, and 2B3 (Alkharfy et al., 2008) and SULT1A1, 1B1, and 1C1 (Shimada et al., 1999). In mice, LPS administration resulted in the downregulation of 10 of 13 P450 mRNAs studied, with the exception of two that were induced (Chaluvadi et al., 2009). Other enzymes down-regulated in LPS-treated mice include Ugt1a1 (Ghose et al., 2008), Sult 2a1 (Kim et al., 2004), carboxylesterases 1 and 2 (Mao et al., 2011), and flavin monooxygenses Fmo1, 3, and 5 but not Fmo4 (Zhang et al., 2009). These effects were blocked in C3H/HeJ mice harboring a naturally occurring null mutation of TLR4 (Ghose et al., 2008; Chaluvadi et al., 2009; Zhang et al., 2009). The estrogen sulfotransferase Sult2e1 was shown to be induced in mice treated with LPS (Jiang et al., 2015), and this enzyme is involved in the regulation of the inflammatory response (Chai et al., 2015).

As shown in Fig. 2.1, the adaptor protein MyD88 adapter-like (MAL, also known as TIRAP) couples MyD88-dependent signaling to TLR4 (De Nardo, 2015). Downregulation of Cyp3a11 and Ugt1A1 after LPS treatment was normal in $Tirap^{-/-}$ and $Trif^{-/-}$ mice, suggesting that the MyD88- and TRIF-dependent pathways can function redundantly in P450 downregulation or that the MyD88 pathway can proceed without MAL/TIRAP (Ghose et al., 2008; Shah et al., 2016).

Toll-Like Receptor 2

Ligands for TLR2 include the yeast cell wall product mannan and lipoteichoic acid, a major component of the cell walls of gram-positive bacteria. Lipoteichoic acid injection in mice downregulated several DMEs Cyp2b10 > Sultn > Cyp2a4 > Cyp3a11, without affecting Ugt1a1 or Sult1a1 (Ghose et al., 2009), which was partially KC dependent. The different specificity from the response to LPS is not unexpected, since TLR2 signals specifically through the MyD88 pathway (Fig. 2.1). These effects were ablated in $Tlr2^{-/-}$ mice (Ghose et al., 2011). TLR2- and MAL-dependent downregulation could be recapitulated in cultured primary hepatocytes, suggesting that lipoteichoic acid downregulates DMEs via a direct action on hepatocytes (Ghose et al., 2011).

Toll-Like Receptor 3

TLR3 is an endosomal receptor that senses double-stranded viral mRNAs. TLR3 can interact directly with TRIF without the need for TRAM and it signals only via this pathway

(De Nardo, 2015). Therefore, type I IFNs (α, β) are the proximate mediators in response to TLR3 activation. Renton and Mannering (1976) first described the reduction of hepatic P450–associated activities in rat liver by IFN inducers, including the synthetic double-stranded RNA poly rI.rC. This was subsequently shown to occur via downregulation of specific P450 mRNAs (Morgan and Norman, 1990; Morgan, 1991). However, the downregulation of Cyp3a11 and Cyp1a2 by poly rI.rC treatment in mice was shown to occur independently of IFN induction (Ghaffari et al., 2011). DME downregulation is also independent of TRIF (Shah et al., 2016). Cytosolic PRRs for double-stranded RNAs also participate in immune responses to viral infection (RIG-1 and MDA5), and it is possible that the TRIF-independent effects occur via those receptors (Ghaffari et al., 2011).

Proinflammatory Cytokines

Because of their roles in regulation of APPs, IL-1, IL-6, and TNFα were the first cytokines to be tested for their abilities to affect activities and expression of P450 enzymes in animals (Ghezzi et al., 1986; Ferrari et al., 1993; Nadin et al., 1995). Studies in cultured primary rat hepatocytes demonstrated that cytokines could downregulate P450 expression with some specificity. Thus, IL-1, TNFα, and IL-6 all downregulated the mRNA of the major P450 in male rat liver, CYP2C11 (Chen et al., 1995). IFNγ was ineffective in CYP2C11 downregulation (Chen et al., 1995), whereas it was able to downregulate constitutive and inducible rat CYP3A mRNAs (Tapner et al., 1996). In human hepatocytes, CYP1A2, CYP2C, CYP2E1, and CYP3A were each downregulated by IL-1β, IL-6, or TNFα after 72 h of treatment, whereas IFNγ only downregulated CYP1A2 and CYP2E1 (Abdel-Razzak et al., 1993). Later studies in hepatocytes treated for 24 h with high concentrations of cytokines essentially confirmed these findings and provided further evidence that human P450s differ in their susceptibility to cytokines (Aitken and Morgan, 2007). Interestingly, IL-6 downregulated all human P450 mRNAs studied (CYP2B6, 2C8, 2C9, 2C18, 2C19, and 3A4), albeit with different efficacies (Fig. 2.3; Aitken and Morgan, 2007). LPS, IL-1β, and TNFα each showed a similar pattern of P450 regulation, consistent with their use of a common NF-κB-dependent signaling component (Figs. 2.1 and 2.2). In human hepatocytes, IL-6-induced CRP and SAA mRNAs with EC_{50} values of 23 and 73 pg/mL, respectively, whereas downregulation of CYP3A4 after 72 h of treatment occurred with an EC_{50} of only 3 pg/mL. About 20- to 500-fold higher IL-6 concentrations were required for downregulation of other human P450s (Dickmann et al., 2011). This marks CYP3A4 as a highly sensitive target for IL-6, whereas the relevance of downregulation of other P450s by higher concentrations of IL-6 would depend more on local concentrations of IL-6 and other patient-specific factors.

Caveats to Primary Hepatocyte Work

Most studies in hepatocytes have used preparations in which KCs are present in small numbers that may contribute to indirect effects of applied cytokines as observed for KC-dependent downregulation of CYP3A4 by IL-2 in human hepatocytes (Sunman et al., 2004). KC-hepatocyte cocultures showed enhanced responses of CYP3A4 to IL-1, but not IL-6 (Nguyen et al., 2015). Cocultures may be a better model than highly purified hepatocytes for studying the cytokine regulation of hepatic drug metabolism. However, it remains to be seen which model best reflects quantitative responses observed in vivo.

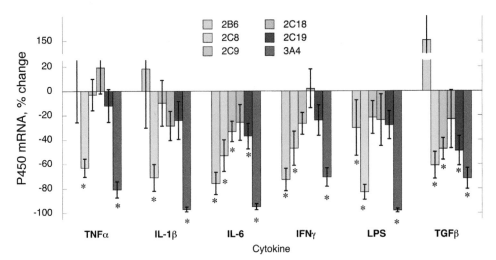

Hepatocytes in culture rapidly change to a less differentiated phenotype that includes drastically reduced expression of P450s and other DMEs (Sidhu et al., 1993). Although current culture techniques help restore the adult hepatic phenotype, there are likely to be at least quantitative differences in responses compared with the liver. It is also possible that some observed responses could be due to cytokine-evoked changes in the cell's phenotype. This is especially true if long (72 h) incubation times are used, e.g., in studies conducted to address Food and Drug Administration concerns about new drugs (Evers et al., 2013).

Participation of Cytokines in DME Regulation In Vivo

The importance of a particular cytokine for DME regulation in any given disease state will depend on many factors, including its concentration in the vicinity of the hepatocytes, time course of its production, modulation of and by other cytokines, natural antagonists (e.g., IL-1-ra), and facilitators (e.g., soluble receptors). To address this question, investigators have used cytokine or cytokine receptor knockout mice, as well as neutralizing antibodies. In interpreting these results, one must remember that if deletion or neutralization of a cytokine attenuates an effect of inflammation on hepatic DMEs, the effect could be caused indirectly via an effect on other inflammatory mediators.

INTERLEUKIN-6

The absence of IL-6 in null mice had no effect on the downregulation of multiple P450 mRNAs in the LPS model (Siewert et al., 2000). This probably indicates that in this model of global inflammation, redundant pathways function to downregulate P450 expression. In mice injected with turpentine (a model of sterile inflammation) or Bacillus Calmette–Guerin (BCG, tuberculosis) vaccine, downregulation of several P450s was blocked in IL-6$^{-/-}$ animals consistent with a role of IL-6 in DME regulation (Siewert et al., 2000; Ashino et al., 2004) in these models. Injection of polyclonal IL-6 antibodies reversed the downregulation of hepatic Cyp3a enzymes in arthritic mice (Ashino et al., 2007). The downregulation of Cyp3a11 (but not other P450s) in mice with infectious colitis was blocked in IL-6$^{-/-}$ mice, although this may have been at least partially due to the absence of an IFNγ response (Nyagode et al., 2010).

TUMOR NECROSIS FACTOR α

Like IL-6 knockout mice, TNFR1 and TNFR2 double knockout (Warren et al., 1999) or TNFα$^{-/-}$ (Ashino et al., 2004) mice also displayed little change in their downregulations of P450 expression in response to LPS. However, the downregulation of Cyp2c29, but not Cyp3a11, by BCG vaccine was attenuated in TNFα$^{-/-}$ mice (Ashino et al., 2004). A role for TNFα in a model of preadjuvant arthritis was demonstrated by the partial blockade of Cyp1a and Cyp3a downregulation by infliximab, a therapeutic TNFα monoclonal antibody (Ling and Jamali, 2009). Our experiments in IL-6$^{-/-}$, TNFR1$^{-/-}$, and IFNγ$^{-/-}$ mice infected with *Citrobacter rodentium* suggested that TNFα is the most important cytokine for Cyp3a downregulation in this infectious colitis model (Nyagode et al., 2010; Kinloch et al., 2011). This conclusion was supported by subsequent experiments using a dominant-negative form of TNFα (Nyagode et al., 2014).

INTERLEUKIN-1β

Studies in IL-1β-deficient mice have not revealed an in vivo role for IL-1β in the downregulation of Cyp2c29 or Cyp3a11 in BCG-induced inflammation (Ashino et al., 2004), or for any P450s studied in the infectious colitis model (Kinloch et al., 2011).

Other Cytokines

Studies on regulation of human P450 enzymes by other cytokines are summarized in Table 2.1. Much more needs to be done in this area. IL-2 is a T-cell-derived cytokine used for treatment of melanoma and renal cancer. A study in patients with cancer suggests that P450 enzymes may be downregulated during IL-2 therapy. However, studies in human hepatocytes have yielded conflicting results. Since human hepatocytes were found not to express the IL-2 receptor β subunit (Nguyen et al., 2015), any in vivo effects on hepatic P450 may be indirect (Sunman et al., 2004). IL-4 is a T helper cell-2-type cytokine, which was shown to induce CYP2E1 in human hepatocytes without affecting CYP3A mRNA (Abdel-Razzak et al., 1993). Whether this occurs in vivo has yet to be determined. P450-dependent activities have been measured in healthy people treated with the antiinflammatory cytokine IL-10, and its effects, if any, were small. IL-12 and IL-23, involved in the pathophysiology of psoriasis, did not affect the regulation of several P450 enzymes in hepatocyte cultures, nor of CYP3A4 in hepatocyte–KC cocultures.

TABLE 2.1   Evidence for Regulation of Human P450 Enzymes by Various Cytokines

Cytokine	Humans/Model System	Effect	References
IL-2	Patients with cancer	Decreased CYP1A2, 2C, 2E1, 3A4 protein and activity	Elkahwaji et al. (1999)
	Hepatocytes	Decreased CYP3A4 mRNA, KC dependent	Sunman et al. (2004)
	Hepatocytes	Minimal effect on CYP3A4 with or without KC (no IL-2 receptor detected)	Nguyen et al. (2015)
IL-4	Hepatocytes, hepatoma cells	Induced CYP2E1 mRNA	Abdel-Razzak et al. (1993), Abdel-Razzak et al. (2004), and Wang et al. (2010a)
IL-10	Healthy humans	12% decrease in CYP3A4 activity, no effect on CYP1A2, 2D6, 2C9	Gorski et al. (2000)
	Healthy humans	No effect on CYP3A4 activity	Chakraborty et al. (1999)
IL-12	Hepatocytes	No effect on CYP2B6, 2C9, 2C19, 3A4	Dallas et al. (2013)
IL-23	Hepatocytes	Minimal effect on CYP3A4 with or without KC	Nguyen et al. (2015)
	Hepatocytes	No effect on CYP2B6, 2C9, 2C19, 3A4	Dallas et al. (2013)

REGULATION OF P450 ENZYMES IN SPECIFIC DISEASE STATES AND MODELS

In this section, we will focus on diseases for which there are clinical human data. Most such studies have been done in adults. There are no well-documented reports of racial or ethnic differences in these responses, and although a few studies have reported small gender differences, these have not been large. However, reports of larger effects of schistosomiasis and hepatitis A virus (HAV) infection on pharmacokinetics in children (see subsequently) than in adults highlight the need for more clinical studies in pediatric populations and suggest that other special populations such as geriatrics or pregnant women should also be studied.

Liver Disease

CYP1A2 and 2E1 protein levels in biopsies of cirrhotic livers were 47% and 41% of controls, respectively (Guengerich and Turvy, 1991). CYP3A and CYP2C protein levels were not significantly affected. The expression of UGTs 1A4, 2B4, and 2B7 was significantly downregulated in biopsies from patients with high inflammation scores, as was that of CYP1A2, whereas UGT expression was not affected by the degree of fibrosis (Congiu et al., 2002).

In vivo phenotyping of patients with mild and moderate liver disease revealed a 79% reduction in CYP2C19 activity (mephenytoin) compared with healthy controls, whereas

CYP2D6 activities were not affected (Adedoyin et al., 1998). Another study found reduced activities of CYP2C19 (37%), CYP1A2 (caffeine, 69%), CYP2D6 (debrisoquine, 71%), and CYP2E1 (chlorzoxazone, 60%) that were negatively correlated with severity of disease (Frye et al., 2006).

Viral Infections

Influenza

The serum half-life of theophylline, a CYP1A2 substrate, was almost 70% increased in five asthmatic children with influenza and one with adenoviral infection (Chang et al., 1978). Soon thereafter, it was reported that 11 children with influenza B infection and theophylline toxicity had elevated plasma levels of theophylline (Kraemer et al., 1982). In 10 people with an acute viral respiratory tract infection, antipyrine clearance (mediated by at least six P450 enzymes) was reduced by 22%, concomitant with elevations in plasma IFNα and IFNγ levels (Brockmeyer et al., 1998). A 50% reduction in antipyrine clearance in saliva was found in six children with respiratory tract infections of unspecified origin (Forsyth et al., 1982). There have been no other reported studies on influenza infection on drug pharmacokinetics, although there have been additional case reports on theophylline levels or clearance.

Human Immunodeficiency Virus

Due to previous observations that adverse reactions to trimethoprim–sulfamethoxazole were more prevalent in patients with AIDS, or patients who were slow acetylators, several groups tested N-acetyltransferase 2 (NAT2) activity in human immunodeficiency virus (HIV)-infected patients. Three different studies reported that NAT2 activity was reduced only in patients with advanced AIDS (Lee et al., 1993; Jones et al., 2010), by which genotypic fast acetylators acquire a slow acetylator phenotype with disease progression (O'Neil et al., 1997). One contrary study in 40 patients with HIV infection reported that there was 96% concordance of phenotype and genotype, even in the 20 patients with advanced AIDS (Kaufmann et al., 1996).

The impact of HIV on hepatic CYP3A4 activity, if any, is small (Slain et al., 2000; Jetter et al., 2010; Jones et al., 2010), but CYP2D6 may be dramatically affected in HIV infection. In 17 drug-naive patients with HIV infection, there was a 15% discordance of genotype and phenotype, associated with a 90% reduction in CYP2D6 activity in the infected group measured by the urinary ratio of dextromethorphan to its N-demethylated metabolite (Jones et al., 2010).

Hepatitis C Virus

There is considerable evidence that chronic hepatitis C virus (HCV) infection is associated with reduced activity of CYP3A4. Several studies reported higher steady-state levels of the CYP3A4 substrate cyclosporine A (CsA) and/or lower titrated doses in HCV$^+$ transplant patients than in HCV$^-$ (Tuncer et al., 2000; Latorre et al., 2002; Wolffenbuttel et al., 2003). Pharmacokinetic studies confirmed reduced clearance and increased exposure to CYP3A4 substrates in HCV$^+$ patients (Reesink et al., 2010; Morcos et al., 2013), even those who are asymptomatic (Wolffenbuttel et al., 2004). These findings are consistent with a report of increased toxicity of CsA in HCV$^+$ transplant patients (Horina et al., 1993).

Information is scarce on pharmacokinetics of drugs metabolized by other enzymes in HCV infection. Aminopyrine demethylation (catalyzed primarily by CYP2C19) was reduced by 57% and 30%, respectively, in patients with HCV infection with or without cirrhosis (Giannini et al., 2002). Liver biopsies from Japanese patients with HCV infection showed downregulations of multiple P450 mRNAs as well as those of the xenobiotic receptors CAR, pregnane X receptor (PXR), and aryl hydrocarbon receptor (AhR), which were dependent on the fibrosis stage (Nakai et al., 2008; Hanada et al., 2012). Only CYP1A2 correlated with the degree of inflammation. Two biopsy studies reported CYP2E1 mRNA downregulation correlated with fibrosis stage (Asselah et al., 2005; Bieche et al., 2005), whereas another found 37% upregulation of CYP2E1 in patients with HCV infection with steatosis but no correlation with degree of fibrosis or inflammation (Gochee et al., 2003).

Kirby et al. studied the impact of HCV and hepatitis B virus (HBV) infection on the expression of CYP2A6 by immunohistochemical analysis. In livers of patients with HBV and HCV infection, CYP2A6 expression was higher in hepatocytes close to areas with fibrosis and inflammation (Kirby et al., 1996). Smaller elevations were seen with CYP3A4 and CYP2B6. This was a small study of three patients with HBV infection and three with HCV infection.

Minimal effects of HCV infection were observed on the expression or activities of human P450 and drug transporter mRNAs in chimeric mice with humanized livers, except activity of CYP1A2, which was reduced by 50% (Kikuchi et al., 2010). The authors suggest that changes observed in pharmacokinetic parameters in infected humans might be secondary to fibrosis and inflammation. Indeed P450-mediated drug metabolism has been used as a measure of liver impairment during HCV hepatitis (Giannini et al., 2002).

Hepatitis B Virus

In liver samples from surgical patients with HBV infection, CYP3A4 activity and expression, determined by Western blotting, were 66% and 54%, respectively, of those of surgical patients without infection (Li et al., 2006). Plasma phenacetin clearance (CYP1A2) was 47% lower in patients with HBV infection than in normal controls, and O-deethylated metabolites also decreased by 25% (Aitken et al., 2008). Wang et al. phenotyped 106 patients with cirrhosis and 41 with chronic HBV infection for CYP1A2 and SULT1A1 activities using phenacetin. CYP1A2 activity was reduced by 91% and 68%, respectively, in the two cohorts, whereas SULT1A1 activities were not different from control (Wang et al., 2010b).

In mice transgenic for the HBV large envelope polypeptide, liver expression of Cyp2a5 and Cyp3a proteins was elevated (Kirby et al., 1994), consistent with the same group's observation of elevated CYP2A6 and 3A4 in livers of HBV-infected patients (Kirby et al., 1996). Two reports implicate the HBV protein Hbx in P450 regulation. Hbx stimulated expression of CYP3A4 in HepG2 cells via a specific interaction with PXR (Niu et al., 2013). Secondly, Hbx downregulated CYP2E1 expression in HepG2 cells, via downregulation of hepatocyte nuclear factor 4α (HNF4α) (Liu et al., 2014). These reports are difficult to reconcile because HNF4α is also an important regulator of CYP3A4 and its induction is via PXR activation. Hbx causes chronic activation of c-rapidly accelerated fibrosarcoma (c-RAF)/ERK2 signaling in the liver, leading to activation of transcription factors including AP-1 and NF-κB and inflammation and oxidative stress (Hildt et al., 2002; Schaedler et al., 2010; Balmasova et al., 2014).

Hepatitis A Virus

Only one study reported on the impact of HAV infection in humans. 7-OH coumarin excretion was measured as an index of CYP2A6 activity in 11 children and 9 adults with acute jaundice related to HVA infection. Compared with healthy controls, overall CYP2A6 activity was reduced by 37% in adults, but much more so (by 72%) in children.

Bacterial Infections

Sepsis

In a study of 51 children aged 1 day to 18 years with sepsis, there was a 50% reduction in antipyrine clearance (Carcillo et al., 2003), which was greater in children who also had multiple organ failure. Antipyrine clearance correlated with plasma IL-6 and nitrate (a product of NOS2) levels, which suggests that inflammation was a driving factor. In a study of 42 patients with sepsis following visceral surgery, aminopyrine clearance was significantly impaired and inversely correlated with TNFα levels and nitrate levels (Novotny et al., 2007), consistent with a primary role of inflammation in regulating P450 activity.

Lidocaine is metabolized mainly by CYP1A2 via N-deethylation to monoethylglycinexylidide (MEGX) and 3-hydroxylation at therapeutically relevant concentrations (Wang et al., 2000; Orlando et al., 2004). In patients with septic pneumonia, lidocaine N-demethylation in vivo was inversely correlated with IL-6 levels (Igonin et al., 2000). Lidocaine N-demethylation after coronary artery graft bypass surgery in patients with sepsis was only 20–25% that of patients without sepsis (Jakob et al., 2002).

In renal transplant patients, trough CsA (CYP3A4) levels were approximately doubled during gram-negative bacterial or fungal infections, which declined back to the preinfection level after the infection resolved (Hegazy et al., 2015).

Helicobacter pylori

Helicobacter pylori infection of the gastric mucosa is causative of peptic ulcers and is associated with other gastrointestinal diseases. In cirrhotic patients, H. pylori infection was associated with a 45% reduction in MEGX formation from lidocaine (CYP1A2), compared with uninfected patients (Giannini et al., 2001). In cirrhotic patients with HCV infection, H. pylori infection was associated with a 62% decrease in MEGX formation (Giannini et al., 2003). These studies showed that infection can downregulate P450 activity in humans even against a background of impaired liver function. However, CYP2C19 appears to be insensitive to this infection (Sagar et al., 1998).

Parasitic Infections

Malaria

The impact of malaria on the pharmacokinetics of the antimalarial drug quinine is well documented. The major human metabolite is 3-hydroxyquinine, and CYP3A4 is the main enzyme responsible. An early study reported that the ratio of plasma quinine: (quinine + metabolites) was increased in five patients with an experimentally induced infection of

Plasmodium falciparum. Subsequent studies have confirmed that the clearance of quinine is reduced (White et al., 1982; Supanaranond et al., 1991; Pukrittayakamee et al., 1997; Babalola et al., 1998), and its half-life lengthened (White et al., 1982) by factors of 40–70% during acute infection. Some studies indicate that the magnitude of the effect on quinine exposure is proportional to the degree of parasitemia or severity of infection (White et al., 1982; Kloprogge et al., 2014), but none reported an increase in toxicity of quinine. One study reported no difference in quinine pharmacokinetics between pregnant and nonpregnant Sudanese women with malaria (Abdelrahim et al., 2007), whereas another in Ugandan women reported that quinine exposure was proportional to parasite load (Kloprogge et al., 2014) and that quinine exposures in pregnancy were lower than those measured in nonpregnant patients, possibly due to the induction of CYP3A4 during pregnancy.

Clinical studies on the impact of malaria on other DMEs are few. Although the overall clearance of caffeine was unaffected by infection in Nigerian adults, CYP1A2 activity (paraxanthine:caffeine ratio) was reduced by 31% (Akinyinka et al., 2000a,b). A much larger effect was found in children, in whom oral clearance of caffeine was reduced to 36% of control and CYP1A2 activity was only 10–20% of control.

Plasmodium berghei malaria in mice was associated with downregulation of Cyp3a11, 2e1, and 1a2 mRNAs and associated activities (Carvalho et al., 2009), whereas coumarin hydroxylase activity associated with Cyp2a5 was induced (De-Oliveira et al., 2006). The cytosolic PRR Mda5 in hepatocytes recognizes plasmodium RNA as a PAMP (Liehl et al., 2014), and it would be interesting to know if Mda5 is involved in DME modulation in malaria.

Schistosomiasis

Schistosomiasis is caused by infection with trematode worms. More than 200 million people are infected annually, of whom less than 20% receive treatment. The worms mature in the portal venous system, during which time the infection is asymptomatic. The female adult worms begin to produce eggs about 4–6 weeks after infection (Gotardo et al., 2011), and the chronic disease is a result of the host's immune response to the eggs around which granulomas are formed. In the liver, this can eventually result in hepatosplenomegaly, liver fibrosis, and portal hypertension.

Fourteen published articles with pharmacokinetic data were found in a review (Wilby et al., 2013). In general, schistosomal infection tended only to impact pharmacokinetics in patients with liver disease (Wilby et al., 2013). The largest effects were observed with propranolol and the antischistosomal drug praziquantel, both of which have high hepatic extraction ratios. The C_{max} and AUC for propranolol, which is metabolized mainly by CYP2D6 and 1A2, were elevated 2.5-fold compared with uninfected controls (Homeida et al., 1987). About 2.5- to 5-fold increases in half-life or AUC of praziquantel (a CYP3A4 and 2D6 substrate) have been reported (Watt et al., 1988; Mandour et al., 1990). Significant findings were also reported for drugs with low hepatic extraction such as metronidazole (CYP2C9 and 2D6), antipyrine, and acetaminophen (UGTs). Two studies reported significant clinical responses associated with the altered pharmacokinetics (Wilby et al., 2013).

Reduced hepatic blood flow likely contributes to the observed changes especially for high extraction drugs (Wilby et al., 2013). However, the downregulation of hepatic cytochrome P450 mRNAs, proteins, and associated activities has been documented in animal studies, and again this occurs mainly in the stage when granulomas form in the liver (Gotardo et al., 2011; Mimche et al., 2014). Of the 33 DME mRNAs studied, 20 (P450, Ugt, and Sult as well as Fmo3) were downregulated to 1–50% of control levels during the granulomatous stage of infection in mice (Mimche et al., 2014), suggesting that downregulation of multiple DMEs may occur in people with liver involvement, which could contribute to the reported pharmacokinetic changes. Cyp1a2, 2c29, 2e1, 2j25, 3a11, 4f13, and 4f18 as well as Sult1a1mRNAs were upregulated by 27–67% before egg laying commenced (Mimche et al., 2014), suggesting that some drugs could have increased clearance in humans without liver involvement. Th2 cytokine expressions (IL-4, IL-5, and IL-13) in the granulomatous livers were much higher than those of the proinflammatory cytokines (Mimche et al., 2014), suggesting that the Th2 cytokines should be considered as possible regulators of DME expression.

Leishmaniasis

Leishmaniasis is a parasitic disease that afflicts 0.2–0.4 million people each year. Visceral leishmaniasis is the most serious infection, involving infection of liver, spleen, and bone marrow with *Leishmania donovani* or *Leishmania infantum*. In 18 infected Brazilian men and 6 women who were phenotyped, significant increases (on the order of 35–100%) in CYP3A4 (midazolam) and CYP2C19 (omeprazole) activities were found at completion of curative therapy and 3–6 months later, compared with activities before treatment. Plasma IL-6 levels were 6- to 26-fold higher in the patients during therapy than after therapy, which the authors proposed might contribute to the observed changes in P450 activities.

Liver Flukes

Opisthorchiasis viverrini is a liver fluke parasite that establishes in the bile ducts. Infected individuals with biliary fibrosis and dosed with coumarin had a significantly increased (45%) excretion of 7-hydroxycoumarin, an index of CYP2A6 activity, compared with uninfected subjects (Satarug et al., 1996). Infected subjects without biliary fibrosis had a similar trend, which was not significant. Significant reductions in CYP2A6 activity in both infected groups were observed after treatment with praziquantel.

Amebiasis

In patients with amebic liver abscesses with or without jaundice, the half-life of antipyrine was approximately double that of healthy controls (Narang et al., 1982) and was correlated with serum albumin, a negative APP. On the other hand, bilirubin glucuronyltransferase activity (UGT1A1) was unaffected.

Sterile Inflammation

Vaccination

The effects of influenza vaccination on pharmacokinetics or levels of drugs have been studied extensively (Grabenstein, 1990; Pellegrino et al., 2015). These studies have tended to focus on drugs with a low therapeutic index, for which relatively small changes in clearance could have important clinical consequences.

Two studies have found that influenza vaccination reduces theophylline clearance or elevates steady-state theophylline levels (Renton et al., 1980; Meredith et al., 1985) 24 h later. Meredith et al. (1985) reported a return to prevaccination values by 7 days. A larger number of studies concluded no effect of influenza vaccine (Pellegrino et al., 2015). Overall it appears that there is no consistent effect of vaccination on CYP1A2 activity and theophylline clearance. However, most of the above-mentioned studies used different vaccines or batches of vaccine, and it is possible that the response could be batch specific.

Due to the low therapeutic index of warfarin (metabolized by CYP2C9), there have been a number of studies to determine whether influenza vaccination affects the therapeutic efficacy or frequency of adverse reactions to the anticoagulant, and there is no consistent evidence that vaccination affects warfarin pharmacodynamics (Kuo et al., 2012; Pellegrino et al., 2015).

Other studies reported no effect of influenza vaccination on pharmacokinetics of erythromycin or alprazolam (CYP3A4) (Scavone et al., 1989; Hayney et al., 2002) or chlorzoxazone (CYP2E1) (Kim and Wilkinson, 1996). However, in a study of 22 healthy young subjects of whom 12 were vaccinated, there was a 40% decrease in CYP2C19-catalyzed (Niwa et al., 1999) aminopyrine metabolism 7 days after vaccination, with partial recovery by day 21 (Kramer and McClain, 1981).

BCG (tuberculosis) vaccine caused a 20% increase in theophylline half-life and a 28% reduction in clearance 14 days after vaccination in nine healthy young females with a positive skin test (Gray et al., 1983). A study of four patients with cancer and four volunteers reported no effect of BCG vaccination on phenytoin (CYP2C9) AUC in either group. Another small study of aminopyrine (CYP2C19) clearance in patients with extrahepatic cancers found that one-third of the patients treated with BCG had 40–60% reductions in clearance. In rats, downregulation of P450s was observed following BCG injection and was blocked with the KC toxicant gadolinium chloride (Kim et al., 2011).

Arthritis

Rheumatoid arthritis (RA) is a chronic inflammatory disease of the joints that afflicts 1.5 million US adults at any given time. Proinflammatory cytokines including IL-1, IL-6, IL-17, and TNFα are key drivers of the inflammatory cascade that ultimately results in degradation of bone and cartilage. There is little direct evidence that drug clearance is reduced in humans with RA. However, IL-6 antagonism can increase drug clearance in patients with RA (Schmitt et al., 2011), suggesting a reversal of inflammatory IL-6-mediated suppression. Moreover, simvastatin plasma levels in these patients with RA were higher than those reported in the literature for healthy volunteers (Schmitt et al., 2011). CYP2D6 activity may be unaffected in RA, as a study of patients with RA found no discordance of genotype and phenotype (Beyeler et al., 1994).

In human T-cell leukemia virus type I transgenic mice, the presence of arthritis downregulated Cyp3a11 mRNA but not those of Cyp2e1 or Cyp2c9 (Ashino et al., 2007). Collagen antibody-induced arthritis caused the downregulation of many P450 mRNAs, as well as Ugt1a1, 1a9, 2a3, and 2b5, whereas Cyp3a13 was induced (Dickmann et al., 2012). Notably, CAR and PXR were upregulated in this model. Adjuvant-induced RA in rats caused downregulation of CYP3A and CYP1A1 proteins (Ling and Jamali, 2009), and in another such model CYP2B1, 2B2, 3A1, and 3A2 mRNAs were all markedly suppressed (Sanada et al., 2011)

Cancer

Cancer is a group of chronic heterogeneous diseases that have in common an inflammatory component. Indeed the degree of inflammation, as indicated by the ratio of CRP to albumin in the plasma is a predictor of outcome in several different cancers (Coutant et al., 2015). A large number of anticancer drugs are cleared or activated by cytochrome P450 enzymes, and the possibility that their metabolism is influenced by the patient's inflammatory response has profound implications for the efficacy and toxicity of cancer chemotherapeutics and comedications.

A body of evidence is accumulating that cancer is associated with altered expression (usually downregulation) of CYP3A4 in human liver (Table 2.2). A retrospective study of clinical trial data found that the clearances of two CYP3A4 substrates, midazolam (54 patients) and enzastaurin (1065 patients), were reduced by 28% and 33%, respectively, in patients with cancer compared with healthy controls (Coutant et al., 2015). Advanced cancer was associated with sixfold elevation of plasma IL-6, whereas TNFα levels were only 24% higher in patients with cancer (Coutant et al., 2015). The variability of each cytokine was high in patients with cancer, reflecting heterogeneity of the inflammatory responses in this group.

Consistent with variability of the inflammatory response in patients with cancer, and a role of this response in the downregulation of CYP3A4, several clinical studies have reported an inverse association of CYP3A4 substrate clearance with CRP (Fig. 2.4) (Rivory et al., 2002), AAG (Bruno et al., 1996; Hirth et al., 2000), and/or a positive correlation with albumin (Hirth et al., 2000). IL-6 levels, but not those of TNFα or IL-1β, were correlated with CRP levels (Rivory et al., 2002), which suggests that IL-6 may have contributed to the observed suppression of CYP3A4-mediated erythromycin clearance. The sixfold variability in CYP3A4-mediated clearance and >100-fold variability in CRP in individual patients with cancer (Rivory et al., 2002) show that some patients with cancer have much lower CYP3A4 activity than others, with predicted adverse effects on drug toxicity. Two studies found that aspects of the toxicity of docetaxel, a CYP3A4 substrate, were predicted by plasma levels of AAG (Bruno et al., 2003), or AAG and CRP (Charles et al., 2006b) before treatment.

Two small studies on pharmacokinetics of two CYP2C9 substrates suggested no effect (tolbutamide; Shord et al., 2008) or increased activity (phenytoin; Wan et al., 1979) in patients with cancer. Conversely, 25% of patients with cancer studied who had a CYP2C19 extensive metabolizer genotype were phenotypic poor metabolizers (Williams et al., 2000), and the rest of the patients had phenotypic activities that trended toward slow metabolizer levels. This suggests that CYP2C19 may be downregulated or inhibited during cancer.

The CYP1A2 and NAT2 activities of 174 young Caucasian patients were determined using caffeine phenotyping. CYP1A2 activities were 10% lower in patients with cancer, whereas NAT2 activities were the same in both populations (Vistisen et al., 2004). The activity of the sulfotransferase SULT1A1, as measured by the ratio of phenacetin sulfate to glucuronide, was increased ninefold in patients with liver cancer with chronic HBV infection (Wang et al., 2010b), but not in patients with chronic HBV infection without cancer. This is the largest effect of cancer reported on drug metabolism, which needs to be further studied.

Suppression of Cyp3a expression in mice bearing the Engelbreth–Holm–Swarm sarcoma was unaffected in IL-6 knockout mice, but was inhibited by antibody to IL-6, indicating that the source of IL-6 responsible for the downregulation is the tumor itself (Kacevska et al., 2013). Downregulation was accompanied by activation of the JAK-STAT and MAPK

TABLE 2.2   Impact of Cancer on Drug Metabolism in Humans

Type of Cancer	Enzymes Studied	Population/Study	Findings	References
Miscellaneous	CYP3A4	521 patients with cancer in phase 1 and phase 2 studies of docetaxel CL	AAG level was a predictor of docetaxel CL (along with hepatic function)	Bruno et al. (1996)
Non–small-cell lung carcinoma	CYP3A4	Phenotyped 30 patients with cancer by determination of 6β-hydroxycortisol to cortisol urinary ratio and by docetaxel PK	Significant correlation of docetaxel CL and AAG levels was observed, as well as with age.	Yamamoto et al. (2000)
Metastatic sarcoma	CYP3A4	21 patients underwent the erythromycin breath test and also docetaxel PK analysis	Relatively weak inverse correlation of docetaxel CL with AAG, and also weak direct correlation with albumin	Hirth et al. (2000)
Lung, breast	CYP3A4	40 patients with cancer, mostly with lung or breast cancer, were administered the erythromycin breath test to estimate CYP3A4 activity	CYP3A4 activity was negatively correlated with both CRP and AAG levels in plasma. IL-6 levels, but not TNFα or IL-1β, were also well correlated with CRP	Rivory et al. (2002)
Miscellaneous	CYP3A4	PBPK model to study midazolam clearance in database of cancer drug studies at Eli Lilly. 54 patients with cancer and 205 healthy subjects	Cancer was the main predictor of midazolam CL, with cancer predicted to reduce CL by 28%. CRP and AAG were measured in small subsets, and no conclusion could be drawn about their abilities to predict	Coutant et al. (2015)
Miscellaneous	CYP3A4	PBPK model to study enzastaurin clearance in database of cancer drug studies at Eli Lilly. 1065 patients with cancer and 121 healthy subjects	Approximately 33% decrease in enzastaurin (CYP3A4) CL in patients with cancer versus healthy subjects. Correlated with albumin levels in plasma	Coutant et al. (2015)
Miscellaneous	CYP3A4	640 patients in 24 phase 2 studies	Docetaxel CL was the best predictor of toxicity	Bruno et al. (1998)
Non–small-cell lung carcinoma	CYP3A4	180 patients in 6 phase 2 trials	Docetaxel AUC was the only predictor of severe toxicity during the first course of drug therapy. Elevated AAG was a predictor of both poor response and patient survival	Bruno et al. (2003)

TABLE 2.2   Impact of Cancer on Drug Metabolism in Humans—cont'd

Type of Cancer	Enzymes Studied	Population/Study	Findings	References
Miscellaneous	CYP3A4	Studied predictors of docetaxel toxicity in 68 patients with advanced cancer (lung, breast, head and neck, and prostate)	Hematological toxicity was predicted by docetaxel clearance. Nonhematological toxicity was not predicted by pharmacokinetic parameters, but was predicted by baseline CRP and AAG levels before treatment	Charles et al. (2006b)
Melanoma	CYP2C9	Measured phenytoin PK in 8 patients with cancer and compared with 4 healthy volunteers	AUC of phenytoin in volunteers was almost double that in patients with cancer. This suggests that cancer (6 of 8 patients had melanoma) induces CYP2C9	Wan et al. (1979)
Miscellaneous	CYP2C9	Measured tolbutamide CL in 10 patients and 10 matched controls	Tolbutamide clearance and urinary metabolic ratios were not different in the two groups, although mean IL-6 and TNFα levels in the plasma were elevated 5- and 17-fold, respectively (not statistically significant)	Shord et al. (2008)
Miscellaneous	CYP2C19	Measured omeprazole hydroxylation (plasma single time point) and 2C19 genotype in 16 patients with metastatic cancers of various origins	Although all 16 patients were genotypic extensive metabolizers, 4 were phenotypic poor metabolizers and the other 12 had activities that were lower than expected	Williams et al. (2000)
Testicular	CYP1A2 NAT2	Phenotyped 174 young (<45) Caucasian patients and 183 controls for CYP1A2 and NAT2 activity using urinary metabolites of caffeine	Median CYP1A2 activity was 10% lower than in controls. No differences in NAT2 activity. This was not tested statistically	Vistisen et al. (2004)
Liver	CYP1A1 SULT1A1	Phenotyped 41 patients with chronic HBV infection, 148 hepatic carcinoma patients (secondary to HBV), 106 cirrhotic patients and 82 controls for CYP1A2 and SULT1A1 using phenacetin as probe (deethylation and sulfate/glucuronide ratio)	Patients with cancer had ninefold higher SULT1A1 activity compared with healthy controls, but no change in 1A2 activity. Patients with HBV infection had 67% reduction in CYP1A1 activity, but normal SULT1A1 activity	Wang et al. (2010b)

AAG, α1-Acid glycoprotein; *AUC*, area under the curve; *CL*, clearance; *CRP*, C-reactive protein; *HBV*, hepatitis B virus; *IL*, interleukin; *NAT*, N-acetyltransferase; *PBPK*, physiologically based pharmacokinetic modeling; *PK*, pharmacokinetics; *TNF*, tumor necrosis factor.

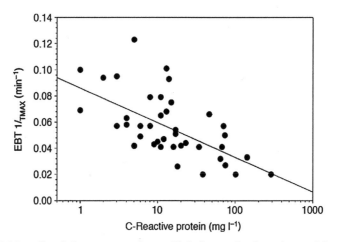

FIGURE 2.4 **CYP3A4-mediated clearance correlates with inflammation in patients with advanced cancer.** The relationship between the 1/TMAX parameter of the erythromycin breath test and serum C-reactive protein in 40 patients with advanced cancer. The upper limit of normal of C-reactive protein (CRP) is 10 mg/L. *Reprinted from Rivory, L.P., Slaviero, K.A., Clarke, S.J., 2002. Hepatic cytochrome P450 3A drug metabolism is reduced in cancer patients who have an acute-phase response. Br. J. Cancer 87:277–280, with permission.*

pathways in the liver, and this was also attenuated by the antibody (Kacevska et al., 2013). Tumor presence was associated with a downregulation of a β-galactosidase transgene under the regulation of the CYP3A4 promoter, demonstrating transcriptional regulation of CYP3A4 in cancer (Charles et al., 2006a).

Lupus Erythematosus

Systemic lupus erythematosus (SLE) is an autoimmune inflammatory disease. Based on a high prevalence of the CYP2D6 poor metabolizer phenotype in patients with SLE, Baer et al. (1986) suggested that CYP2D6 might be involved in disease susceptibility. Another study found that CYP2D6 allele frequency was not different in patients with SLE (Sabbagh et al., 1998), suggesting that the reason CYP2D6 PM phenotype is more frequent may be phenoconversion, i.e., CYP2D6 is downregulated during SLE. Interestingly, Lahita et al. (1981) reported that the extent of estradiol 16α-hydroxylation (CYP3A4 and CYP1A2) was approximately 70% higher in patients with SLE than in controls, regardless of gender, suggesting that CYP3A4 and/or CYP1A2 may be induced during SLE.

Behçet Disease

Behçet disease is a chronic relapsing inflammatory disorder associated with elevated plasma levels of IL-6 and other Th2-related cytokines (Goktas et al., 2015). In 52 patients with Behçet disease, a 75-fold increase in metabolic ratio of losartan was found, indicating downregulation of CYP2C9 (Goktas et al., 2015). More studies are needed to determine the impact of this disease on other P450 enzymes.

Critical Illness

There have been several studies describing the extensive impairment of drug metabolism in critically ill patients. This includes reduced metabolism of midazolam by both CYP3A4 (Shelly et al., 1987; Ince et al., 2012) and UGTs (Ince et al., 2012). There is no substantive evidence that inflammation is involved in the response, although this is considered likely. In children, reduced midazolam clearance was negatively correlated to disease severity, whereas there was no correlation with the degree of inflammation as measured by plasma CRP concentrations (Vet et al., 2012).

Congestive Heart Failure

Congestive heart failure (CHF) is associated with inflammation and a rise in plasma levels of proinflammatory cytokines. In 16 patients with CHF, Frye et al. (2002) found an unexpectedly high fraction of phenotypic CYP2C19 poor metabolizers, and a striking negative correlation of CYP2C19 activity with plasma levels of IL-6 and TNFα, suggestive of inflammation-mediated downregulation of CYP2C19. CYP1A2 activities were negatively associated with IL-6 concentrations, but not with TNFα. In contrast, no evidence was found for inflammatory regulation of CYP2E1 or CYP2D6 in these patients (Frye et al., 2002). CHF is characterized by a slow decline in hepatic blood flow with disease progression, and a decrease in carvedilol clearance (a CYP2D6 substrate) in CHF has been attributed to reduced hepatic blood flow (Saito et al., 2010; Rasool et al., 2015).

To detect whether the changes in drug clearance in heart failure are due to changes in hepatic enzyme content, liver hypoxia, or liver congestion, Ng et al. (2000) studied the clearance of propranolol in rats with right ventricular heart failure. They found that a 97% reduction in propranolol intrinsic clearance could only be partially accounted for by reduced hepatic P450 contents.

Bone Marrow Transplantation

There have been two small studies of CsA (CYP3A4) clearance in patients receiving the immunosuppressant following a bone marrow transplant. In one study, the clearance of CsA was reduced by 50% in the period between 3 and 7 days after transplant and 14—20 days (Schwinghammer et al., 1991). In another study of six patients, serum IL-6 levels increased and peaked on average at 11 days after transplantation, with CRP behaving similarly (Chen et al., 1994). Plasma levels of CsA also rose, peaking slightly after IL-6, implicating inflammation and possibly IL-6 in the reduced clearance of CsA.

DISEASE-DEPENDENT DRUG—DRUG INTERACTIONS

In a clinical trial of tocilizumab, an IL-6 receptor antibody developed for the treatment of arthritis (Schmitt et al., 2011), exposure to simvastatin (a CYP3A4 substrate) in patients with RA was reduced by 57% 1 week after a single dose of tocilizumab, presumably due to reversal of CYP3A4 downregulation by IL-6. Exposure was still reduced 6 weeks after treatment. This is termed a disease-dependent drug—drug interaction (DDDI) because the effect of tocilizumab would not be seen in a healthy patient. In a probe cocktail study of the anti-IL-6 antibody sirukumab in patients with RA, CYP 2C19-catalyzed clearance of omeprazole was most affected (37–45% increase), whereas CYP2C9 (S-warfarin) was least affected (18–19%) (Zhuang et al., 2015). The impact of sirukumab on CYP3A4-mediated midazolam exposure was slightly less than that reported for tocilizumab on simvastatin. Caffeine clearance was increased by sirukumab treatment, suggesting that RA may induce CYP1A2 in humans.

The principle of DDDI had been demonstrated in rodents sometime before the clinical studies. The downregulation of hepatic CYP3A mRNAs, proteins, and activities in two arthritis models was reversed by polyclonal IL-6 antibodies (Ashino et al., 2007) and by the TNFα antibody infliximab (Ling and Jamali, 2009). Later, a dominant-negative form of TNFα was shown to attenuate the downregulation of mouse Cyp3a mRNAs in the *C. rodentium* model of infectious colitis (Nyagode et al., 2014). One might postulate that any therapy that reduces inflammation, regardless of mechanism, has the same effect as cytokine antibodies on DME downregulation. This remains to be tested.

MECHANISMS OF REGULATION

Inflammatory stimuli cause the downregulation of mRNA expression of many DMEs. Transcriptional regulation has been confirmed in vivo via transcription run-on assays (Cheng et al., 2003) and reporter gene expression in vitro (Chen et al., 1995) and in vivo (Charles et al., 2006a). Although this may be the dominant mechanism in most cases, several other levels of regulation have been demonstrated. The great diversity of mechanisms clarifies why DMEs, like APPs, are not coordinately regulated during inflammation and that this depends on the disease or inflammatory stimulus.

Transcriptional Mechanisms

When evaluating mechanisms of regulation, it is important to distinguish correlative studies from those for which direct mechanistic evidence has been presented.

Direct Repression via Negative Response Elements

NF-κB plays a central role in inflammation responses (Figs. 2.1 and 2.2). It can also downregulate DME transcription via binding to negative control elements of the rat *CYP2C11* (Iber et al., 2000) and human *UGT1A1* (Shiu et al., 2013) genes. Binding sites for NF-κB have been identified by electrophoretic mobility shift assay in the rat *CYP1A1*, *CYP2B1/2*, and *CYP2D5* promoters (Zordoky and El-Kadi, 2009), but whether they mediate transcriptional suppression is not known. Two direct mechanisms for repression of the CYP3A4 gene by IL-6 have been described. IL-6 stimulates the selective translation of liver-enriched inhibitory protein (LIP), a short form of C/EBPβ that is a dominant inhibitor, resulting in antagonism of the transcriptionally active forms of C/EBP and downregulation of CYP3A4 transcription (Jover et al., 2002). Differentially expressed in chondrocytes 1 (DEC1) is rapidly induced by IL-6 in hepatocytes, and actively represses CYP3A4 transcription in response to IL-6 (Mao et al., 2012).

Downregulation of Positive Transcription Factors

C/EBP isoforms and HNFs are transcription factors that contribute to the basal expression of many P450 genes. In rodent livers, HNF1α, HNF3β, and HNF4α DNA binding activities are rapidly downregulated in response to LPS injection (Chen et al., 1995; Li and Klaassen, 2004). Repression of a CYP3A4 reporter transgene in mice with extrahepatic cancers was associated with decreased levels of both the LIP and active forms of C/EBPβ (Kacevska et al., 2011). One would predict that the downregulation of multiple positive factors is likely to contribute to downregulation. Studies in HNF1α knockout mice demonstrated the importance of reduced HNF1α binding for downregulation of the drug transporter (Li and Klaassen, 2004).

Nuclear receptors PXR and CAR mediate the selective induction of subsets of DME genes by xenobiotics, and retinoid X receptor-α (RXRα) is their obligatory dimerization partner. Numerous studies have demonstrated the downregulation of each of these receptors by inflammatory stimuli (Beigneux et al., 2000; Pascussi et al., 2000; Assenat et al., 2004; Ghose et al., 2008, 2011; Ghaffari et al., 2011; Kacevska et al., 2011) and that this causes suppression of drug-induced expression of target genes (Muntane-Relat et al., 1995; Pascussi et al., 2000; Assenat et al., 2004; Moriya et al., 2012). IL-1 downregulates CAR in an NF-κB-dependent mechanism (Assenat et al., 2004). The degree to which downregulation (or inhibition, see later discussion) of nuclear receptors contributes to the downregulation of DME expression in the absence of drug inducers is less clear. In $PXR^{-/-}$ or $CAR^{-/-}$ mice, downregulation of DME genes by LPS was not impaired (Richardson and Morgan, 2005; Shah et al., 2014). However, the downregulation of Cyp3a11 and some drug transporters by IL-6 injection was attenuated (Teng and Piquette-Miller, 2005) in $PXR^{-/-}$ mice, and the downregulation of DME genes by the TLR2 ligand lipoteichoic acid was attenuated in $CAR^{-/-}$ mice (Shah et al., 2014). In human hepatocytes, downregulation of CYP3A4 could be inhibited by knockdown of PXR with small interfering RNA (Yang et al., 2010a). Taken together, these results suggest that modulation of nuclear receptor expression or activity contributes to the downregulation of constitutive DME expression, the magnitude of the contribution depending on the nature of the inflammatory stimulus. Diet may also affect their contributions, given that dietary components are activators of PXR and CAR (Gao and Xie, 2010).

Inhibitory Binding to Positive Transcription Factors

NF-κB can bind to RXR, and this inhibits the binding of PXR to the CYP3A4 promoter and subsequent induction of this enzyme (Gu et al., 2006). It seems likely that this mechanism could also affect CAR function. The AhR mediates the induction of many DMEs, notably the CYP1A and CYP1B subfamilies, by polycyclic and polyhalogenated aromatic hydrocarbons, and its interaction with NF-κB can inhibit ligand-mediated induction of these genes (Tian et al., 1999). On the other hand, NF-κB activation can induce AhR via an NF-κB response element, and thereby potentiate CYP1B1 induction by AhR agonists (Smerdova et al., 2014; Vogel et al., 2014).

Induction Mechanisms

The mechanism of induction of CYP2E1 in human hepatocytes by IL-4 was studied in HepG2 cells (Abdel-Razzak et al., 2004). The IL-4 responsive region of the gene contained putative binding sites for STAT6, AP-1, NF-κB, nuclear factor of activated T cells (NFAT), and C/EBP, to which the binding of AP-1 and NFAT in a protein kinase C–dependent manner was demonstrated (Abdel-Razzak et al., 2004). The functional roles of STAT6 and NFATc1 were determined by Wang et al. (2010a). Sult1e1 (estrogen sulfotransferase) is induced in mouse liver following LPS treatment or cecal ligation and puncture, and this depends on NF-κB binding to a response element in its promoter (Gu et al., 2006).

As noted earlier, human CYP2A6 is upregulated in some inflammatory diseases, and this is also true of its mouse counterpart Cyp2a5 (Su and Ding, 2004). Both are targets of nuclear factor (erythroid-derived 2)-like 2 (Nrf2), which is activated in response to oxidative stress (Su and Ding, 2004; Abu-Bakar et al., 2007; Yokota et al., 2010). HBV can induce Nrf2 target genes via activation of RAF and mitogen-extracellular signaling-regulated kinase signaling pathways by the viral proteins HBx and LHBs. Whether cytokines can upregulate CYP2A5 or Cyp2a5 via Nrf2 remains to be determined.

Epigenetic Mechanisms

The study of epigenetic mechanisms in regulation of DME gene expression is a relatively new field. In rats with experimentally induced chronic kidney diseases, the downregulation of CYP2C11 and CYP3A2 is accompanied by decreases in histone acetylation in the regions necessary for nuclear receptor activation (Velenosi et al., 2014). However, any contribution of inflammation to this is speculative.

Posttranscriptional Mechanisms

Nitric Oxide

During an inflammatory response, hepatocytes and KC produce nitric oxide, due to the induction of NOS2 by inflammatory cytokines. Therefore, the contribution of NO to DME downregulation during inflammation has been studied intensively. NO binds to the prosthetic group of hemoproteins and as such NO produces both reversible and irreversible inhibition of P450 enzymes (Wink et al., 1993; Kim et al., 1995; Takemura et al., 1999). In vivo, this has particular importance in the early phase of the inflammatory response (Barakat et al., 2001).

There have been several reports that NOS inhibition could attenuate the downregulation of P450 mRNAs by inflammatory stimuli. Most of these studies were conducted in vivo and it is possible that inhibition of NOS in vivo indirectly affects P450 expression via modulation of the inflammatory response itself. Moreover, these reports are matched by a similar number of negative findings.

The evidence for downregulation of P450 protein levels by NO is stronger and more consistent. The downregulation of some P450 proteins is attenuated or blocked when NOS2 is inhibited (Carlson and Billings, 1996; Khatsenko et al., 1997; Ferrari et al., 2001; Eum et al., 2006). In response to IL-1β or LPS, which induces NOS2 in hepatocytes, rat CYP2B1 is downregulated by NO- and ubiquitin-dependent proteasomal degradation of the protein (Ferrari et al., 2001; Lee et al., 2008). This is much faster than downregulation of its mRNA, which is NO independent (Ferrari et al., 2001). Rat CYP3A2 undergoes the same regulation (Lee et al., 2008), whereas CYP2C11 is not sensitive to NO (Sewer and Morgan, 1997). CYP2B1 inhibition by peroxynitrite in vitro is due to stoichiometric nitration of Tyr190 (Lin et al., 2003), but the contribution of this modification to NO-directed degradation has not been shown. Human CYP2B6 protein is also downregulated in an NO-dependent manner, under conditions where the mRNA is not affected (Aitken et al., 2008). Other NO-dependent proteolytic mechanisms may exist, because the downregulation of CYP2C22 occurs in the presence of proteasome inhibitors (Lee et al., 2014).

MicroRNAs

MicroRNAs (miRNAs) regulate the translation and/or stability of cellular mRNAs, thereby providing a mechanism of posttranscriptional control of gene expression. Rieger et al. found that of several miRNAs elevated in cholestatic and inflamed livers, miR-130b transfection into HepaRG cells caused decreases in CAR, farnesoid X receptor, and CYP1A1, 1A2, 2A6, 2C8, 2C9, and 2C19 expression. A functional role for miR-130b was confirmed by regulation of a reporter gene coupled to the 3′-untranslated region of the CYP2C9 promoter.

The potential roles of other miRNAs in the inflammatory downregulation of P450 protein and mRNA expression are largely unexplored. Correlative evidence and in silico exploration of miRNA-binding sites suggests a role for several miRNAs, especially miR-155, in regulation of CYP3A4 expression in cirrhotic livers (Vuppalanchi et al., 2013), but this awaits functional confirmation and elucidation of the role of inflammation.

CONCLUSION

Inflammatory regulation of DMEs is broadly applicable to a spectrum of human diseases, and cell and animal experiments have provided clear evidence for the involvement of proinflammatory cytokines in this regulation. The relative importance of individual cytokines in specific disease states is not well understood, although IL-6 appears to be a major factor in some situations. Cytokine-independent regulation via TLRs is also possible. Understanding the contribution of inflammatory regulation to interindividual variation in drug metabolism, and predicting the impact of disease (or its amelioration by therapy) in individuals will require a better understanding of the mechanisms behind these responses. More clinical studies analyzing the correlative and predictive value of biomarkers are needed, including the cytokines themselves, APPs, or other inflammatory outputs.

References

Abdelrahim, I.I., Adam, I., Elghazali, G., Gustafsson, L.L., Elbashir, M.I., Mirghani, R.A., 2007. Pharmacokinetics of quinine and its metabolites in pregnant Sudanese women with uncomplicated *Plasmodium falciparum* malaria. J. Clin. Pharm. Ther. 32, 15–19.

Abdel-Razzak, Z., Loyer, P., Fautrel, A., Gautier, J.C., Corcos, L., Turlin, B., Beaune, P., Guillouzo, A., 1993. Cytokines down-regulate expression of major cytochrome P-450 enzymes in adult human hepatocytes in primary culture. Mol. Pharmacol. 44, 707–715.

Abdel-Razzak, Z., Garlatti, M., Aggerbeck, M., Barouki, R., 2004. Determination of interleukin-4-responsive region in the human cytochrome P450 2E1 gene promoter. Biochem. Pharmacol. 68, 1371–1381.

Abu-Bakar, A., Lamsa, V., Arpiainen, S., Moore, M.R., Lang, M.A., Hakkola, J., 2007. Regulation of CYP2A5 gene by the transcription factor nuclear factor (erythroid-derived 2)-like 2. Drug Metab. Dispos. 35, 787–794.

Adedoyin, A., Arns, P.A., Richards, W.O., Wilkinson, G.R., Branch, R.A., 1998. Selective effect of liver disease on the activities of specific metabolizing enzymes: investigation of cytochromes P450 2C19 and 2D6. Clin. Pharmacol. Ther. 64, 8–17.

Aitken, A.E., Morgan, E.T., 2007. Gene-specific effects of inflammatory cytokines on cytochrome P450 2C, 2B6 and 3A4 mRNA levels in human hepatocytes. Drug Metab. Dispos. 35, 1687–1693.

Aitken, A.E., Richardson, T.A., Morgan, E.T., 2006. Regulation of drug-metabolizing enzymes and transporters in inflammation. Annu. Rev. Pharmacol. Toxicol. 46, 123–149.

Aitken, A.E., Lee, C.M., Morgan, E.T., 2008. Roles of nitric oxide in inflammatory downregulation of human cytochromes P450. Free Radic. Biol. Med. 44, 1161–1168.

Akinyinka, O.O., Sowunmi, A., Honeywell, R., Renwick, A.G., 2000a. The effects of acute falciparum malaria on the disposition of caffeine and the comparison of saliva and plasma-derived pharmacokinetic parameters in adult Nigerians. Eur. J. Clin. Pharmacol. 56, 159–165.

Akinyinka, O.O., Sowunmi, A., Honeywell, R., Renwick, A.G., 2000b. The pharmacokinetics of caffeine in Nigerian children suffering from malaria and kwashiorkor. Eur. J. Clin. Pharmacol. 56, 153–158.

Akira, S., Isshiki, H., Sugita, T., Tanabe, O., Kinoshita, S., Nishio, Y., Nakajima, T., Hirano, T., Kishimoto, T., 1990. A nuclear factor for IL-6 expression (NF-IL6) is a member of a C/EBP family. EMBO J. 9, 1897–1906.

Alkharfy, K.M., Poloyac, S.M., Congiu, M., Desmond, P.V., Frye, R.F., 2008. Effect of the acute phase response induced by endotoxin administration on the expression and activity of UGT isoforms in rats. Drug Metab. Lett. 2, 248–255.

Ashino, T., Oguro, T., Shioda, S., Horai, R., Asano, M., 2004. Involvement of interleukin-6 and tumor necrosis factor alpha in CYP3A11 and 2C29 down-regulation by Bacillus Calmette–Guerin and lipopolysaccharide in mouse liver. Drug Metab. Dispos. 32, 707–714.

Ashino, T., Arima, Y., Shioda, S., Iwakura, Y., Numazawa, S., Yoshida, T., 2007. Effect of interleukin-6 neutralization on CYP3A11 and metallothionein-1/2 expressions in arthritic mouse liver. Eur. J. Pharmacol. 558, 199–207.

Asselah, T., Bieche, I., Laurendeau, I., Paradis, V., Vidaud, D., Degott, C., Martinot, M., Bedossa, P., Valla, D., Vidaud, M., Marcellin, P., 2005. Liver gene expression signature of mild fibrosis in patients with chronic hepatitis C. Gastroenterology 129, 2064–2075.

Assenat, E., Gerbal-Chaloin, S., Larrey, D., Saric, J., Fabre, J.M., Maurel, P., Vilarem, M.J., Pascussi, J.M., 2004. Interleukin 1beta inhibits CAR-induced expression of hepatic genes involved in drug and bilirubin clearance. Hepatology 40, 951–960.

Babalola, C.P., Bolaji, O.O., Ogunbona, F.A., Sowunmi, A., Walker, O., 1998. Pharmacokinetics of quinine in African patients with acute falciparum malaria. Pharm. World Sci. 20, 118–122.

Baer, A.N., McAllister, C.B., Wilkinson, G.R., Woosley, R.L., Pincus, T., 1986. Altered distribution of debrisoquine oxidation phenotypes in patients with systemic lupus erythematosus. Arthritis Rheum. 29, 843–850.

Balmasova, I.P., Yushchuk, N.D., Mynbaev, O.A., Alla, N.R., Malova, E.S., Shi, Z., Gao, C.L., 2014. Immunopathogenesis of chronic hepatitis B. World J. Gastroenterol. 20, 14156–14171.

Barakat, M.M., El-Kadi, A.O., du Souich, P., 2001. L-NAME prevents in vivo the inactivation but not the downregulation of hepatic cytochrome P450 caused by an acute inflammatory reaction. Life Sci. 69, 1559–1571.

Baumann, H., Gauldie, J., 1994. The acute phase response. Immunol. Today 15, 74–80.

Beigneux, A., Moser, A., Shigenaga, J., Grunfeld, C., Feingold, K., 2000. The acute phase response is associated with retinoid X receptor repression in rodent liver. J. Biol. Chem. 275, 16390–16399.

Betts, J.C., Cheshire, J.K., Akira, S., Kishimoto, T., Woo, P., 1993. The role of NF-kappa B and NF-IL6 transactivating factors in the synergistic activation of human serum amyloid A gene expression by interleukin-1 and interleukin-6. J. Biol. Chem. 268, 25624–25631.

Beyeler, C., Daly, A.K., Armstrong, M., Astbury, C., Bird, H.A., Idle, J.R., 1994. Phenotype/genotype relationships for the cytochrome P450 enzyme CYP2D6 in rheumatoid arthritis: influence of drug therapy and disease activity. J. Rheumatol. 21, 1034–1039.

Bieche, I., Asselah, T., Laurendeau, I., Vidaud, D., Degot, C., Paradis, V., Bedossa, P., Valla, D.C., Marcellin, P., Vidaud, M., 2005. Molecular profiling of early stage liver fibrosis in patients with chronic hepatitis C virus infection. Virology 332, 130–144.

Bilzer, M., Roggel, F., Gerbes, A.L., 2006. Role of Kupffer cells in host defense and liver disease. Liver Int. 26, 1175–1186.

Brenner, D., Blaser, H., Mak, T.W., 2015. Regulation of tumour necrosis factor signalling: live or let die. Nat. Rev. Immunol. 15, 362–374.

Brockmeyer, N.H., Barthel, B., Mertins, L., Goos, M., 1998. Changes of antipyrine pharmacokinetics during influenza and after administration of interferon-alpha and -beta. Int. J. Clin. Pharmacol. Ther. 36, 309–311.

Bruno, R., Vivier, N., Vergniol, J.C., De Phillips, S.L., Montay, G., Sheiner, L.B., 1996. A population pharmacokinetic model for docetaxel (Taxotere): model building and validation. J. Pharmacokinet. Biopharm. 24, 153–172.

Bruno, R., Hille, D., Riva, A., Vivier, N., ten Bokkel Huinnink, W.W., van Oosterom, A.T., Kaye, S.B., Verweij, J., Fossella, F.V., Valero, V., Rigas, J.R., Seidman, A.D., Chevallier, B., Fumoleau, P., Burris, H.A., Ravdin, P.M., Sheiner, L.B., 1998. Population pharmacokinetics/pharmacodynamics of docetaxel in phase II studies in patients with cancer. J. Clin. Oncol. 16, 187–196.

Bruno, R., Olivares, R., Berille, J., Chaikin, P., Vivier, N., Hammershaimb, L., Rhodes, G.R., Rigas, J.R., 2003. Alpha-1-acid glycoprotein as an independent predictor for treatment effects and a prognostic factor of survival in patients with non-small cell lung cancer treated with docetaxel. Clin. Cancer Res. 9, 1077–1082.

Carcillo, J.A., Doughty, L., Kofos, D., Frye, R.F., Kaplan, S.S., Sasser, H., Burckart, G.J., 2003. Cytochrome P450 mediated-drug metabolism is reduced in children with sepsis-induced multiple organ failure. Intensive Care Med. 29, 980–984.

Carlson, T.J., Billings, R.E., 1996. Role of nitric oxide in the cytokine-mediated regulation of cytochrome P-450. Mol-Pharmacol. 49, 796–801.

Carvalho, R.S., Friedrich, K., De-Oliveira, A.C., Suarez-Kurtz, G., Paumgartten, F.J., 2009. Malaria downmodulates mRNA expression and catalytic activities of CYP1A2, 2E1 and 3A11 in mouse liver. Eur. J. Pharmacol. 616, 265–269.

Celsus A.C. De Medicina. In: ca. 100 BC.

Chai, X., Guo, Y., Jiang, M., Hu, B., Li, Z., Fan, J., Deng, M., Billiar, T.R., Kucera, H.R., Gaikwad, N.W., Xu, M., Lu, P., Yan, J., Fu, H., Liu, Y., Yu, L., Huang, M., Zeng, S., Xie, W., 2015. Oestrogen sulfotransferase ablation sensitizes mice to sepsis. Nat. Commun. 6, 7979.

Chakraborty, A., Blum, R.A., Mis, S.M., Cutler, D.L., Jusko, W.J., 1999. Pharmacokinetic and adrenal interactions of IL-10 and prednisone in healthy volunteers. J. Clin. Pharmacol. 39, 624–635.

Chaluvadi, M.R., Nyagode, B.A., Kinloch, R.D., Morgan, E.T., 2009. TLR4-dependent and -independent regulation of hepatic cytochrome P450 in mice with chemically induced inflammatory bowel disease. Biochem. Pharmacol. 77, 464–471.

Chang, K.C., Bell, T.D., Lauer, B.A., Chai, H., 1978. Altered theophylline pharmacokinetics during acute respiratory viral illness. Lancet 1, 1132–1133.

Charles, K.A., Rivory, L.P., Brown, S.L., Liddle, C., Clarke, S.J., Robertson, G.R., 2006a. Transcriptional repression of hepatic cytochrome P450 3A4 gene in the presence of cancer. Clin. Cancer Res. 12, 7492–7497.

Charles, K.A., Rivory, L.P., Stockler, M.R., Beale, P., Beith, J., Boyer, M., Clarke, S.J., 2006b. Predicting the toxicity of weekly docetaxel in advanced cancer. Clin. Pharmacokinet. 45, 611–622.

Chen, Y.L., Le Vraux, V., Leneveu, A., Dreyfus, F., Stheneur, A., Florentin, I., De Sousa, M., Giroud, J.P., Flouvat, B., Chauvelot-Moachon, L., 1994. Acute-phase response, interleukin-6, and alteration of cyclosporine pharmacokinetics. Clin. Pharmacol. Ther. 55, 649–660.

Chen, J.Q., Strom, A., Gustafsson, J.A., Morgan, E.T., 1995. Suppression of the constitutive expression of cytochrome P-450 2C11 by cytokines and interferons in primary cultures of rat hepatocytes: comparison with induction of acute-phase genes and demonstration that CYP2C11 promoter sequences are involved in the suppressive response to interleukins 1 and 6. Mol. Pharmacol. 47, 940–947.

Cheng, P., Wang, M., Morgan, E., 2003. Rapid transcriptional suppression of rat cytochrome P450 genes by endotoxin treatment and its inhibition by curcumin. J. Pharmacol. Exp. Ther. 307, 1205–1212.

Congiu, M., Mashford, M.L., Slavin, J.L., Desmond, P.V., 2002. UDP glucuronosyltransferase mRNA levels in human liver disease. Drug Metab. Dispos. 30, 129–134.

Coutant, D.E., Kulanthaivel, P., Turner, P.K., Bell, R.L., Baldwin, J., Wijayawardana, S.R., Pitou, C., Hall, S.D., 2015. Understanding disease-drug interactions in Cancer patients: implications for dosing within the therapeutic window. Clin. Pharmacol. Ther. 98, 76–86.

Dallas, S., Chattopadhyay, S., Sensenhauser, C., Batheja, A., Singer, M., Silva, J., 2013. Interleukins-12 and -23 do not alter expression or activity of multiple cytochrome P450 enzymes in cryopreserved human hepatocytes. Drug Metab. Dispos. 41, 689–693.

De Nardo, D., 2015. Toll-like receptors: activation, signalling and transcriptional modulation. Cytokine 74, 181–189.

De-Oliveira, A.C., Da-Matta, A.C., Paumgartten, F.J., 2006. *Plasmodium berghei* (ANKA): infection induces CYP2A5 and 2E1 while depressing other CYP isoforms in the mouse liver. Exp. Parasitol. 113, 256–261.

Dickmann, L.J., Patel, S.K., Rock, D.A., Wienkers, L.C., Slatter, J.G., 2011. Effects of interleukin-6 (IL-6) and an anti-IL-6 monoclonal antibody on drug-metabolizing enzymes in human hepatocyte culture. Drug Metab. Dispos. 39, 1415–1422.

Dickmann, L.J., McBride, H.J., Patel, S.K., Miner, K., Wienkers, L.C., Slatter, J.G., 2012. Murine collagen antibody induced arthritis (CAIA) and primary mouse hepatocyte culture as models to study cytochrome P450 suppression. Biochem. Pharmacol. 83, 1682–1689.

Eklund, C.M., 2009. Proinflammatory cytokines in CRP baseline regulation. Adv. Clin. Chem. 48, 111–136.

Elkahwaji, J., Robin, M.A., Berson, A., Tinel, M., Letteron, P., Labbe, G., Beaune, P., Elias, D., Rougier, P., Escudier, B., Duvillard, P., Pessayre, D., 1999. Decrease in hepatic cytochrome P450 after interleukin-2 immunotherapy. Biochem. Pharmacol. 57, 951–954.

Eum, H.A., Yeom, D.H., Lee, S.M., 2006. Role of nitric oxide in the inhibition of liver cytochrome P450 during sepsis. Nitric Oxide 15, 423–431.

Evers, R., Dallas, S., Dickmann, L.J., Fahmi, O.A., Kenny, J.R., Kraynov, E., Nguyen, T., Patel, A.H., Slatter, J.G., Zhang, L., 2013. Critical review of preclinical approaches to investigate cytochrome p450-mediated therapeutic protein drug-drug interactions and recommendations for best practices: a white paper. Drug Metab. Dispos. 41, 1598–1609.

Ferrari, L., Herber, R., Batt, A.M., Siest, G., 1993. Differential effects of human recombinant interleukin-1 beta and dexamethasone on hepatic drug-metabolizing enzymes in male and female rats. Biochem. Pharmacol. 45, 2269–2277.

Ferrari, L., Peng, N., Halpert, J.R., Morgan, E.T., 2001. Role of nitric oxide in down-regulation of CYP2B1 protein, but not RNA, in primary cultures of rat hepatocytes. Mol. Pharmacol. 60, 209–216.

Forsyth, J.S., Moreland, T.A., Rylance, G.W., 1982. The effect of fever on antipyrine metabolism in children. Br. J. Clin. Pharmacol. 13, 811–815.

Frye, R.F., Schneider, V.M., Frye, C.S., Feldman, A.M., 2002. Plasma levels of TNF-alpha and IL-6 are inversely related to cytochrome P450-dependent drug metabolism in patients with congestive heart failure. J. Card. Fail. 8, 315–319.

Frye, R.F., Zgheib, N.K., Matzke, G.R., Chaves-Gnecco, D., Rabinovitz, M., Shaikh, O.S., Branch, R.A., 2006. Liver disease selectively modulates cytochrome P450–mediated metabolism. Clin. Pharmacol. Ther. 80, 235–245.

Gaffen, S.L., Jain, R., Garg, A.V., Cua, D.J., 2014. The IL-23-IL-17 immune axis: from mechanisms to therapeutic testing. Nat. Rev. Immunol. 14, 585–600.

Gandhi, A., Moorthy, B., Ghose, R., 2012. Drug disposition in pathophysiological conditions. Curr. Drug Metab. 13, 1327–1344.

Gao, J., Xie, W., 2010. Pregnane X receptor and constitutive androstane receptor at the crossroads of drug metabolism and energy metabolism. Drug Metab. Dispos. 38, 2091–2095.

Ghaffari, A.A., Chow, E.K., Iyer, S.S., Deng, J.C., Cheng, G., 2011. Polyinosinic-polycytidylic acid suppresses acetaminophen-induced hepatotoxicity independent of type I interferons and toll-like receptor 3. Hepatology 53, 2042–2052.

Ghezzi, P., Saccardo, B., Villa, P., Rossi, V., Bianchi, M., Dinarello, C.A., 1986. Role of interleukin-1 in the depression of liver drug metabolism by endotoxin. Infect. Immun. 54, 837–840.

Ghose, R., White, D., Guo, T., Vallejo, J., Karpen, S.J., 2008. Regulation of hepatic drug-metabolizing enzyme genes by Toll-like receptor 4 signaling is independent of Toll-interleukin 1 receptor domain-containing adaptor protein. Drug Metab. Dispos. 36, 95–101.

Ghose, R., Guo, T., Haque, N., 2009. Regulation of gene expression of hepatic drug metabolizing enzymes and transporters by the Toll-like receptor 2 ligand, lipoteichoic acid. Arch. Biochem. Biophys. 481, 123–130.

Ghose, R., Guo, T., Vallejo, J.G., Gandhi, A., 2011. Differential role of Toll-interleukin 1 receptor domain-containing adaptor protein in Toll-like receptor 2-mediated regulation of gene expression of hepatic cytokines and drug-metabolizing enzymes. Drug Metab. Dispos. 39, 874–881.

Giannini, E., Fasoli, A., Borro, P., Chiarbonello, B., Malfatti, F., Romagnoli, P., Botta, F., Testa, E., Fumagalli, A., Polegato, S., Savarino, V., Testa, R., 2001. Impairment of cytochrome P-450-dependent liver activity in cirrhotic patients with *Helicobacter pylori* infection. Aliment. Pharmacol. Ther. 15, 1967–1973.

Giannini, E., Fasoli, A., Chiarbonello, B., Malfatti, F., Romagnoli, P., Botta, F., Testa, E., Polegato, S., Fumagalli, A., Testa, R., 2002. 13C-aminopyrine breath test to evaluate severity of disease in patients with chronic hepatitis C virus infection. Aliment. Pharmacol. Ther. 16, 717–725.

Giannini, E., Fasoli, A., Botta, F., Romagnoli, P., Malfatti, F., Chiarbonello, B., Mamone, M., Savarino, V., Testa, R., 2003. *Helicobacter pylori* infection is associated with greater impairment of cytochrome P-450 liver metabolic activity in anti-HCV positive cirrhotic patients. Dig. Dis. Sci. 48, 802−808.

Gochee, P.A., Jonsson, J.R., Clouston, A.D., Pandeya, N., Purdie, D.M., Powell, E.E., 2003. Steatosis in chronic hepatitis C: association with increased messenger RNA expression of collagen I, tumor necrosis factor-alpha and cytochrome P450 2E1. J. Gastroenterol. Hepatol. 18, 386−392.

Goktas, M.T., Hatta, F., Karaca, O., Kalkisim, S., Kilic, L., Akdogan, A., Babaoglu, M.O., Bozkurt, A., Hellden, A., Bertilsson, L., Yasar, U., 2015. Lower CYP2C9 activity in Turkish patients with Behcet's disease compared to healthy subjects: a down-regulation due to inflammation? Eur. J. Clin. Pharmacol. 71, 1223−1228.

Gorski, J.C., Hall, S.D., Becker, P., Affrime, M.B., Cutler, D.L., Haehner-Daniels, B., 2000. In vivo effects of interleukin-10 on human cytochrome P450 activity. Clin. Pharmacol. Ther. 67, 32−43.

Gotardo, M.A., Hyssa, J.T., Carvalho, R.S., De-Carvalho, R.R., Gueiros, L.S., Siqueira, C.M., Sarpa, M., De-Oliveira, A.C., Paumgartten Jr., F., 2011. Modulation of expression and activity of cytochrome P450s and alteration of praziquantel kinetics during murine schistosomiasis. Mem. Inst. Oswaldo Cruz 106, 212−219.

Grabenstein, J.D., 1990. Drug interactions involving immunologic agents. Part I. Vaccine-vaccine, vaccine-immunoglobulin, and vaccine-drug interactions. DICP: Ann. Pharmacother. 24, 67−81.

Gray, J.D., Renton, K.W., Hung, O.R., 1983. Depression of theophylline elimination following BCG vaccination. Br. J. Clin. Pharmacol. 16, 735−737.

Gu, X., Ke, S., Liu, D., Sheng, T., Thomas, P.E., Rabson, A.B., Gallo, M.A., Xie, W., Tian, Y., 2006. Role of NF-kappaB in regulation of PXR-mediated gene expression: a mechanism for the suppression of cytochrome P-450 3A4 by proinflammatory agents. J. Biol. Chem. 281, 17882−17889.

Guengerich, F.P., Turvy, C.G., 1991. Comparison of levels of several human microsomal cytochrome P-450 enzymes and epoxide hydrolase in normal and disease states using immunochemical analysis of surgical liver samples. J. Pharmacol. Exp. Ther. 256, 1189−1194.

Hagihara, K., Nishikawa, T., Sugamata, Y., Song, J., Isobe, T., Taga, T., Yoshizaki, K., 2005. Essential role of STAT3 in cytokine-driven NF-kappaB-mediated serum amyloid A gene expression. Genes Cells 10, 1051−1063.

Hanada, K., Nakai, K., Tanaka, H., Suzuki, F., Kumada, H., Ohno, Y., Ozawa, S., Ogata, H., 2012. Effect of nuclear receptor downregulation on hepatic expression of cytochrome P450 and transporters in chronic hepatitis C in association with fibrosis development. Drug Metab. Pharmacokinet. 27, 301−306.

Hayney, M.S., Hammes, R.J., Fine, J.P., Bianco, J.A., 2002. Effect of influenza immunization on CYP3A4 activity. Vaccine 20, 858−861.

Hegazy, S.K., Adam, A.G., Hamdy, N.A., Khalafallah, N.M., 2015. Effect of active infection on cytochrome P450-mediated metabolism of cyclosporine in renal transplant patients. Transpl. Infect. Dis. 17, 350−360.

Heinrich, P.C., Behrmann, I., Haan, S., Hermanns, H.M., Muller-Newen, G., Schaper, F., 2003. Principles of interleukin (IL)-6-type cytokine signalling and its regulation. Biochem. J. 374, 1−20.

Hildt, E., Munz, B., Saher, G., Reifenberg, K., Hofschneider, P.H., 2002. The PreS2 activator MHBs(t) of hepatitis B virus activates c-raf-1/Erk2 signaling in transgenic mice. EMBO J. 21, 525−535.

Hirth, J., Watkins, P.B., Strawderman, M., Schott, A., Bruno, R., Baker, L.H., 2000. The effect of an individual's cytochrome CYP3A4 activity on docetaxel clearance. Clin. Cancer Res. 6, 1255−1258.

Homeida, M.M., Ali, H.M., Arbab, B.M., Harron, D.W., 1987. Propranolol disposition in patients with hepatosplenic schistosomiasis. Br. J. Clin. Pharmacol. 24, 393−396.

Horina, J.H., Wirnsberger, G.H., Kenner, L., Holzer, H., Krejs, G.J., 1993. Increased susceptibility for CsA-induced hepatotoxicity in kidney graft recipients with chronic viral hepatitis C. Transplantation 56, 1091−1094.

Iber, H., Chen, Q., Cheng, P.Y., Morgan, E.T., 2000. Suppression of CYP2C11 gene transcription by interleukin-1 mediated by NF-kappaB binding at the transcription start site. Arch. Biochem. Biophys. 377, 187−194.

Igonin, A.A., Armstrong, V.W., Shipkova, M., Kukes, V.G., Oellerich, M., 2000. The monoethylglycinexylidide (MEGX) test as a marker of hepatic dysfunction in septic patients with pneumonia. Clin. Chem. Lab. Med. 38, 1125−1128.

Ince, I., de Wildt, S.N., Peeters, M.Y., Murry, D.J., Tibboel, D., Danhof, M., Knibbe, C.A., 2012. Critical illness is a major determinant of midazolam clearance in children aged 1 month to 17 years. Ther. Drug Monit. 34, 381−389.

Jakob, S.M., Ruokonen, E., Rosenberg, P.H., Takala, J., 2002. Effect of dopamine-induced changes in splanchnic blood flow on MEGX production from lidocaine in septic and cardiac surgery patients. Shock 18, 1−7.

Jetter, A., Fatkenheuer, G., Frank, D., Klaassen, T., Seeringer, A., Doroshyenko, O., Kirchheiner, J., Hein, W., Schomig, E., Fuhr, U., Wyen, C., 2010. Do activities of cytochrome P450 (CYP)3A, CYP2D6 and P-glycoprotein differ between healthy volunteers and HIV-infected patients? Antivir. Ther. 15, 975–983.

Jiang, M., Klein, M., Zanger, U.M., Mohammad, M.K., Cave, M.C., Gaikwad, N.W., Dias, N.J., Selcer, K.W., Guo, Y., He, J., Zhang, X., Shen, Q., Qin, W., Li, J., Li, S., Xie, W., 2015. Inflammatory regulation of steroid sulfatase: a novel mechanism to control estrogen homeostasis and inflammation in chronic liver disease. J. Hepatol.

Jones, A.E., Brown, K.C., Werner, R.E., Gotzkowsky, K., Gaedigk, A., Blake, M., Hein, D.W., van der Horst, C., Kashuba, A.D., 2010. Variability in drug metabolizing enzyme activity in HIV-infected patients. Eur. J. Clin. Pharmacol. 66, 475–485.

Jover, R., Bort, R., Gmez-Lechn, M., Castell, J., 2002. Down-regulation of human CYP3A4 by the inflammatory signal interleukin 6: molecular mechanism and transcription factors involved. FASEB J. 16, 1799.

Kacevska, M., Downes, M.R., Sharma, R., Evans, R.M., Clarke, S.J., Liddle, C., Robertson, G.R., 2011. Extrahepatic cancer suppresses nuclear receptor-regulated drug metabolism. Clin. Cancer Res. 17, 3170–3180.

Kacevska, M., Mahns, A., Sharma, R., Clarke, S.J., Robertson, G.R., Liddle, C., 2013. Extra-hepatic cancer represses hepatic drug metabolism via interleukin (IL)-6 signalling. Pharm. Res. 30, 2270–2278.

Kaufmann, G.R., Wenk, M., Taeschner, W., Peterli, B., Gyr, K., Meyer, U.A., Haefeli, W.E., 1996. N-acetyltransferase 2 polymorphism in patients infected with human immunodeficiency virus. Clin. Pharmacol. Ther. 60, 62–67.

Khatsenko, O.G., Boobis, A.R., Gross, S.S., 1997. Evidence for nitric oxide participation in down-regulation of CYP2B1/2 gene expression at the pretranslational level. Toxicol. Lett. 90, 207–216.

Kikuchi, R., McCown, M., Olson, P., Tateno, C., Morikawa, Y., Katoh, Y., Bourdet, D.L., Monshouwer, M., Fretland, A.J., 2010. Effect of hepatitis C virus infection on the mRNA expression of drug transporters and cytochrome p450 enzymes in chimeric mice with humanized liver. Drug Metab. Dispos. 38, 1954–1961.

Kim, R.B., Wilkinson, G.R., 1996. CYP2E1 activity is not altered by influenza vaccination. Br. J. Clin. Pharmacol. 42, 529–530.

Kim, Y.M., Bergonia, H.A., Muller, C., Pitt, B.R., Watkins, W.D., Lancaster Jr., J.R., 1995. Loss and degradation of enzyme-bound heme induced by cellular nitric oxide synthesis. J. Biol. Chem. 270, 5710–5713.

Kim, M.S., Shigenaga, J., Moser, A., Grunfeld, C., Feingold, K.R., 2004. Suppression of DHEA sulfotransferase (Sult2A1) during the acute-phase response. Am. J. Physiol. 287, E731–E738.

Kim, T.H., Lee, S.H., Lee, S.M., 2011. Role of Kupffer cells in pathogenesis of sepsis-induced drug metabolizing dysfunction. FEBS J. 278, 2307–2317.

Kinloch, R.D., Lee, C.M., van Rooijen, N., Morgan, E.T., 2011. Selective role for tumor necrosis factor-alpha, but not interleukin-1 or Kupffer cells, in down-regulation of CYP3A11 and CYP3A25 in livers of mice infected with a noninvasive intestinal pathogen. Biochem. Pharmacol. 82, 312–321.

Kirby, G.M., Chemin, I., Montesano, R., Chisari, F.V., Lang, M.A., Wild, C.P., 1994. Induction of specific cytochrome P450s involved in aflatoxin B1 metabolism in hepatitis B virus transgenic mice. Mol. Carcinog. 11, 74–80.

Kirby, G.M., Batist, G., Alpert, L., Lamoureux, E., Cameron, R.G., Alaoui-Jamali, M.A., 1996. Overexpression of cytochrome P-450 isoforms involved in aflatoxin B1 bioactivation in human liver with cirrhosis and hepatitis. Toxicol. Pathol. 24, 458–467.

Klein, K., Winter, S., Turpeinen, M., Schwab, M., Zanger, U.M., 2010. Pathway-targeted pharmacogenomics of CYP1A2 in human liver. Front. Pharmacol. 1, 129.

Kloprogge, F., Jullien, V., Piola, P., Dhorda, M., Muwanga, S., Nosten, F., Day, N.P., White, N.J., Guerin, P.J., Tarning, J., 2014. Population pharmacokinetics of quinine in pregnant women with uncomplicated *Plasmodium falciparum* malaria in Uganda. J. Antimicrob. Chemother. 69, 3033–3040.

Kraemer, M.J., Furukawa, C.T., Koup, J.R., Shapiro, G.G., Pierson, W.E., Bierman, C.W., 1982. Altered theophylline clearance during an influenza B outbreak. Pediatrics 69, 476–480.

Kramer, P., McClain, C.J., 1981. Depression of aminopyrine metabolism by influenza vaccination. New Engl. J. Med. 305, 1262–1264.

Kuo, A.M., Brown, J.N., Clinard, V., 2012. Effect of influenza vaccination on international normalized ratio during chronic warfarin therapy. J. Clin. Pharm. Ther. 37, 505–509.

Lahita, R.G., Bradlow, H.L., Kunkel, H.G., Fishman, J., 1981. Increased 16 alpha-hydroxylation of estradiol in systemic lupus erythematosus. J. Clin. Endocrinol. Metab. 53, 174–178.

Latorre, A., Morales, E., Gonzalez, E., Herrero, J.C., Ortiz, M., Sierra, P., Dominguez-Gil, B., Torres, A., Munoz, M.A., Andres, A., Manzanares, C., Morales, J.M., 2002. Clinical management of renal transplant patients with hepatitis C virus infection treated with cyclosporine or tacrolimus. Transplant. Proc. 34, 63–64.

Lee, B.L., Wong, D., Benowitz, N.L., Sullam, P.M., 1993. Altered patterns of drug metabolism in patients with acquired immunodeficiency syndrome. Clin. Pharmacol. Ther. 53, 529–535.

Lee, C.M., Kim, B.Y., Li, L., Morgan, E.T., 2008. Nitric oxide-dependent proteasomal degradation of cytochrome P450 2B proteins. J. Biol. Chem. 283, 889–898.

Lee, C.M., Lee, B.S., Arnold, S.L., Isoherranen, N., Morgan, E.T., 2014. Nitric oxide and interleukin-1beta stimulate the proteasome-independent degradation of the retinoic acid hydroxylase CYP2C22 in primary rat hepatocytes. J. Pharmacol. Exp. Ther. 348, 141–152.

Li, N., Klaassen, C.D., 2004. Role of liver-enriched transcription factors in the down-regulation of organic anion transporting polypeptide 4 (oatp4; oatplb2; slc21a10) by lipopolysaccharide. Mol. Pharmacol. 66, 694–701.

Li, S., Hu, Z.H., Miao, X.H., 2006. Effects of chronic HBV infection on human hepatic cytochrome P450 3A4. Zhonghua yi xue za zhi 86, 2703–2706.

Liehl, P., Zuzarte-Luis, V., Chan, J., Zillinger, T., Baptista, F., Carapau, D., Konert, M., Hanson, K.K., Carret, C., Lassnig, C., Muller, M., Kalinke, U., Saeed, M., Chora, A.F., Golenbock, D.T., Strobl, B., Prudencio, M., Coelho, L.P., Kappe, S.H., Superti-Furga, G., Pichlmair, A., Vigario, A.M., Rice, C.M., Fitzgerald, K.A., Barchet, W., Mota, M.M., 2014. Host-cell sensors for *Plasmodium* activate innate immunity against liver-stage infection. Nat. Med. 20, 47–53.

Lin, H.L., Kent, U.M., Zhang, H., Waskell, L., Hollenberg, P.F., 2003. Mutation of tyrosine 190 to alanine eliminates the inactivation of cytochrome P450 2B1 by peroxynitrite. Chem. Res. Toxicol. 16, 129–136.

Ling, S., Jamali, F., 2009. The effect of infliximab on hepatic cytochrome P450 and pharmacokinetics of verapamil in rats with pre-adjuvant arthritis: a drug-disease and drug-drug interaction. Basic Clin. Pharmacol. Toxicol. 105, 24–29.

Liu, J., Sendelbach, L.E., Parkinson, A., Klaassen, C.D., 2000. Endotoxin pretreatment protects against the hepatotoxicity of acetaminophen and carbon tetrachloride: role of cytochrome P450 suppression. Toxicology 147, 167–176.

Liu, H., Lou, G., Li, C., Wang, X., Cederbaum, A.I., Gan, L., Xie, B., 2014. HBx inhibits CYP2E1 gene expression via downregulating HNF4alpha in human hepatoma cells. PLoS ONE 9, e107913.

Mandour, M.E., el Turabi, H., Homeida, M.M., el Sadig, T., Ali, H.M., Bennett, J.L., Leahey, W.J., Harron, D.W., 1990. Pharmacokinetics of praziquantel in healthy volunteers and patients with schistosomiasis. Trans. R. Soc. Trop. Med. Hyg. 84, 389–393.

Mao, Z., Li, Y., Peng, Y., Luan, X., Gui, H., Feng, X., Hu, G., Shen, J., Yan, B., Yang, J., 2011. Lipopolysaccharide down-regulates carbolesterases 1 and 2 and reduces hydrolysis activity in vitro and in vivo via p38MAPK-NF-kappaB pathway. Toxicol. Lett. 201, 213–220.

Mao, Z., Luan, X., Cao, G., Liu, W., Xiong, J., Hu, G., Chen, R., Ning, R., Shang, W., Yang, J., Yan, B., 2012. DEC1 binding to the proximal promoter of CYP3A4 ascribes to the downregulation of CYP3A4 expression by IL-6 in primary human hepatocytes. Biochem. Pharmacol. 84, 701–711.

Medzhitov, R., 2008. Origin and physiological roles of inflammation. Nature 454, 428–435.

Meredith, C.G., Christian, C.D., Johnson, R.F., Troxell, R., Davis, G.L., Schenker, S., 1985. Effects of influenza virus vaccine on hepatic drug metabolism. Clin. Pharmacol. Ther. 37, 396–401.

Mimche, S.M., Nyagode, B.A., Merrell, M.D., Lee, C.M., Prasanphanich, N.S., Cummings, R.D., Morgan, E.T., 2014. Hepatic cytochrome P450s, phase II enzymes and nuclear receptors are downregulated in a Th2 environment during *Schistosoma mansoni* infection. Drug Metab. Dispos. 42, 134–140.

Morcos, P.N., Moreira, S.A., Brennan, B.J., Blotner, S., Shulman, N.S., Smith, P.F., 2013. Influence of chronic hepatitis C infection on cytochrome P450 3A4 activity using midazolam as an in vivo probe substrate. Eur. J. Clin. Pharmacol. 69, 1777–1784.

Morgan, E.T., Norman, C.A., 1990. Pretranslational suppression of cytochrome P-450h (IIC11) gene expression in rat liver after administration of interferon inducers. Drug Metab. Dispos. 18, 649–653.

Morgan, E.T., Lee, C.M., Nyagode, B.A., 2012. Regulation of drug metabolizing enzymes and transporters in infection, inflammation, and cancer. In: Lyubimov, A.V. (Ed.), Encyclopedia of Drug Metabolism and Interactions. Wiley, Hoboken, NJ, pp. 1–45.

Morgan, E.T., 1991. Suppression of P450IIC12 gene expression and elevation of actin messenger ribonucleic acid levels in the livers of female rats after injection of the interferon inducer poly rI.poly rC. Biochem. Pharmacol. 42, 51–57.

Moriya, N., Kataoka, H., Fujino, H., Nishikawa, J., Kugawa, F., 2012. Effect of lipopolysaccharide on the xenobiotic-induced expression and activity of hepatic cytochrome P450 in mice. Biol. Pharm. Bull. 35, 473–480.

Moshage, H.J., Roelofs, H.M., van Pelt, J.F., Hazenberg, B.P., van Leeuwen, M.A., Limburg, P.C., Aarden, L.A., Yap, S.H., 1988. The effect of interleukin-1, interleukin-6 and its interrelationship on the synthesis of serum amyloid A and C-reactive protein in primary cultures of adult human hepatocytes. Biochem. Biophys. Res. Commun. 155, 112–117.

Muntane-Relat, J., Ourlin, J.C., Domergue, J., Maurel, P., 1995. Differential effects of cytokines on the inducible expression of CYP1A1, CYP1A2, and CYP3A4 in human hepatocytes in primary culture. Hepatology 22, 1143–1153.

Nadin, L., Butler, A.M., Farrell, G.C., Murray, M., 1995. Pretranslational down-regulation of cytochromes P450 2C11 and 3A2 in male rat liver by tumor necrosis factor alpha. Gastroenterology 109, 198–205.

Nakai, K., Tanaka, H., Hanada, K., Ogata, H., Suzuki, F., Kumada, H., Miyajima, A., Ishida, S., Sunouchi, M., Habano, W., Kamikawa, Y., Kubota, K., Kita, J., Ozawa, S., Ohno, Y., 2008. Decreased expression of cytochromes P450 1A2, 2E1, and 3A4 and drug transporters Na^+-taurocholate-cotransporting polypeptide, organic cation transporter 1, and organic anion-transporting peptide-C correlates with the progression of liver fibrosis in chronic hepatitis C patients. Drug Metab. Dispos. 36, 1786–1793.

Narang, A.P., Datta, D.V., Mathur, V.S., 1982. Antipyrine clearance, aminopyrine N-demethylase, and bilirubin UDP-glucuronyl transferase activity in patients with amoebic liver abscess. Biopharm. Drug Dispos. 3, 39–45.

Ng, C.Y., Ghabrial, H., Morgan, D.J., Ching, M.S., Smallwood, R.A., Angus, P.W., 2000. Impaired elimination of propranolol due to right heart failure: drug clearance in the isolated liver and its relationship to intrinsic metabolic capacity. Drug Metab. Dispos. 28, 1217–1221.

Nguyen, T.V., Ukairo, O., Khetani, S.R., McVay, M., Kanchagar, C., Seghezzi, W., Ayanoglu, G., Irrechukwu, O., Evers, R., 2015. Establishment of a hepatocyte-Kupffer cell coculture model for assessment of proinflammatory cytokine effects on metabolizing enzymes and drug transporters. Drug Metab. Dispos. 43, 774–785.

Niu, Y., Wu, Z., Shen, Q., Song, J., Luo, Q., You, H., Shi, G., Qin, W., 2013. Hepatitis B virus X protein co-activates pregnane X receptor to induce the cytochrome P450 3A4 enzyme, a potential implication in hepatocarcinogenesis. Dig. Liver Dis. 45, 1041–1048.

Niwa, T., Sato, R., Yabusaki, Y., Ishibashi, F., Katagiri, M., 1999. Contribution of human hepatic cytochrome P450s and steroidogenic CYP17 to the N-demethylation of aminopyrine. Xenobiotica 29, 187–193.

Novotny, A.R., Emmanuel, K., Maier, S., Westerholt, A., Weighardt, H., Stadler, J., Bartels, H., Schwaiger, M., Siewert, J.R., Holzmann, B., Heidecke, C.D., 2007. Cytochrome P450 activity mirrors nitric oxide levels in postoperative sepsis: predictive indicators of lethal outcome. Surgery 141, 376–384.

Nyagode, B.A., Lee, C.M., Morgan, E.T., 2010. Modulation of hepatic cytochrome P450s by *Citrobacter rodentium* infection in interleukin-6- and interferon-{gamma}-null mice. J. Pharmacol. Exp. Ther. 335, 480–488.

Nyagode, B.A., Jahangardi, R., Merrell, M.D., Tansey, M.G., Morgan, E.T., 2014. Selective effects of a therapeutic protein targeting tumor necrosis factor-alpha on cytochrome P450 regulation during infectious colitis: implications for disease-dependent drug–drug interactions. Pharmacol. Res. Perspect. 2, e00027.

O'Neil, W.M., Gilfix, B.M., DiGirolamo, A., Tsoukas, C.M., Wainer, I.W., 1997. N-acetylation among HIV-positive patients and patients with AIDS: when is fast, fast and slow, slow? Clin. Pharmacol. Ther. 62, 261–271.

Onishi, R.M., Gaffen, S.L., 2010. Interleukin-17 and its target genes: mechanisms of interleukin-17 function in disease. Immunology 129, 311–321.

Orlando, R., Piccoli, P., De Martin, S., Padrini, R., Floreani, M., Palatini, P., 2004. Cytochrome P450 1A2 is a major determinant of lidocaine metabolism in vivo: effects of liver function. Clin. Pharmacol. Ther. 75, 80–88.

Pascussi, J.M., Gerbal-Chaloin, S., Pichard-Garcia, L., Daujat, M., Fabre, J.M., Maurel, P., Vilarem, M.J., 2000. Interleukin-6 negatively regulates the expression of pregnane X receptor and constitutively activated receptor in primary human hepatocytes. Biochem. Biophys. Res. Commun. 274, 707–713.

Patel, D.N., King, C.A., Bailey, S.R., Holt, J.W., Venkatachalam, K., Agrawal, A., Valente, A.J., Chandrasekar, B., 2007. Interleukin-17 stimulates C-reactive protein expression in hepatocytes and smooth muscle cells via p38 MAPK and ERK1/2-dependent NF-kappaB and C/EBPbeta activation. J. Biol. Chem. 282, 27229–27238.

Pellegrino, P., Clementi, E., Capuano, A., Radice, S., 2015. Can vaccines interact with drug metabolism? Pharmacol. Res. 92, 13–17.

Pukrittayakamee, S., Looareesuwan, S., Keeratithakul, D., Davis, T.M., Teja-Isavadharm, P., Nagachinta, B., Weber, A., Smith, A.L., Kyle, D., White, N.J., 1997. A study of the factors affecting the metabolic clearance of quinine in malaria. Eur. J. Clin. Pharmacol. 52, 487–493.

Rasool, M.F., Khalil, F., Laer, S., 2015. A physiologically based pharmacokinetic drug-disease model to predict carvedilol exposure in adult and paediatric heart failure patients by incorporating pathophysiological changes in hepatic and renal blood flows. Clin. Pharmacokinet. 54, 943–962.

Reesink, H.W., Fanning, G.C., Farha, K.A., Weegink, C., Van Vliet, A., Van 't Klooster, G., Lenz, O., Aharchi, F., Marien, K., Van Remoortere, P., de Kock, H., Broeckaert, F., Meyvisch, P., Van Beirendonck, E., Simmen, K., Verloes, R., 2010. Rapid HCV-RNA decline with once daily TMC435: a phase I study in healthy volunteers and hepatitis C patients. Gastroenterology 138, 913—921.

Renton, K.W., Mannering, G.J., 1976. Depression of hepatic cytochrome P-450-dependent monooxygenase systems with administered interferon inducing agents. Biochem. Biophys. Res. Commun. 73, 343—348.

Renton, K.W., Gray, J.D., Hall, R.I., 1980. Decreased elimination of theophylline after influenza vaccination. Can. Med. Assoc. J. 123, 288—290.

Renton, K.W., 2005. Regulation of drug metabolism and disposition during inflammation and infection. Expert Opin. Drug Metab. Toxicol. 1, 629—640.

Richardson, T., Morgan, E., 2005. Hepatic cytochrome P450 gene regulation during endotoxin-induced inflammation in nuclear receptor knockout mice. J. Pharmacol. Exp. Ther. 314, 703—709.

Rieger, J.K., Klein, K., Winter, S., Zanger, U.M., 2013. Expression variability of absorption, distribution, metabolism, excretion-related microRNAs in human liver: influence of nongenetic factors and association with gene expression. Drug Metab. Dispos. 41, 1752—1762.

Rivory, L.P., Slaviero, K.A., Clarke, S.J., 2002. Hepatic cytochrome P450 3A drug metabolism is reduced in cancer patients who have an acute-phase response. Br. J. Cancer 87, 277—280.

Sabbagh, N., Marez, D., Queyrel, V., Lo Guidice, J.M., Spire, C., Vanhille, P., Jorgensen, C., Hachulla, E., Broly, F., 1998. Genetic analysis of the cytochrome P450 CYP2D6 polymorphism in patients with systemic lupus erythematosus. Pharmacogenetics 8, 191—194.

Sagar, M., Seensalu, R., Tybring, G., Dahl, M.L., Bertilsson, L., 1998. CYP2C19 genotype and phenotype determined with omeprazole in patients with acid-related disorders with and without Helicobacter pylori infection. Scand. J. Gastroenterol. 33, 1034—1038.

Saito, M., Kawana, J., Ohno, T., Hanada, K., Kaneko, M., Mihara, K., Shiomi, M., Nagayama, M., Sumiyoshi, T., Ogata, H., 2010. Population pharmacokinetics of R- and S-carvedilol in Japanese patients with chronic heart failure. Biol. Pharm. Bull. 33, 1378—1384.

Salazar-Mather, T.P., Hokeness, K.L., 2003. Calling in the troops: regulation of inflammatory cell trafficking through innate cytokine/chemokine networks. Viral Immunol. 16, 291—306.

Sanada, H., Sekimoto, M., Kamoshita, A., Degawa, M., 2011. Changes in expression of hepatic cytochrome P450 subfamily enzymes during development of adjuvant-induced arthritis in rats. J. Toxicol. Sci. 36, 181—190.

Satarug, S., Lang, M.A., Yongvanit, P., Sithithaworn, P., Mairiang, E., Mairiang, P., Pelkonen, P., Bartsch, H., Haswell-Elkins, M.R., 1996. Induction of cytochrome P450 2A6 expression in humans by the carcinogenic parasite infection, Opisthorchiasis viverrini. Cancer Epidemiol. Biomarkers Prev. 5, 795—800.

Scavone, J.M., Blyden, G.T., Greenblatt, D.J., 1989. Lack of effect of influenza vaccine on the pharmacokinetics of antipyrine, alprazolam, paracetamol (acetaminophen) and lorazepam. Clin. Pharmacokinet. 16, 180—185.

Schaedler, S., Krause, J., Himmelsbach, K., Carvajal-Yepes, M., Lieder, F., Klingel, K., Nassal, M., Weiss, T.S., Werner, S., Hildt, E., 2010. Hepatitis B virus induces expression of antioxidant response element-regulated genes by activation of Nrf2. J. Biol. Chem. 285, 41074—41086.

Schmitt, C., Kuhn, B., Zhang, X., Kivitz, A.J., Grange, S., 2011. Disease—drug—drug interaction involving tocilizumab and simvastatin in patients with rheumatoid arthritis. Clin. Pharmacol. Ther. 89, 735—740.

Schroder, A., Klein, K., Winter, S., Schwab, M., Bonin, M., Zell, A., Zanger, U.M., 2013. Genomics of ADME gene expression: mapping expression quantitative trait loci relevant for absorption, distribution, metabolism and excretion of drugs in human liver. Pharmacogenomics J. 13, 12—20.

Schwinghammer, T.L., Przepiorka, D., Venkataramanan, R., Wang, C.P., Burckart, G.J., Rosenfeld, C.S., Shadduck, R.K., 1991. The kinetics of cyclosporine and its metabolites in bone marrow transplant patients. Br. J. Clin. Pharmacol. 32, 323—328.

Sewer, M.B., Morgan, E.T., 1997. Nitric oxide-independent suppression of P450 2C11 expression by interleukin-1beta and endotoxin in primary rat hepatocytes. Biochem. Pharmacol. 54, 729—737.

Shah, R.R., Smith, R.L., 2015. Inflammation-induced phenoconversion of polymorphic drug metabolizing enzymes: hypothesis with implications for personalized medicine. Drug Metab. Dispos. 43, 400—410.

Shah, P., Guo, T., Moore, D.D., Ghose, R., 2014. Role of constitutive androstane receptor in Toll-like receptor-mediated regulation of gene expression of hepatic drug-metabolizing enzymes and transporters. Drug Metab. Dispos. 42, 172—181.

Shah, P., Omoluabi, O., Moorthy, B., Ghose, R., 2016. Role of adaptor protein Toll-like interleukin domain containing adaptor inducing interferon b in toll-like receptor 3- and 4-mediated regulation of hepatic drug metabolizing enzyme and transporter genes. Drug Metab. Dispos. 44, 61—67.

Shedlofsky, S.I., Israel, B.C., McClain, C.J., Hill, D.B., Blouin, R.A., 1994. Endotoxin administration to humans inhibits hepatic cytochrome P450-mediated drug metabolism. J. Clin. Invest. 94, 2209—2214.

Shedlofsky, S.I., Israel, B.C., Tosheva, R., Blouin, R.A., 1997. Endotoxin depresses hepatic cytochrome P450-mediated drug metabolism in women. Br. J. Clin. Pharmacol. 43, 627—632.

Shelly, M.P., Mendel, L., Park, G.R., 1987. Failure of critically ill patients to metabolise midazolam. Anaesthesia 42, 619—626.

Shimada, M., Watanabe, E., Iida, Y., Nagata, K., Yamazoe, Y., 1999. Alteration of hepatic sulfation by endotoxin. Jpn. J. Pharmacol. 80, 371—373.

Shiu, T.Y., Huang, T.Y., Huang, S.M., Shih, Y.L., Chu, H.C., Chang, W.K., Hsieh, T.Y., 2013. Nuclear factor kappaB down-regulates human UDP-glucuronosyltransferase 1A1: a novel mechanism involved in inflammation-associated hyperbilirubinaemia. Biochem. J. 449, 761—770.

Shord, S.S., Cavallari, L.H., Viana, M.A., Momary, K., Neceskas, J., Molokie, R.E., Deyo, K., Patel, S.R., 2008. Cytochrome P450 2C9 mediated metabolism in people with and without cancer. Int. J. Clin. Pharmacol. Ther. 46, 365—374.

Sidhu, J.S., Farin, F.M., Omiecinski, C.J., 1993. Influence of extracellular matrix overlay on phenobarbital-mediated induction of CYP2B1, 2B2, and 3A1 genes in primary adult rat hepatocyte culture. Arch. Biochem. Biophys. 301, 103—113.

Siewert, E., Bort, R., Kluge, R., Heinrich, P., Castell, J., Jover, R., 2000. Hepatic cytochrome P450 down-regulation during aseptic inflammation in the mouse is interleukin 6 dependent. Hepatology 32, 49—55.

Slain, D., Pakyz, A., Israel, D.S., Monroe, S., Polk, R.E., 2000. Variability in activity of hepatic CYP3A4 in patients infected with HIV. Pharmacotherapy 20, 898—907.

Smerdova, L., Smerdova, J., Kabatkova, M., Kohoutek, J., Blazek, D., Machala, M., Vondracek, J., 2014. Upregulation of CYP1B1 expression by inflammatory cytokines is mediated by the p38 MAP kinase signal transduction pathway. Carcinogenesis 35, 2534—2543.

Su, T., Ding, X., 2004. Regulation of the cytochrome P450 2A genes. Toxicol. Appl. Pharmacol. 199, 285—294.

Sunman, J.A., Hawke, R.L., LeCluyse, E.L., Kashuba, A.D., 2004. Kupffer cell-mediated IL-2 suppression of CYP3A activity in human hepatocytes. Drug Metab. Dispos. 32, 359—363.

Supanaranond, W., Davis, T.M., Pukrittayakamee, S., Silamut, K., Karbwang, J., Molunto, P., Chanond, L., White, N.J., 1991. Disposition of oral quinine in acute falciparum malaria. Eur. J. Clin. Pharmacol. 40, 49—52.

Takemura, S., Minamiyama, Y., Imaoka, S., Funae, Y., Hirohashi, K., Inoue, M., Kinoshita, H., 1999. Hepatic cytochrome P450 is directly inactivated by nitric oxide, not by inflammatory cytokines, in the early phase of endotoxemia. J. Hepatol. 30, 1035—1044.

Takeuchi, O., Akira, S., 2010. Pattern recognition receptors and inflammation. Cell 140, 805—820.

Tapner, M., Liddle, C., Goodwin, B., George, J., Farrell, G.C., 1996. Interferon gamma down-regulates cytochrome P450 3A genes in primary cultures of well-differentiated rat hepatocytes. Hepatology 24, 367—373.

Teng, S., Piquette-Miller, M., 2005. The involvement of the pregnane X receptor in hepatic gene regulation during inflammation in mice. J. Pharmacol. Exp. Ther. 312, 841—848.

Tian, Y., Ke, S., Denison, M.S., Rabson, A.B., Gallo, M.A., 1999. Ah receptor and NF-kappaB interactions, a potential mechanism for dioxin toxicity. J. Biol. Chem. 274, 510—515.

Tsutsui, H., Cai, X., Hayashi, S., 2015. Interleukin-1 family cytokines in liver diseases. Mediators Inflamm. 630265, 2015.

Tuncer, M., Suleymanlar, G., Ersoy, F.F., Yakupoglu, G., 2000. Effects of hepatitis C virus infection on cyclosporine trough levels in renal transplant patients. Transplant. Proc. 32, 569—571.

Velenosi, T.J., Feere, D.A., Sohi, G., Hardy, D.B., Urquhart, B.L., 2014. Decreased nuclear receptor activity and epigenetic modulation associates with down-regulation of hepatic drug-metabolizing enzymes in chronic kidney disease. FASEB J. 28, 5388—5397.

Vet, N.J., de Hoog, M., Tibboel, D., de Wildt, S.N., 2012. The effect of critical illness and inflammation on midazolam therapy in children. Pediatr. Crit. Care Med. 13, e48—e50.

Vistisen, K., Loft, S., Olsen, J.H., Vallentin, S., Ottesen, S., Hirsch, F.R., Poulsen, H.E., 2004. Low CYP1A2 activity associated with testicular cancer. Carcinogenesis 25, 923—929.

Vogel, C.F., Khan, E.M., Leung, P.S., Gershwin, M.E., Chang, W.L., Wu, D., Haarmann-Stemmann, T., Hoffmann, A., Denison, M.S., 2014. Cross-talk between aryl hydrocarbon receptor and the inflammatory response: a role for nuclear factor-kappaB. J. Biol. Chem. 289, 1866–1875.

Voleti, B., Agrawal, A., 2005. Regulation of basal and induced expression of C-reactive protein through an overlapping element for OCT-1 and NF-kappaB on the proximal promoter. J. Immunol. 175, 3386–3390.

Vuppalanchi, R., Liang, T., Goswami, C.P., Nalamasu, R., Li, L., Jones, D., Wei, R., Liu, W., Sarasani, V., Janga, S.C., Chalasani, N., 2013. Relationship between differential hepatic microRNA expression and decreased hepatic cytochrome P450 3A activity in cirrhosis. PLoS ONE 8, e74471.

Wan, H.H., Thatcher, N., Mullen, P.W., Smith, G.N., Wilkinson, P.M., 1979. Lack of effect of immunotherapy with BCG and *Corynebacterium parvum* on hepatic drug hydroxylation in man. Br. J. Cancer 39, 441–444.

Wang, J.S., Backman, J.T., Taavitsainen, P., Neuvonen, P.J., Kivisto, K.T., 2000. Involvement of CYP1A2 and CYP3A4 in lidocaine N-deethylation and 3-hydroxylation in humans. Drug Metab. Dispos. 28, 959–965.

Wang, J., Hu, Y., Nekvindova, J., Ingelman-Sundberg, M., Neve, E.P., 2010a. IL-4-mediated transcriptional regulation of human CYP2E1 by two independent signaling pathways. Biochem. Pharmacol. 80, 1592–1600.

Wang, X.R., Qu, Z.Q., Li, X.D., Liu, H.L., He, P., Fang, B.X., Xiao, J., Huang, W., Wu, M.C., 2010b. Activity of sulfotransferase 1A1 is dramatically upregulated in patients with hepatocellular carcinoma secondary to chronic hepatitis B virus infection. Cancer Sci. 101, 412–415.

Warren, G., Poloyac, S., Gary, D., Mattson, M., Blouin, R., 1999. Hepatic cytochrome P-450 expression in tumor necrosis factor-a receptor (p55/p75) knockout mice after endotoxin administration. J. Pharmacol. Exp. Ther. 288, 945–950.

Watt, G., White, N.J., Padre, L., Ritter, W., Fernando, M.T., Ranoa, C.P., Laughlin, L.W., 1988. Praziquantel pharmacokinetics and side effects in *Schistosoma japonicum*-infected patients with liver disease. J. Infect. Dis. 157, 530–535.

Weber, A., Wasiliew, P., Kracht, M., 2010. Interleukin-1 (IL-1) pathway. Sci. Signal. 3, cm1.

White, N.J., Looareesuwan, S., Warrell, D.A., Warrell, M.J., Bunnag, D., Harinasuta, T., 1982. Quinine pharmacokinetics and toxicity in cerebral and uncomplicated falciparum malaria. Am. J. Med. 73, 564–572.

Wilby, K.J., Gilchrist, S.E., Ensom, M.H., 2013. A review of the pharmacokinetic implications of schistosomiasis. Clin. Pharmacokinet. 52, 647–656.

Williams, M.L., Bhargava, P., Cherrouk, I., Marshall, J.L., Flockhart, D.A., Wainer, I.W., 2000. A discordance of the cytochrome P450 2C19 genotype and phenotype in patients with advanced cancer. Br. J. Clin. Pharmacol. 49, 485–488.

Wink, D.A., Osawa, Y., Darbyshire, J.F., Jones, C.R., Eshenaur, S.C., Nims, R.W., 1993. Inhibition of cytochromes P450 by nitric oxide and a nitric oxide-releasing agent. Arch. Biochem. Biophys. 300, 115–123.

Wolffenbuttel, L., Goncalves, E.A., Manfro, R.C., Goncalves, L.F., 2003. Elevated cyclosporine A trough levels in HCV positive kidney transplant recipients. Rev. Ass. Med. Bras. 49, 141–144.

Wolffenbuttel, L., Poli, D.D., Manfro, R.C., Goncalves, L.F., 2004. Cyclosporine pharmacokinetics in anti-HCV[+] patients. Clin. Transplant. 18, 654–660.

Woolbright, B.L., Jaeschke, H., 2015. Xenobiotic and endobiotic mediated interactions between the cytochrome P450 system and the inflammatory response in the liver. Adv. Pharmacol. 74, 131–161.

Wu, J., Meng, Z., Jiang, M., Zhang, E., Trippler, M., Broering, R., Bucchi, A., Krux, F., Dittmer, U., Yang, D., Roggendorf, M., Gerken, G., Lu, M., Schlaak, J.F., 2010. Toll-like receptor-induced innate immune responses in non-parenchymal liver cells are cell type-specific. Immunology 129, 363–374.

Xu, D.X., Wei, W., Sun, M.F., Wu, C.Y., Wang, J.P., Wei, L.Z., Zhou, C.F., 2004. Kupffer cells and reactive oxygen species partially mediate lipopolysaccharide-induced downregulation of nuclear receptor pregnane x receptor and its target gene CYP3a in mouse liver. Free Radic. Biol. Med. 37, 10–22.

Xu, Z., Karlsson, J.O.M., Huan, Z., 2015. Modeling the dynamics of acute phase protein expression in human hepatoma cells stimulated by IL-6. Processes 3, 50–70.

Yamamoto, N., Tamura, T., Kamiya, Y., Sekine, I., Kunitoh, H., Saijo, N., 2000. Correlation between docetaxel clearance and estimated cytochrome P450 activity by urinary metabolite of exogenous cortisol. J. Clin. Oncol. 18, 2301–2308.

Yang, J., Hao, C., Yang, D., Shi, D., Song, X., Luan, X., Hu, G., Yan, B., 2010a. Pregnane X receptor is required for interleukin-6-mediated down-regulation of cytochrome P450 3A4 in human hepatocytes. Toxicol. Lett. 197, 219–226.

Yang, X., Zhang, B., Molony, C., Chudin, E., Hao, K., Zhu, J., Gaedigk, A., Suver, C., Zhong, H., Leeder, J.S., Guengerich, F.P., Strom, S.C., Schuetz, E., Rushmore, T.H., Ulrich, R.G., Slatter, J.G., Schadt, E.E., Kasarskis, A., Lum, P.Y., 2010b. Systematic genetic and genomic analysis of cytochrome P450 enzyme activities in human liver. Genome Res. 20, 1020–1036.

Yokota, S., Higashi, E., Fukami, T., Yokoi, T., Nakajima, M., 2010. Human CYP2A6 is regulated by nuclear factor-erythroid 2 related factor 2. Biochem. Pharmacol. 81, 289–294.

Zhang, D., Jiang, S.L., Rzewnicki, D., Samols, D., Kushner, I., 1995. The effect of interleukin-1 on C-reactive protein expression in Hep3B cells is exerted at the transcriptional level. Biochem. J. 310 (Pt 1), 143–148.

Zhang, D., Sun, M., Samols, D., Kushner, I., 1996. STAT3 participates in transcriptional activation of the C-reactive protein gene by interleukin-6. J. Biol. Chem. 271, 9503–9509.

Zhang, J., Chaluvadi, M.R., Reddy, R., Motika, M.S., Richardson, T.A., Cashman, J.R., Morgan, E.T., 2009. Hepatic flavin-containing monooxygenase gene regulation in different mouse inflammation models. Drug Metab. Dispos. 37, 462–468.

Zhuang, Y., de Vries, D.E., Xu, Z., Marciniak Jr., S.J., Chen, D., Leon, F., Davis, H.M., Zhou, H., 2015. Evaluation of disease-mediated therapeutic protein-drug interactions between an anti-interleukin-6 monoclonal antibody (sirukumab) and cytochrome P450 activities in a phase 1 study in patients with rheumatoid arthritis using a cocktail approach. J. Clin. Pharmacol.

Zordoky, B.N., El-Kadi, A.O., 2009. Role of NF-kappaB in the regulation of cytochrome P450 enzymes. Curr. Drug Metab. 10, 164–178.

Regulation of Drug Transporters by Inflammation

D. Kojovic, M. Piquette-Miller

University of Toronto, Toronto, ON, Canada

O U T L I N E

Introduction	59	Solute Carrier Uptake Transporting Family	73
Acute Inflammation	60		
Models of Acute Inflammation	61	Chronic Inflammation	75
Effect of Acute Inflammation on Drug Transporters	62	Impact of Chronic Inflammation on Drug Transporters	75
ABC Efflux Transporters	62	Rheumatoid Arthritis	75
P-Glycoprotein (MDR1/ABCB1)	63	Inflammatory Bowel Disease	77
Breast Cancer Resistance Protein (BCRP/ABCG2)	68	Chronic Renal Failure	79
Multidrug Resistance-Associated Proteins	70	Cholestasis	79
Bile Salt Export Pump (BSEP/ABCB11)	72	Conclusion	80
		References	80

INTRODUCTION

For many years, inflammation was considered to be a completely beneficial response for host defense and rehabilitation. However, in recent decades, it has been discovered that inflammation can also play a part in pathogenesis and has been implicated in a number of disease states. Inflammation is known as a complex biological response that aids in host protection from harmful external stimuli, cell damage, or irritation within the body. This response is thought to be part of our innate immunity that is meant to remove harmful pathogens, irritants, or necrotic cells and to initiate tissue repair in the affected areas. The response to specific physical, biological, or chemical irritation is dynamic, as an insufficient inflammatory response allows continuous destruction and may not allow for tissue repair. On the other hand, excessive or prolonged inflammation may lead to further complications and chronic diseases. Because complications can be caused by a disbalanced inflammatory response, it is closely regulated within the body.

Over four decades ago, studies began to surface indicating increases in plasma concentrations of drugs in patient and animal models of inflammation (Belpaire et al., 1989). As discussed in other chapters within this book, inflammation has been found to induce changes in the expression and activity of drug-metabolizing enzymes. Changes in drug metabolism and plasma binding were believed to be responsible for altered plasma drug concentrations. More recent studies have revealed that inflammation-mediated changes in the expression and activity of drug transporters may also contribute to interindividual variability in drug disposition. Examination into the impact of inflammation on the expression of drug transporters is a fairly recent field of study and is thus evolving as new work emerges. There are two major groups of transporters, the active ATP-binding cassette (ABC) family of efflux transporters, and the SCL family of uptake transporters. This chapter focuses on changes in the expression of transporters that have been identified by the International Transporter Consortium as clinically important in drug absorption and disposition and hence drug development. Overall, the changes seen in the expression of ABC and SLC transporters in the liver, kidney, intestine, brain, and placenta have been best characterized during acute inflammation and thus the chapter primarily focuses on the acute inflammatory response.

ACUTE INFLAMMATION

Acute inflammation is the first line of defense against infectious microorganisms and immunological stressors such as trauma, burn, and malignant growths (Gabay and Kushner, 1999; Haslett, 1992). It is a nonspecific immediate response that changes the microenvironment, increasing blood flow to recruit and accumulate fluid, and recruiting immune cells such as leukocytes, lymphocytes, and neutrophils (Gruys et al., 2005; Feghali and Wright, 1997). It is characterized by redness, heat, swelling, pain, and loss of function. Other physiological changes include increased production of the positive acute phase proteins. The induction in plasma concentrations can range from the 2- to 10-fold increase observed with alpha-1 acid glycoprotein upward to a 1000-fold increase in levels of C-reactive protein and amyloid A (Gruys et al., 2005; Cray et al., 2009). These proteins have various functions including, but not limited to, binding foreign and damaged cells, enhancing phagocytosis by macrophages, and recruitment of immune cells. These acute phase proteins are often used as markers of inflammation. At the same time, there is a decreased production of many other hepatic proteins that are referred to as the negative acute phase proteins. Examples include albumin, transferrin, and antithrombin. It is important to note that interpatient variability plays a role and inflammation-mediated changes in plasma protein concentrations of both the positive and negative acute phase proteins are not uniform throughout the population.

The acute phase reaction also elicits the release of several proinflammatory cytokines, including interleukin (IL) 1α and 1β, IL-6, IL-8, tumor necrosis factor (TNF)-α, and interferon (IFN). These small and short-lived molecules are involved in communication between cells by the interaction of cell surface receptors and epithelial cells of many organs. They are released by macrophages at the site of inflammation, and they play an important role in the acute inflammatory reactions through a complex network of cellular interactions. These cytokines are also involved in the activation of inflammatory transcriptional factors such as NF-κB, which in turn regulates the expression of a vast number of genes (Petrovic et al., 2007). Therefore the onset of inflammation can affect the regulation of many target genes including drug-metabolizing enzymes, membrane transporters, and their transcription factors. Changes that occur during an acute inflammatory response are generally transient, lasting only a few days once the inflammatory response is resolved.

MODELS OF ACUTE INFLAMMATION

Both in vivo and in vitro models have been used to examine the impact of inflammation on the regulation of drug transporters. Most frequently, rodent models of acute inflammation are employed due to practical and ethical concerns, and they have been well characterized in the past. Physiological changes similar to humans can be achieved in these models by administration of bacterial, viral, protozoal, or chemical agents or by direct exposure to proinflammatory cytokines.

Administration of lipopolysaccharide (LPS), a bacterial endotoxin, is one of the most extensively characterized models of acute inflammation. It is used to model bacterial infections or sepsis and is known to result in a highly reproducible induction of proinflammatory cytokines, as well as physical symptoms such as fever and hypotension (Copeland et al., 2005). On the other hand, viral infections are most commonly modeled through administration of poly-Inosinic:poly-Cytidilic acid (poly I:C), a synthetic double-stranded RNA, which is a potent inducer of IFN (Fortier et al., 2004; Gandhi et al., 2007). Administration of poly I:C also induces a number of other proinflammatory cytokines such as IL-6, IL-12, and TNF-α, and produces symptoms such as malaise and fever (Fortier et al., 2004). The subcutaneous administration of turpentine, an organic solvent distilled from pine resin, is also frequently used to model aseptic acute inflammation or trauma in rodents. The subcutaneous injection of other irritants such as carrageenan or magnesium silicate (talc) has also been used to model acute inflammation.

As inflammation-mediated changes in gene expression are thought to be attributed through cytokine-mediated pathways, cytokines can often be directly administered in vitro, and in vivo, to initiate the inflammatory response. Several studies have suggested that IL-6 is directly linked to the transcriptional changes of P-glycoprotein (P-gp) in the liver of rodents (Sukhai et al., 2000, 2001; Hartmann et al., 2001; Lee and Piquette-Miller, 2001). Other cytokines such as TNF-α and IL-1β have also been linked to transcriptional changes in several of the ABC family of proteins in vitro and in vivo, and thus these proinflammatory cytokines likely play a fundamental role in the regulation of transporters

(Hartmann et al., 2001; Fardel and Le Vée, 2009). Indeed, cytokine levels are frequently measured to monitor the inflammatory response to bacterial and viral mimetics. Although it is difficult to directly translate rodent models to the clinical setting due to species differences in drug disposition and gene isoforms, it has been shown that there are similarities in the release of cytokines, activation of transcriptional factors, and gene expression changes in humans and rodents during an acute inflammatory response (Copeland et al., 2005; Roe et al., 1998; Poloyac et al., 1999).

EFFECT OF ACUTE INFLAMMATION ON DRUG TRANSPORTERS

Interest in the area of altered drug disposition in inflammation was generated when it was observed that various inflammatory conditions in humans such as Crohn's disease (CD) or rheumatoid arthritis (RA) were associated with large increases in plasma concentrations of oxyprenolol and propranolol (Kendall et al., 1979; Schneider et al., 1976) Historically, inflammation-mediated changes in drug disposition, elimination, and clearance were primarily ascribed to altered drug metabolism and protein binding. However, emerging evidence in the last two decades has revealed the association of altered drug transporter expression due to an inflammatory response. As many therapeutic agents are transferred across epithelial membranes via transporter proteins, they play a pivotal role in altered pharmacokinetics during inflammation.

Some of the first studies to describe inflammatory-mediated changes on drug transporters examined changes in the hepatic expression of the ABC efflux transporter P-gp and multidrug resistance-associated protein 2 (MRP2) in models of acute inflammation. Since then, the regulation of many other transporters has been explored. Subsequent studies also expanded to examine inflammatory-mediated changes in other epithelial membrane barriers. Although the acute inflammatory response is known to alter the expression of many liver-derived proteins, the effect of inflammation is not limited to the liver, and changes can be seen in epithelial tissues of the intestine, kidney, brain, and placenta. Moreover, as many ABC and SLC transporters have overlapping substrates, it is also believed that the combined changes in the expression and activity of these two families of transporters will further alter the transepithelial transfer of substrates across membrane barriers, and in this manner have great potential to impact the absorption, distribution, and excretion of drugs (Jaisue et al., 2010; Yang et al., 2009).

ABC Efflux Transporters

ABC drug efflux transporters are a superfamily of membrane proteins found within all living organisms, facilitating the transport of exogenous and endogenous substrates across epithelial membranes. These transporters are ubiquitously expressed in the apical or basolateral membranes of numerous organs such as the liver, kidney, intestine, brain, heart, lungs, placenta, uterus, mammary gland, and testis among others. The localization of ABC and SLC transporters in epithelial membranes of brain, liver, kidney, and intestine can be seen in Figs. 3.1—3.4. They are involved in the transport of a broad range of substrates and, although there are some conformational differences across the 48 functional ABC transporters in the

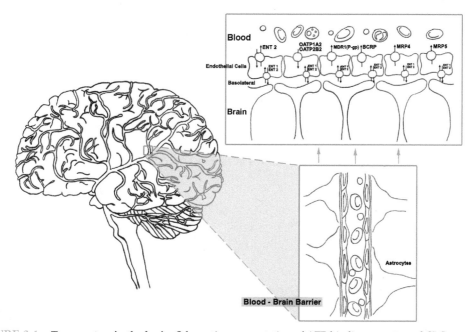

FIGURE 3.1 Transporters in the brain. Schematic representation of ATP-binding cassette and SLC transporters in brain capillary endothelial cells. *BCRP*, breast cancer resistance protein; *MDR*, multidrug resistance protein; *OATP*, organic anion transporting polypeptides; *P-gp*, P-glycoprotein. *Illustration by Nathan Piquette-Miller.*

human genome, there is considerable overlap of their substrates. The ABC superfamily is a highly conserved group of transporters, sharing a specific gene sequence that encodes the ATP-binding cassette. This conserved domain, also termed the nucleotide-binding domain (NBD), is the site of substrate binding and subsequent ATP hydrolysis, providing the energy needed for the translocation of substrates across cellular membranes.

Within this group of transporters, a few are of particular importance, as they are also known to transport clinically important drugs. Among these key transporters are the multidrug resistance protein 1, also known as P-gp (MDR1, encoded by the ABCB1 gene in humans and *Abcb1a* and *Abcb1b* gene in rodents), the MRP group (encoded by the ABCC genes in humans and *Abcc* genes in rodents), breast cancer resistance protein (BCRP, encoded by ABCG2 gene in humans and *Abcg2* gene in rodents), and the bile salt export pump (BSEP, encoded by the ABCB11 gene in humans and *Abcb11* gene in rodents). The following is a brief description of the key drug transporters in this family; their expression, classification, localization, and function have been the focus of many review articles and much of this information can be found on the University of California, San Francisco (UCSF)-US Food and Drug Administration (FDA) transportal website (http://dbts.ucsf.edu/fdatransportal).

P-Glycoprotein (MDR1/ABCB1)

P-gp is a 170-kDa protein consisting of two NBDs, each occurring after six transmembrane helices. It is thought to play a protective role by secreting potentially toxic endogenous and exogenous compounds across epithelial membranes, thereby preventing drug entry or

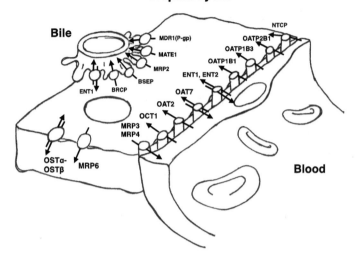

FIGURE 3.2 Transporters in the liver. Schematic representation of ATP-binding cassette and SLC transporters in the basolateral and canalicular membrane of hepatocytes. *BCRP*, breast cancer resistance protein; *BSEP*, bile salt export pump; *MDR*, multidrug resistance protein; *MRP*, multidrug resistance-associated protein; *OAT*, organic anion transporters; *OATP*, organic anion transporting polypeptides; *OCT*, organic cation transporters; *P-gp*, P-glycoprotein. *Illustration by Nathan Piquette-Miller.*

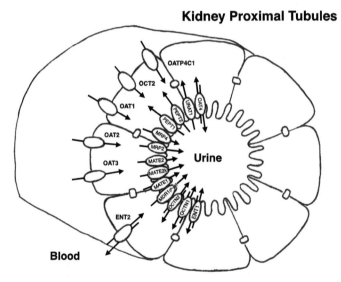

FIGURE 3.3 Transporters in the kidney. Schematic representation of ATP-binding cassette and SLC transporter localization in the apical and basolateral membranes of the proximal renal tubules. *MDR*, multidrug resistance protein; *MRP*, multidrug resistance-associated protein; *OAT*, organic anion transporters; *OATP*, organic anion transporting polypeptides; *OCT*, organic cation transporters; *OCTN*, organic cation/carnitine transporters. *Illustration by Nathan Piquette-Miller.*

Intestinal Epithelia

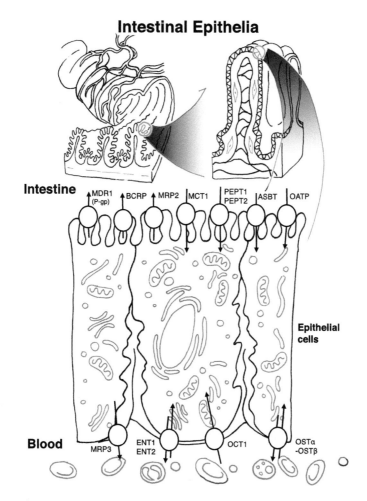

FIGURE 3.4 **Transporters in the intestines.** Schematic representation of ATP-binding cassette and SLC transporter localization in the apical and basolateral membranes of intestinal enterocytes. *BCRP*, breast cancer resistance protein; *MDR*, multidrug resistance protein; *MRP*, multidrug resistance-associated protein; *OATP*, organic anion transporting polypeptides; *OCT*, organic cation transporters; *P-gp*, P-glycoprotein. *Illustration by Nathan Piquette-Miller.*

promoting drug secretion. Specifically, it is located at the endothelium of the blood–brain barrier and testis, on the apical surface of hepatocytes, intestinal enterocytes, proximal renal tubules, and placental syncytiotrophoblasts. It transports a broad range of chemically diverse substrates, including many chemotherapeutic agents. Indeed, overexpression of P-gp at the cell surface of tumors is an important contributor to multidrug resistance.

LIVER

P-gp was the first drug transporter to be discovered and cloned; therefore it remains one of the most extensively characterized transporters. To date, many research groups have examined the impact of inflammation on the expression and activity of P-gp. One of the first in vivo reports demonstrated an inflammation-mediated downregulation of P-gp in both the turpentine and endotoxin models of acute inflammation. As compared with controls, a significant 70–80% decrease in the hepatic protein expression of P-gp was seen in turpentine- or endotoxin-treated male rats. Furthermore, P-gp-mediated efflux of rhodamine 123 (a known P-gp substrate) was decreased by 45–60% in hepatocytes isolated from these rats (Belliard et al., 2004). A decrease in the hepatic mRNA and protein expression of P-gp are also seen in mice after administration of turpentine, endotoxin, or IL-6 (Berengue et al., 2003).

As there are two isoforms that encode for P-gp in rodents, differences in their regulation have been observed in several instances. Although endotoxin-induced inflammation reportedly decreases the expression of both isoforms in mice, results from rat models generally show a significant decrease in the *Abcb1a* isoform, but a marked increase in mRNA levels of the *Abcb1b* isoform (Cherrington et al., 2004; Vos et al., 1998; Petrovic and Piquette-Miller, 2010). On the other hand, hepatic protein expression is downregulated in both species (Sukhai et al., 2000, 2001; Hartmann et al., 2001, 2005; Piquette-Miller et al., 1998). These findings are in line with pharmacokinetic studies that have demonstrated that changes in transporter expression leads to functional changes of the protein. Studies in mice have shown that the endotoxin-mediated downregulation of *Abcb1a* in liver is associated with a 50% decrease in biliary clearance of the P-gp substrate doxorubicin as well as reduced systemic clearance of the drug (Hartmann et al., 2005). Likewise, the endotoxin-mediated downregulation of *Abcb1a* in rat liver is associated with corresponding increases in the hepatic accumulation of 99m Tc-sestamibi and decreased biliary secretion of digoxin, both of which are substrates of P-gp (Wang et al., 2005; Goralski et al., 2003). Administration of shiga-like toxin II, a toxin that is released by some strains of *Escherichia coli*, has also been reported to decrease the hepatobiliary clearance of doxorubicin due to P-gp downregulation (Hidemura et al., 2003; Ando et al., 2001). Endotoxin isolated from sources other than *E. coli*, such as *Klebsiella pneumoniae*, has also been found to decrease hepatic P-gp expression in rats along with diminished biliary clearance of rhodamine 123 (Ando et al., 2001). The acute inflammatory response as modeled using the viral mimetic poly I:C has been reported to decrease the hepatic expression of *Abcb1a* mRNA in pregnant rats along with a corresponding increase in hepatic accumulation of lopinavir, a substrate of P-gp (Petrovic and Piquette-Miller, 2010).

INTESTINE

The intestine acts as an important physiological barrier and is involved in the absorption of all orally administered drugs. Efflux transporters such as P-gp, which are highly expressed in the intestinal epithelium, play a role in limiting absorption of many clinically important compounds. As such, it is critical to understand the alterations that are imposed during inflammation. An inflammation-mediated decrease in the jejunal and ileal expression of *Abcb1a* along with a corresponding decline in the basolateral to apical efflux of the P-gp substrates, amiodarone and rhodamine 123, has been reported in endotoxin-treated rats (Kalitsky-Szirtes et al., 2004). There is also evidence that similar changes occur in humans. Increased plasma concentrations of tacrolimus in transplant patients suffering from infectious diarrhea (Berengue et al., 2003) have been linked to a decreased intestinal activity of P-gp in these patients (Lemahieu et al., 2005). Administration of cytokines can also impose changes. Several studies have reported that administration of IL-2 leads to a decrease in the expression and functional activity of intestinal P-gp in mice (Bonhomme-Faivre et al., 2002; Veau et al., 2002; Castagne et al., 2004). Likewise, in vitro incubation of human intestinal Caco-2 cells with TNF-α or IL-2 imposes a strong time-dependent attenuation of ABCB1 mRNA levels along with significant decreases in rhodamine 123 transport (Belliard et al., 2002, 2004). Cytokine-dependent decreases in ABCB1 expression have been reported in human intestinal biopsies treated with the inflammatory cytokines TNF-α, IL-1β, or IFN-γ (Blokzijl et al., 2007). On the other hand, Bertilsson et al. (2001) reported an induction in ABCB1 mRNA levels but increased permeability in Caco-2 cells after incubation with IL-1β, IL-6, or IFN-γ (Bertilsson et al., 2001). The discrepancy between results is not clear at present; however, different methods, cytokines, or cell lines may play a role.

KIDNEY

Information regarding renal P-gp expression during acute inflammation is limited. Work conducted in rat kidney proximal tubule cell lines treated with LPS, alone or in conjunction with TNF-α, resulted in an increase in the expression and activity of P-gp after 24 h (Heemskerk et al., 2010). The in vivo administration of E. coli–derived endotoxin was reported to elicit an increase in renal Abcb1b mRNA and P-gp protein levels, resulting in a 2.5-fold increase in renal clearance of doxorubicin in mice (Wang et al., 2005). Significant increases in the renal expression of Abcb1a and Abc1b along with increased P-gp protein expression have also been reported in LPS-treated rats (Heemskerk et al., 2007). Likewise, an increased mRNA and protein expression of P-gp is observed in the kidneys of pregnant mice infected with the malaria parasite Plasmodium berghei (Cressman et al., 2014). On the other hand, administration of endotoxin isolated from K. pneumoniae imposed a reduction in the renal expression of Abcb1a and Abcb1b transcripts along with a corresponding decrease in net tubular secretion of rhodamine 123 in rats after 6 h (Ando et al., 2001). The discrepancy between results is not clear at present; however, different methods, species, and models of inflammation may play a role.

BRAIN

P-gp is also highly expressed in the brain facilitating active efflux of substrates from neural and glial cells and regulation of transcellular traffic across endothelial cells that form the blood—brain barrier. In brain-derived continuous and primary cell lines, administration of proinflammatory cytokines elicited opposing effects on P-gp expression, inducing a slight decrease in mRNA levels after IL-6 administration, and significant increases after TNF-α treatment at both the gene and protein levels (Poller et al., 2010; Ronaldson and Bendayan, 2006). These changes, however, did not affect the functionality of the protein, as the uptake of the P-gp substrate rhodamine 123 was unaffected (Poller et al., 2010). Another in vitro work has similarly shown induction of P-gp in cultured porcine brain capillary endothelial cells after a 6-h exposure to TNF-α; however, this effect was transient and P-gp expression was significantly decreased at 24 and 48 h after cytokine exposure (von Wedel-Parlow et al., 2009). Incubation of cultured rat astrocytes with gp120, an HIV-1 viral envelope glycoprotein, was observed to stimulate an inflammatory response along with a 4.7-fold downregulation of P-gp protein levels, leading to significantly increased intracellular accumulation of the substrates digoxin and saquinavir (Ronaldson and Bendayan, 2006). Inflammation-mediated changes in P-gp have also been reported in vivo. In rodent models, both intracranial and intraperitoneal administration of LPS resulted in a reduction in the expression of *Abcb1a* mRNA in brain tissues, with a concordant increase in the CNS accumulation of digoxin and 99m Tc-sestamibi (Wang et al., 2005; Goralski et al., 2003). Intravenous administration of endotoxin derived from *K. pneumoniae* to mice also produced a significant decrease in P-gp protein levels in brain homogenates 6 h after endotoxin exposure; however, levels were found to return to control levels after 24 h (Zhao et al., 2002a). The transient change in protein expression was not found to alter the transport of doxorubicin across the blood−brain barrier. On the other hand, shiga-like toxin II was found to increase rather than decrease the expression of P-gp in the brains of mice within 6 h of injection and levels remained higher at 24 h (Zhao et al., 2002b).

PLACENTA

The placenta is the frontline barrier between the mother and developing fetus, expressing numerous clinically relevant drug transporters in the apical and basolateral membranes. These transporters are believed to play a protective role by preventing entry or facilitating efflux of potentially harmful endogenous and exogenous substrates from the fetal compartment. In vitro work using primary term trophoblasts demonstrated that treatment of cells with the proinflammatory cytokines, TNF-α or IL-1β, significantly decreases the expression of *Abcb1* at the gene and protein level (Evseenko et al., 2007). Incubation of first but not third trimester placental villous explants with endotoxin has been found to impose a reduction in the mRNA and protein expression of *ABCB1* (Lye et al., 2015). In contrast, incubations with poly I:C decreased expression of ABCB1 in third trimester but not in first trimester explants. This suggests that inflammatory triggers may depend on gestational age. Nevertheless, both endotoxin and poly I:C elicited an increase in IL-8 mRNA levels in the explants regardless of term. Preclinical studies conducted in pregnant rats treated with endotoxin and poly I:C have demonstrated induction of proinflammatory cytokines along with time- and dose-dependent decreases in *Abcb1a* and *Abcb1b* placental gene expression (Petrovic and Piquette-Miller, 2010; Wang et al., 2005; Petrovic et al., 2008). Changes in P-gp expression were also associated with an increased accumulation of the substrates digoxin, Tc-sestamibi, and lopinavir in the fetal compartment of pregnant rodents, suggesting comprised function of this transporter under inflammatory stress (Petrovic and Piquette-Miller, 2010; Wang et al., 2005; Bloise et al., 2013). Likewise, decreased mRNA and protein expression of *Abcb1a* and *Abcb1b* mRNA have been reported in placental tissues isolated from *P. berghei*–infected mice (Cressman et al., 2014). Interestingly, observed changes in fetal livers were similar to those seen in maternal liver. Studies examining human placental tissues isolated from women with chorioamnionitis, a bacterial infection of placental membranes, detected increased but highly variable mRNA levels of *Abcb1* in preterm chorioamnionitis placentas as compared with healthy controls (Mason et al., 2011; Petrovic et al., 2015). Interestingly, mRNA levels of Abcb1 were highly and positively correlated to IL-6 expression (Petrovic et al., 2015). However, due to the nature of human studies, neither was sufficiently powered to detect changes in protein expression or at term, and thus additional studies are needed.

Breast Cancer Resistance Protein (BCRP/ABCG2)

The structure of the 72-kDa ABCG2 is unique from other ABC transporters in that it is a half transporter with a single NBD and six transmembrane domains. It is thought that

BCRP forms a homodimer to become functional (Ni et al., 2010). Originally discovered in a breast cancer cell line exhibiting multidrug resistance to chemotherapeutic agents, it is now known to transport a wide array of drugs as well as endogenous compounds (Ni et al., 2010). Although the range of substrates transported by BCRP is less broad than that of P-gp, it is involved in the transport of a number of clinically important antiretroviral and anti-cancer drugs. BCRP is highly expressed in tissue barriers of the placenta, blood—brain barrier, mammary tissue, and intestine, where it may play a role in limiting exposure to xenobiotics. Expression in mammary glands is thought to additionally play a role in vitamin excretion into milk. BCRP is also expressed in the liver and kidney, enhancing excretion of substrates into bile and urine, respectively. The regulation of BCRP has gained much attention in recent years. Many in vitro and in vivo studies have detected inflammation-mediated changes in the expression and activity of BCRP. Similar to what has been observed with respect to P-gp, there is evidence pointing to cytokine-mediated regulation of BCRP.

LIVER

Treatment of primary human hepatocytes with IL-6 and IFN but not TNF-α has been reported to decrease the mRNA and protein expression of BCRP (Fardel and Le Vée, 2009; Le Vee et al., 2009, 2011a). These findings are in line with what has been reported in animal models, in which significant decreases in the mRNA and protein expression of *Abcg2* are seen in the livers of pregnant rats within 24 h after administration of either LPS or poly I:C; models with are associated with the systemic release of IL-6 and IFN (Petrovic and Piquette-Miller, 2010). Decreased immunodetectable levels of BCRP are also seen in hepatic membrane fractions isolated from adjuvant-treated rats at both acute and chronic stages of inflammation (Smolen and Steiner, 2003). Moreover, decreased mRNA expression of Bcrp has been reported in the livers of pregnant mice infected with the malaria parasite *P. berghei* (Cressman et al., 2014). Interestingly, the expression of Bcrp is similarly decreased in the fetal livers of these infected mice.

INTESTINE

There are several reports of altered intestinal expression of BCRP in chronic conditions, whereas there are no reports to date in acute models of inflammation.

BRAIN

In general, although there have been a few in vitro studies that have examined the effects of inflammatory mediators on the expression and function of BCRP at the blood—brain barrier, in vivo information is relatively sparse. Treatment of the human brain capillary endothelial hCMEC/D3 cell line with TNF-α, IL-1β, or IL-6 has been reported to decrease the mRNA and protein expression of BCRP along with a corresponding increase in mitroxantrone accumulation, signifying impaired BCRP efflux activity (Poller et al., 2010; von Wedel-Parlow et al., 2009; Evseenko et al., 2007). Likewise, an inflammatory-mediated decrease in the expression and activity of BCRP was observed in LPS-treated mouse BV-2 microglial cells (Gibson et al., 2012). On the other hand, intracerebroventricular injection of the HIV-1 viral protein gp120 to rats, which induced an inflammatory response, was reported to increase the protein expression of Bcrp specifically in the frontal cortex, while remaining unchanged in brain capillaries and other brain regions (Ashraf et al., 2014).

Of note, intracerebroventricular injection of endothelin-1, a cytokine that is released in brain in response to CNS inflammatory disorders, was found to increase the in vivo BCRP-mediated transport of prazosin in adult rat brain but tended to reduce efflux activity in juvenile brain, indicating that inflammation-mediated changes may be altered during development (Harati et al., 2012). Indeed, age-related differences were seen in the expression of endothelin-1-induced cytokines.

PLACENTA

As BCRP expression is highest in the placenta, it plays an important role in protecting the fetus from potentially toxic endogenous and exogenous substrates. In pregnant rats, administration of endotoxin was found to downregulate placental *Abcg2* gene expression and protein levels in a time- and dose-dependent manner. A corresponding increase in placental and fetal accumulation of the ABCG2 substrate glyburide was also seen, indicating that inflammation has an impact on the functional activity of ABCG2 (Petrovic et al., 2008). Likewise, a significant dose-dependent downregulation of placental Abcg2 is observed in rats after administration of poly I:C (Petrovic and Piquette-Miller, 2010). Similar regulation may occur in humans as in vitro treatments of primary human placental trophoblasts with TNF-α or IL-1β cells have been reported to impose a 40–50% decrease in the mRNA and protein expression of ABCG2 along with a decrease in efflux activity (Evseenko et al., 2007). Likewise, 24-h incubations of first trimester human placental explants with endotoxin were found to significantly decrease the mRNA and protein expression of ABCG2 (Lye et al., 2015). On the other hand, incubation with poly I:C was not found to have a significant effect. Inconsistency regarding the effect of disease on ABCG2 regulation exists in the literature. For example, both an induction and reduction of BCRP have been reported in human placental tissues isolated from women with chorioamnionitis, as compared with healthy controls. In one study, significant reductions in BCRP transcript and protein levels were seen when placentas were obtained at either term or preterm parturition alongside markedly elevated levels of IL-6, IL-1β, and TNF-α (Petrovic et al., 2015). Alternatively, an increase in mRNA levels of BCRP was earlier reported in human placentas obtained from chorioamnionitis cases with preterm labor (Mason et al., 2011). As expression of IL-6 and TNF-α was not seen in this study, it is plausible that differences in disease severity, drug administration or gestational stage could be responsible for this discrepancy.

Multidrug Resistance-Associated Proteins

There are currently nine identified members of the MRP family, MRP1–9. They are all characterized as unidirectional efflux pumps and depend on ATP as an energy source for translocation. MRPs can be found at either the apical or basal membranes of tissues (Keppler, 2011). For example, MRP1 is expressed on the basolateral surface of bronchial epithelium, but at the apical surface of trophoblast cells of the placenta (Wright et al., 1998; Brechot et al., 1998; Kozłowska-Rup et al., 2014). Several members of this family of transporters are considered important contributors of drug disposition as well as multidrug resistance (MRP1–5). Numerous in vitro and in vivo studies have reported inflammation-mediated changes in the expression of members of the MRP family of transporters.

The first MRP that was discovered, MRP1, is expressed in many tissues with highest detection in the intestinal epithelium, lung, kidney, liver, testis, and placenta among others

(Cherrington, 2002; Nishimura and Naito, 2005). The expression of MRP1 is relatively low in liver; however, its expression can be induced by conditions such as cholestasis (Cherrington, 2002). MRP1 has broad substrate specificity and plays a role in conferring resistance to numerous chemotherapeutic agents. MRP1 also transporters an array of hydrophobic and anionic molecules, glutathione conjugates, endogenous glutathione, bilirubin, folic acid, dietary compounds, and inflammatory mediators such as leukotrienes and prostaglandins.

MRP2 is a 174-kDa protein localized in the apical membrane of the liver, kidney, intestine, lung, mammary gland, gallbladder, and placenta. MRP2 plays an important role in excretion of endogenous and exogenous substrates into bile, urine, and intestinal lumen. Furthermore, MRP2 has the ability to transport many glutathione, glucuronate, or sulfate-conjugated metabolites. Several genetic polymorphisms of MRP2 can cause impairment of bilirubin transport into bile resulting into a state of hyperbilirubinemia known as Dubin–Johnson syndrome (Borst et al., 2000). Although this holds true, loss of MRP2 function is commonly compensated by increased expression of other ATP-efflux transporting proteins (Donner and Keppler, 2001).

MRP3 is a 169-kDa protein with three transmembrane domains as opposed to two, as seen in MRP1 and MRP2. It is most highly expressed in the liver, pancreas, small intestine, and colon, and expressed at lower levels in the bladder, kidney, lung, spleen, and placenta. MRP3 transports both xenobiotics and endogenous substrates; it has a wide substrate specificity similar to that of MRP2. In contrast to MRP2, MRP3 has a higher affinity for glucuronate than glutathione conjugates.

MRP4 is a 150-kDa protein that is found in numerous human tissues, including the liver, kidney, blood–brain barrier, prostate, and placenta. Polarized cells have shown MRP4 expression localized to the apical and basolateral membranes. Important physiological substrates for MRP4 are the cyclic nucleotide signaling molecules cGMP and cAMP, as well as ADP and several eicosanoids. In addition to the endogenous substrates transported by MRP4, it has affinity for several nucleoside- and nucleotide-based antiviral and anticancer agents.

MRP5, a 185-kDa protein consisting of two membrane-spanning domains and two NBDs, is ubiquitously expressed throughout most tissues, such as the liver, blood–brain barrier, heart, lung, placenta, and muscles. MRP5 has some substrate overlap with MRP4, with high affinity to a number of cyclic nucleotides and antiviral agents. As MRP5 is expressed in the heart, studies have suggested it plays a role in the regulation of cardiac cGMP, and thus the regulation of cardiac contractility (Dazert et al., 2003).

Members six to nine of the MRP family have more recently been discovered and have not yet been fully characterized. There have been reports of overlapping substrates with other MRP transporters such as steroids and anticancer drugs. MRP6 has been linked to the pathogenesis of pseudoxanthoma elasticum, through the transport of vitamin K, whereas MRP8 is unique in its ability to transport odorants and their precursors.

LIVER

Numerous in vivo studies in rodents have demonstrated decreases in the hepatic expression and activity of Mrp2 after administration of endotoxin, in active infections or in various models of cholestasis (Cherrington et al., 2004; Vos et al., 1998; Hartmann et al., 2002; Nakamura et al., 1999; Tang et al., 2000; Donner et al., 2004). Although it has been proposed that Mrp2 downregulation may be mediated by IL-1β-dependent pathways, in vivo administration of IL-1β, IL-6, or TNF-α each imposed a downregulation of Mrp2 in mice. Likewise, primary cultures of human or rat hepatocytes treated with TNF-α, IL-6, or IL-1β, all resulted in reduced mRNA and protein expression of MRP2 after 24 or 48 h of treatment (Diao et al., 2010). As such, proinflammatory cytokines are considered key mediators in the transcriptional regulation of Mrp2. On the other hand, Elferink et al. (2004) observed that, although Mrp2 transcript levels were unchanged in LPS-treated human liver slices, protein levels of Mrp2 were virtually obliterated, suggesting that posttranslational regulatory mechanisms may play an important role in humans (Brca-kova et al., 2009). Corresponding with Mrp2 downregulation, an induction in the expression of hepatic Mrp1 and Mrp3 has been seen in rodents in response to endotoxin, poly I:C, or *P. berghei* infection or proinflammatory cytokines (Lee and Piquette-Miller, 2001; Cherrington et al., 2004; Petrovic and Piquette-Miller, 2010; Le Vee et al., 2011a; Donner and Keppler, 2001; Hartmann et al., 2002; Elferink et al., 2004). It is generally thought that these transporters are induced as a compensatory or protective mechanism to remove potentially toxic bile products from the liver. Studies have also reported regulatory effects on Mrp4−6. Administration of endotoxin was found to significantly induce the hepatic mRNA expression of Mrp5 and Mrp6 in rats, whereas there was a strong trend toward Mrp4 downregulation (Donner et al., 2004). The hepatic mRNA expression of Mrp4 and Mrp6 was observed to be decreased in C3H/HeOuJ mice infected by *Citrobacter rodentium* (Merrell et al., 2014). As incubation of primary human hepatocytes with IL-1β has been shown to decrease mRNA levels of Mrp2, Mrp3, and Mrp4, the proinflammatory cytokines likely play an important role in the regulation of these transporters (Le Vee et al., 2008, 2009).

OTHER TISSUES

Decreased expression of Mrp2 has been shown in the intestine of LPS-treated rats, along with an induction in proinflammatory cytokines and impaired Mrp2-mediated transport (Kalitsky-Szirtes et al., 2004). Likewise, inflammation-mediated reductions in the placental expression of Mrp1, 2, 3 and Mrp1, 3 have been observed in pregnant rats following administration of LPS and poly I:C, respectively (Petrovic and Piquette-Miller, 2010). Administration of endotoxin was also found to decrease Mrp3 and Mrp4 protein levels in the kidneys of mice (Brcakova et al., 2009). Decreased protein expression of Mrp4 and increased Mrp5 expression have been reported in vitro in LPS-treated murine microglial cells, along with increased rhodamine 123 accumulation indicating impaired efflux activity (Gibson et al., 2012).

Bile Salt Export Pump (BSEP/ABCB11)

The BSEP is a 160-kDa protein with 12 membrane-spanning domains. It is predominantly expressed in the canalicular membrane of hepatocytes. Although BSEP has low affinity for only a few therapeutic agents, it plays a critical role in the elimination of conjugated bilirubin and bile salts into bile. In humans, there is no known compensatory mechanism for the loss of function for BSEP, and dysfunctional regulation or inhibition can lead to the accumulation of bile salts resulting in hepatotoxicity or cholestasis (Kosters and Karpen, 2008).

Numerous studies have reported endotoxin-mediated downregulation of BSEP expression in rodents (Le Vee et al., 2011a; Su et al., 2014). The impact of endotoxin, inflammation, and various models of cholestasis on the regulation of BSEP and other bile acid transporters has been extensively reviewed by Geier et al. (2007), Klaassen and Aleksunes (2010a), and Hayashi and Sugiyama (2013). Indeed cholestasis associated with endotoxemia is primarily mediated by BSEP downregulation, which results in a pronounced accumulation of bile salts and acids within hepatocytes. The in vivo administration of IL-6 or IL-1β to mice was found to suppress mRNA levels of Abcb11 by 40–60% in a dose-dependent manner (Hartmann et al., 2002). Likewise, primary cultures of human and rat hepatocytes have shown dramatic decreases in BSEP mRNA expression after exposure to IL-6, IL-1β, or TNF-α (Diao et al., 2010). Furthermore, dramatically decreased protein levels of BSEP were observed in human and rat liver slices exposed to LPS, whereas changes in transcript levels were not equally affected (Elferink et al., 2004). Overall this suggests that inflammation and proinflammatory cytokines play an important role in the transcriptional and posttranslational regulation of BSEP.

Solute Carrier Uptake Transporting Family

Another group of transporters that are involved in determining the fate of drug disposition are the Solute Carrier Superfamily. Widely expressed throughout various tissues, this group of transporters is responsible for the uptake of a diverse range of organic, inorganic, charged, and uncharged molecules across epithelial membranes (Hediger et al., 2004). Unlike the ABC superfamily of transporters, SLC proteins do not function by active transport, but are classified as facilitative or secondary active transporters. As many great reviews have been published on the topic of SLC transporters (Hediger et al., 2004; Hagenbuch and Meier, 2003, 2004; Koepsell, 1998; Kusuhara and Sugiyama, 2005; Meier et al., 2007), we will limit our discussion to specific groups within the family relevant to, and involved in, drug transfer across physiological membranes. These include specific members of the organic anion transporting polypeptides (OATP/SLCO), organic anion transporters (OATs/SLC22A), organic cation transporters (OCTs/SLC22A), and organic cation/carnitine transporters (OCTN/SLC22A4). It is important to note that many compounds are substrates of both the SLC uptake and ABC efflux transporters, suggesting vectorial transport across membranes (Liu and Liu, 2016). The following is a brief description of the key drug transporters in this family; their expression, classification, localization, and function have been the focus of many review articles and much of this information can be found on the UCSF-FDA transportal website (http://dbts.ucsf.edu/fdatransportal).

The OATP group of transporters includes 11 identified human genes. This group has a wide range of tissue distribution at the apical and basolateral membranes of the liver, kidney, intestine, brain, testis, and placenta, and functions mainly to facilitate the transfer of organic anions across the cell membrane. Although this holds true, OATP family members transport neutral as well as cationic substances, and numerous endogenous substrates including bile acids, bilirubin, and hormones (Hagenbuch and Meier, 2004). Substrate specificity within the OATP group is variable, as some are highly selective, and some participate in the uptake and clearance of a broad range of endogenous and therapeutic agents. These substrates include statins, antihypertensive agents, anticancers, antibiotics, antidiabetics, as well as glucuronidated and sulfated compounds.

The OATs and OCTs participate in the transfer of endogenous and exogenous substrates of anionic or cationic nature across biological membranes. They belong to a group within the SLC22A family of transporters and are primarily expressed in the liver, kidney, brain, and placenta. The OATs and OCTs play an important role in the excretion of toxins into bile and renal drug elimination, thereby contributing to drug clearance. Clinically relevant members include OAT1–4 and OCT1–3, which transport a range of anionic and cationic drug substrates, which include a number of neurotransmitter, antidiabetic, antiviral, and anticancer agents (Nies et al., 2011; Roth et al., 2012).

LIVER

Inflammation-induced changes in the expression and function of SLC uptake transporters have been documented in various models of acute inflammation in vitro and in vivo. It is well known and accepted that administration of endotoxin and proinflammatory cytokines is associated with decreases in hepatic SLC transporters Ntcp, Oatp1B1, Oatp1B3, Oatp2B1, and some of the Oats and Octs localized to the sinusoidal membrane (Le Vee et al., 2008, 2011b; Siewert et al., 2004). Primary human hepatocytes treated with IL-1β have been shown to impose a substantial decrease in mRNA levels of Oatp1b1, whereas treatments with IL-6 or TNF-α cause dose-dependent reductions in Oatp2b1, Oatp1b1, Oatp1b3, Oct1, and Oat2 mRNA levels (Le Vee et al., 2008, 2009). These effects are also paralleled in rodents, where mouse and rat mRNA expressions of Oatp1a1, Oatp1a4, and Oatp1b2 are decreased after LPS administration or *C. rodentium* infection (Cherrington et al., 2004; Merrell et al., 2014; Geier et al., 2003; Li, 2004). Furthermore, endotoxin treatments have been found to reduce the mRNA expression of Oat2 in mice and Oat3 and Oct1 in rats, with concurrent inductions of proinflammatory cytokines (Cherrington et al., 2004; Lickteig et al., 2007). Interestingly, pretreatment with the steroidal antiinflammatory agent dexamethasone attenuates the effect of endotoxin on these transporters thereby confirming that inflammation or cytokine-mediated pathways are involved in the regulation of these transporters (Cherrington et al., 2004).

KIDNEY

Limited information exists on the expression profiles of SLC transporters during acute inflammation in the kidney. In vivo administration of LPS has been shown to decrease the gene and protein expression of OAT1 and OAT3 in rats, in a dose-dependent manner (Höcherl et al., 2009). Similar downregulation of OAT1 and OAT3 has been observed in various rat models of acute kidney injury, and this was associated with an impaired renal secretion of *para*-aminohippurate and fexofenadine, which are substrates of these transporters (Matsuzaki et al., 2008; Erman et al., 2014; Schneider et al., 2007). Decreases in renal OCT1 and OCT2 expression, along with decreased creatinine clearance, were also observed in this model (Matsuzaki et al., 2008; Erman et al., 2014).

PLACENTA

The placenta expresses numerous transporters within the trophoblast membrane, including several members of the SLC family, where Oatp2b1 and Oatp4a1 are two of the most highly expressed in humans (Nishimura and Naito, 2005). Administration of poly I:C to pregnant rats resulted in a downregulation of placental Oatp1a4, and Oatp4a1 transcript levels as compared with control pregnant animals (Petrovic and Piquette-Miller, 2010). Likewise, mRNA expression of Oatp1a4, Oatp2b1, and Oatp4a1 were reduced in the placentas of endotoxin-treated rats (Petrovic et al., 2008). Similar regulatory mechanisms may occur in humans as significant decreases in OATP2B1 mRNA and protein expression were found in preterm placental tissues taken from women with chorioamnionitis (Nishimura and Naito, 2005). On the other hand, the mRNA and protein expression of OATP4A1 was not significantly altered in the human placentas.

CHRONIC INFLAMMATION

Chronic inflammation arises from unresolved sources of foreign bodies, irritants, infections, or autoimmune disorders. This type of inflammation can be described as unregulated and can last for months or years causing tissue destruction, fibrosis, and necrosis. Some prominent characteristics are the continued release of proinflammatory cytokines by activated macrophages and retention of cytokines at the site of inflammation. This allows for the continuous presence of tissue repair and injury in tandem, perpetuating the inflammatory response. Another important component of chronic inflammation is the presence of interferon. Due to its signaling capabilities, it stimulates continuous monocyte recruitment and thereby plays a role in sustaining the inflammatory response (Lee et al., 2009).

Chronic inflammation is a component of many prevalent diseases, including persistent viral infections, chronic renal failure (CRF), RA, inflammatory bowel disease (IBD), cholestasis, metabolic disorders, and cancer. Research examining the effects of chronic diseases on drug transporters is still relatively in its infancy and much remains unknown. Knowledge in this area will undoubtedly provide critical information, which will enable us to predict the pharmacokinetics and pharmacodynamics of drugs during chronic inflammatory disorders. Many of these disorders have been discussed in other chapters; therefore we will only highlight a few of these conditions.

IMPACT OF CHRONIC INFLAMMATION ON DRUG TRANSPORTERS

Rheumatoid Arthritis

RA is a chronic inflammatory autoimmune disorder that is characterized by joint inflammation and swelling. Due to the aging population, there is rising prevalence in North America (Lawrence et al., 2008; Helmick et al., 2008; Sacks et al., 2010; Smolen and Steiner, 2003). Although the underlying cause of RA remains unknown, it is believed that the immune and inflammatory systems work together in targeting synovial joints thereby destructing cartilage and bone. This leads to a persisting localized inflammatory response mediated by an overproduction and prolonged presence of proinflammatory cytokines, TNF-α, IL-6, and IL-1β (Smolen and Steiner, 2003; Choy and Panayi, 2001). RA is a progressive disease, leading to a loss of function of affected joints and ultimately decreasing the quality of life for individuals suffering from the illness. RA is also associated with cardiovascular and systemic inflammatory complications that pose additional challenges for this population of patients through systemic inflammation leading to negative cardiovascular health outcomes. Although the onset of disease is unclear, infectious agents have been linked with RA as the immune complexes form, inducing autoantibodies (Choy and Panayi, 2001). The current standard of care for RA includes the use of nonsteroidal antiinflammatory drugs, corticosteroids, and biologic inhibitors of TNF-α (Jessica Burch and Mary Onysko, 2012). Methotrexate, a disease-modifying antirheumatic drug, is most commonly prescribed in RA, and interestingly, is a substrate for both ABC and SLC transporters (Takeda et al., 2002).

Adjuvant arthritis (AA), induced by Freund complete adjuvant, is a frequently used and well-characterized model of RA (Wang et al., 2005; Wahba et al., 2015; Hung et al., 2006). Significant alterations in the disposition and clearance of various drugs including propranolol (Piquette-Miller and Jamali, 1993), acebutolol (Piquette-Miller and Jamali, 1992), and pentobarbital (Dipasquale et al., 1974) have been reported in AA rats. Changes in the pharmacokinetics of these drugs have long been attributed to decreases in the expression of phase I and phase II drug-metabolizing enzymes, and altered plasma drug-binding proteins, which are seen in the AA treatment groups (Kawase et al., 2013; Meunier and Verbeeck, 1999; Ferrari et al., 1993; Whitehouse and Beck, 1973; Ling and Jamali, 2005; Sanada et al., 2011). However, as many drugs are also substrates for transporters, inflammation-mediated changes in drug transporters may contribute to the changes seen in the disposition of therapeutic agents.

Research has shown significant decreases in hepatic *Abcb1a* and *Abcb1b* mRNA levels in AA rats compared with controls, with corresponding decreases in immunodetectable levels of P-gp (Kawase et al., 2014; Uno et al., 2009; Achira et al., 2002a). AA imposed a similar downregulation of *Abcc1*, *Abcc2*, and *Abcg2* mRNA along with significantly increased levels of IL-1β and IL-6 (Kawase et al., 2014; Hanafy et al., 2012). Furthermore, pharmacokinetic studies have shown a significant reduction in the biliary clearance of doxorubicin (Achira et al., 2002a,b) and rhodamine 123 (Kawase et al., 2014) in AA rats compared with healthy animals. Likewise, the hepatic mRNA levels of many SLC transporters including *Oct1*, *Oatp1a1*, *Oatp1b2*, *Oatp1a4*, *Oatp1a5*, *Oatp4a1*, and *Oatp2b1* are decreased in AA (Uno et al., 2009; Hanafy et al., 2012). Conversely, ABC drug transporters in the small intestine showed significant decreases in mRNA levels of *Abcb1a*, *Abcc2*, *Abcc3*, and *Abcg2*, 7 days after adjuvant administration, with a reversion to control levels at 21 days (Uno et al., 2009). Contrary to liver and intestine, *Abcb1a* and *Abcc2* mRNA and protein expressions are increased in the kidneys of AA rats, whereas decreases in the renal mRNA expression of *Abcc6*, *Abcc11*, and *Oatp2b1* have been reported (Kawase et al., 2014; Hanafy et al., 2012). Many of the same trends have been observed in murine collagen models of arthritis, with decreases in hepatic *Abcb1a*, *Abcb1b*, *Abcc3*, and *Abcg2* mRNA levels in animals with arthritis (Kawase et al., 2008). Furthermore, similar to AA, collagen-induced arthritis in mice resulted in a significant downregulation of hepatic *Oatp1b1* at the gene and protein levels, resulting in a decreased elimination of bilirubin after intravenous administration (Kawase et al., 2007).

Although experimental methods of arthritis are primarily done in rodents, it is important to note that the disease is examined over a 21-day period in these models, and thus it is possible that it may not fully represent the persistent, chronic inflammatory state and physiological changes seen in human RA. Although this holds true, it has been observed that patients with RA showed increases in verapamil serum concentrations, alongside significantly elevated IL-6 cytokine levels compared with healthy controls (Mayo et al., 2000). Interestingly, verapamil is a known P-gp and cytochrome P450 (CYP450) substrate (Pauli-Magnus et al., 2000), and thus inflammation-mediated reductions of these proteins together may contribute to the increase in serum drug concentrations. These findings may lead us to believe that results from rodent models of AA may be paralleled in human subjects.

Inflammatory Bowel Disease

IBD is characterized by chronic inflammation of the gastrointestinal (GI) tract and is predominantly manifested as ulcerative colitis (UC) and CD. These two conditions together affect more than 5 million people worldwide, with the highest incidence in Northern Europe and the United States (Burisch and Munkholm, 2015; Molodecky et al., 2012). CD can impact any site within the GI tract; however, it is predominantly localized to the terminal ileum, whereas UC is primarily found to affect the colon and rectum (Xavier and Podolsky, 2007). IBD can arise by several means including genetic factors, environmental causes, bacterial origins, and physical damage of the intestinal barrier (Korolkova et al., 2015). A predominant characteristic of IBD is the enhanced presence of immunoregulatory stimuli including cytokines, chemokines, and growth factors. These molecules all contribute to the pathophysiology of the disease and can be found locally in the tissues and systemically in blood. Research has shown increases in serum proinflammatory cytokines, IL-6, IL-8, TNF-α, and INF-γ in patients with UC and CD compared with healthy controls (Korolkova et al., 2015). Furthermore, mucosal biopsies also revealed increased TNF-α, IL-6, and Il-1β levels from inflamed tissues of sick patients compared with healthy individuals (Raddatz et al., 2005). Currently, there are a number of options for treatment of IBD, including intestinal surgery and medications such as antiinflammatory steroids, TNF-α inhibitors, immunosuppressants, and aminosalicylates.

Despite the growing prevalence of IBD and its impact on life quality, very little is known about how this disease impacts the pharmacokinetics and response to drugs. It is known that several transporters are highly expressed throughout the intestines and play a role in drug absorption. Furthermore, transporter proteins within the intestines, along with other proteins, such as tight junctions, are directly responsible in maintaining the barrier function and the selective permeability of the intestinal membrane. Thus a number of studies have looked into the impact of IBD on transporter regulation. The ABC efflux transporters BCRP, P-gp, and MRP2 are found within the intestines in varying proportions throughout the duodenum, jejunum, ileum, and colon (Englund et al., 2006; Oswald et al., 2013). Together these transporters interact with a wide range of substrates including endogenous substances, exogenous xenobiotics, toxins, and food elements. The significance of these transporters has been shown in multiple studies using knockout (KO) mouse models where ablation of P-gp and Bcrp dramatically increased the intestinal permeability of their substrates (Stephens et al., 2002a,b; van Herwaarden et al., 2003, 2006; Vlaming et al., 2014).

There are numerous animal models that exist for studying the effects of IBD in both rats and mice; however, the dextran sulfate sodium (DSS) model is the most commonly employed as it is time- and cost-effective, and most rodent strains are susceptible (Mizoguchi, 2012). KO rodent models are also employed to study IBD, including, but not limited to, the regulatory cytokines IL-10 KO, IL-2 KO, and IL-7 KO. Studies conducted in DSS-treated mice have shown decreased P-gp protein levels and corresponding decreases in functional transport of rhodamine 123 in four different segments of the intestines. A further downregulation of

P-gp was also observed in DSS-treated IL-10 KO mice as compared with wild type (Buyse et al., 2005). Likewise, studies have demonstrated decreased *Abcb1a* mRNA levels in the intestines of mice after DSS administration, with corresponding decreases in P-gp activity (Langmann et al., 2004; Kawauchi et al., 2014). Varying results are seen with respect to DSS-induced transporter changes in the liver. In one study, DSS did not significantly alter the expression of a wide range of hepatic ABC and SLC transporters (Jahnel et al., 2009), whereas Kawauchi et al. (2014) reported that hepatic mRNA levels of *Abcb1a*, *Abcb11*, and *Abcc2* were significantly decreased in a time-dependent manner from 3 to 7 days post-DSS administration (Kawauchi et al., 2014). A significant reduction in the hepatic protein expression of P-gp was also seen in the DSS-treated rats. As serum cytokine levels were not measured in the first study, differences in DDS doses and systemic inflammatory responses may be responsible for these discrepancies. Of note, acute infection with *C. rodentium*, a model of infectious colitis was found to alter the expression of numerous ABC and SLC transporters in liver (Merrell et al., 2014). Interestingly, *Mdr1a* KO mice have also been utilized as an experimental model of UC, as these animals naturally develop intestinal inflammation histologically similar to IBD, unless maintained in a germ-free environment (Staley et al., 2011; Nones et al., 2009; Panwala et al., 1998). Speculation on the causes of this spontaneous onset of localized inflammation includes poor protective function of the epithelium and a buildup of bacterial by-products and dietary toxins. Indeed, P-gp expression has been associated with regulating interactions with commensal microflora of the gut (Collett et al., 2008). Although it is inappropriate to suggest that the lack of P-gp alone is responsible for the onset of disease, authors suggest that it is rather part of a complex mechanism regulating the intestinal environment (Panwala et al., 1998).

These results seen in rodents correspond to the clinical setting where intestinal tissue samples from patients with active IBD were found to have dramatically reduced mRNA and protein expression of P-gp and BCRP along with increased mRNA expression of IL-6 and IL-1β as compared with healthy control subjects (Englund et al., 2007; Gutmann et al., 2008; Ufer et al., 2009). Cytokine level increases in gut mucosa have also been measured in patients with active intestinal inflammation due to IBD, with most pronounced differences seen in IL-6 mRNA levels, deeming it a suitable marker for intestinal inflammation (Raddatz et al., 2005). In contrast to what is seen with P-gp and BCRP, MRP1 mRNA and protein levels were significantly upregulated in the intestines of patients with CD and UC (Blokzijl et al., 2008). It is plausible that MRP1 induction may serve as a compensatory mechanism for protection against harmful pathogens and xenobiotics when other key transporters are compromised.

Much less information exists on the expression profiles of SLC transporters in the intestines of patients with IBD. However, it has been shown that transcript levels of SLC transporters, OATP2B1, OATP4A1, OCTN1, and OCTN2 among others are dysregulated in patients with IBD at the terminal ileum and colon as compared with healthy control subjects (Wojtal et al., 2009). These increases were modulated by the degree of inflammation and more pronounced in the patients suffering from UC than in those with CD. As there is a clear dysregulation of intestinal transporters in animal models of IBD as well as in patients in the clinic, it is reasonable to assume that these changes may impact the transfer of various ABC and SLC substrates across the intestinal epithelium affecting proper drug therapy through absorption, clearance, and distribution of therapeutic agents.

Chronic Renal Failure

CRF is a progressive disease that is characterized by the gradual loss of kidney function ultimately leading to patients requiring dialysis and kidney transplant. The kidneys are an essential organ playing a role in the detoxification of blood from endogenous metabolites and xenobiotics, and also the regulation of electrolytes, and blood pressure. Numerous in vivo studies in rodent models of CRF have demonstrated that CRF affects drug metabolism and clearance due to a reduction in expression and activity of hepatic, intestinal, and renal transporters, as well as alterations in the expression and function of key enzymatic systems in these organs, primarily the CYP450 family (Naud et al., 2008, 2011; Nolin et al., 2008; Pichette and Leblond, 2003; Leblond et al., 2002; Guévin et al., 2002; Sun et al., 2006). This area of research has been extensively reviewed in this book, so only a brief discussion of transporter changes is included in this chapter and readers are directed to Chapter 7 for more information.

It has been shown that the expressions of P-gp mRNA and protein are induced in the livers of rat models with induced CRF with corresponding increases in biliary excretion of rhodamine 123 (Naud et al., 2008). Likewise, CRF imposes an increase in the hepatic expression of Mrp2 and Mrp3 but not BSEP (Naud et al., 2008; Laouari et al., 2001; Gai et al., 2014). In contrast to what is seen in liver, immunodetectable levels of P-gp, Mrp2, and Mrp3 are significantly decreased in the intestine of CRF rats (Naud et al., 2007). Similarly, significant decreases (30—50%) in protein and mRNA levels of Bcrp, Mrp2, Mrp3, Mrp4, Oat3, Oatp2, Oatp3, and P-gp were demonstrated in CRF rat brain biopsies, as well as in astrocytes and brain endothelial cells incubated with CRF serum (Naud et al., 2012). These results did not fully correlate with in vivo studies; the permeability of benzylpenicillin, a substrate of OAT3, decreased in line with expression changes, whereas the permeability of a number of P-gp substrates remained unchanged.

Knowledge is currently evolving on the regulation of transporters within the kidney. Significant reductions in the expression of P-gp, Oat1, Oat2, Oat3, Oct2, and Oatp1 are seen in the kidneys of CRF rats, whereas renal mRNA and protein expressions of Mrp2, Mrp3, Mrp4, Oatp2, and Oatp3 are increased (Naud et al., 2011; Laouari et al., 2001; Ji et al., 2002). Furthermore, in vivo transport studies have shown a ninefold greater accumulation of [^{14}C]benzylpenicillin and a fourfold accumulation of [^{3}H]digoxin in the kidney of CRF rats, indicating impaired renal secretion due to the disease (Naud et al., 2011). In vitro studies in the human kidney-2 cell line have also shown reductions in the protein expression of P-gp, Oatp1, Oatp2, and Oat3 and increases in the protein expression of Mrp2, MRp4, and Oatp2 when cells were incubated with uremic serum. To date only in vitro or animal studies examining the impact of CRF on transporters have been performed. As it is clear that CRF potentially impacts the pharmacokinetics and pharmacodynamics of drugs through the modification of drug transporters, clinical studies are warranted. As such it is important to consider these alterations in drug therapy and dosing for this population of patients and those receiving hemodialysis.

Cholestasis

Biliary cholestasis is a condition consisting of impaired bile flow from the liver to the intestines. This can manifest due to an obstruction, causing physical blockage, or through genetic impairment resulting in improper bile formation. Several ABC transporter proteins are essential for hepatocellular bile excretion at the canalicular membrane, where genetic or acquired defects of these transporters can result in cholestatic liver disorders (Jansen et al., 2001; Jansen and Müller, 2000; Cuperus et al., 2014). Furthermore, improper function or expression of the transporters leads to decreased bile flow and increased bile toxicity due to the hepatocellular accumulation of endogenous and exogenous toxins, eventually leading to a reduction of liver function (Cuperus et al., 2014). The transporters identified as playing a crucial role in the excretion of bile are BSEP, NTCP, MRP2, MRP3, and MDR3 (Trauner and Boyer, 2003; Cuperus et al., 2014). The effects of cholestasis have been extensively reviewed, and many excellent articles have been published on the topic by Kosters and Karpen (2010), Geier et al. (2007), and Klaassen and Aleksunes (2010b).

As we have stated throughout this chapter, inflammation has the potential to decrease the expression of numerous ABC and SLC transporters in the liver as well as in other organs and tissues. It is interesting to note that in the situation of cholestasis, the decrease in transporter expression leads to a pathological condition, and loss of function. Studies conducted in rodent models of inflammatory cholestasis have indeed observed decreases in the expression and function of Bsep, Ntcp, Mrp2, Mrp6, Oatp1, Oatp2, Oatp4, Oct1, and Oat3 (Cherrington et al., 2004; Geier et al., 2003; Kim et al., 2000; Trauner et al., 1998; Gartung et al., 1996). In patients with cholestasis, liver biopsies indicated dramatic reductions of BSEP, NTCP, OATP1B1, OATP1B3, OATP2, and MRP2 levels compared with control livers (Keitel et al., 2005; Zollner et al., 2001). It is important to note that reduced biliary excretion and cholestasis have consistently shown an induction of Mrp3 and Mrp4 (Zollner et al., 2003, 2006; Wagner et al., 2003; Schuetz et al., 2001). It is possible that these changes represent an adaptive mechanism in response to decreased bile flow, to limit the accumulation toxic compounds in hepatocytes.

CONCLUSION

The collection of studies reviewed in this chapter demonstrates that inflammation and inflammatory mediators are key regulators of many transporters that play diverse roles in xeno- and endobiotic transport. Moreover, inflammation impacts their expression in a number of critical epithelial membrane barriers. Many acute and chronic diseases are associated with an inflammatory component, so the diversity and extent of the population potentially affected are vast. As transporters are becoming increasingly recognized as major players in the determination of drug absorption, distribution, and excretion, knowledge on the regulation of transporters in acute and chronic inflammatory disease gives us a better understanding of the mechanisms governing drug disposition and variation in drug response. As such, more studies investigating the impact of inflammation on drug disposition, pharmacokinetics and pharmacodynamics are required to establish a clear understanding of drug–disease interactions.

References

Achira, M., Totsuka, R., Fujimura, H., Kume, T., 2002a. Tissue-specific regulation of expression and activity of P-glycoprotein in adjuvant arthritis rats. Eur. J. Pharm. Sci. 16, 29–36.

Achira, M., Totsuka, R., Kume, T., 2002b. Decreased activity of hepatic P-glycoprotein in the isolated perfused liver of the adjuvant arthritis rat. Xenobiotica 32, 963–973. http://dx.doi.org/10.1080/0049825021000012664.

Ando, H., Nishio, Y., Ito, K., Nakao, A., Wang, L., Zhao, Y.L., et al., 2001. Effect of endotoxin on P-glycoprotein-mediated biliary and renal excretion of rhodamine-123 in rats. Antimicrob. Agents Chemother. 45, 3462–3467. http://dx.doi.org/10.1128/AAC.45.12.3462-3467.2001.

Ashraf, T., Jiang, W., Hoque, M.T., Henderson, J., Wu, C., Bendayan, R., 2014. Role of anti-inflammatory compounds in human immunodeficiency virus-1 glycoprotein120-mediated brain inflammation. J. Neuroinflammation 11, 91. http://dx.doi.org/10.1186/1742-2094-11-91.

Belliard, A.-M., Tardivel, S., Farinotti, R., Lacour, B., Leroy, C., 2002. Effect of hr-IL2 treatment on intestinal P-glycoprotein expression and activity in Caco-2 cells. J. Pharm. Pharmacol. 54, 1103–1109. http://dx.doi.org/10.1211/002235702320266262.

Belliard, A.-M., Lacour, B., Farinotti, R., Leroy, C., 2004. Effect of tumor necrosis factor-alpha and interferon-gamma on intestinal P-glycoprotein expression, activity, and localization in Caco-2 cells. J. Pharm. Sci. 93, 1524–1536. http://dx.doi.org/10.1002/jps.20072.

Belpaire, F.M., Smet, F., Chindavijak, B., Fraeyman, N., Bogaert, M.G., 1989. Effect of turpentine-induced inflammation on the disposition kinetics of propranolol, metoprolol, and antipyrine in the rat. Fundam. Clin. Pharmacol. 3, 79–88. http://dx.doi.org/10.1111/j.1472-8206.1989.tb00667.x.

Berengue, J.I., López-Espinosa, J.A., Ortega-López, J., Sánchez-Sánchez, L., Castilla-Valdes, P., Asensio-Llorente, M., et al., 2003. Two- to three-fold increase in blood tacrolimus (FK506) levels during diarrhea in liver-transplanted children. Clin. Transplant. 17, 249–253.

Bertilsson, P.M., Olsson, P., Magnusson, K.E., 2001. Cytokines influence mRNA expression of cytochrome P450 3A4 and MDRI in intestinal cells. J. Pharm. Sci. 90, 638–646.

Bloise, E., Bhuiyan, M., Audette, M.C., Petropoulos, S., Javam, M., Gibb, W., et al., 2013. Prenatal endotoxemia and placental drug transport in the mouse: placental size-specific effects. PLoS ONE 8, e65728. http://dx.doi.org/10.1371/journal.pone.0065728.

Blokzijl, H., Vander Borght, S., Bok, L.I.H., Libbrecht, L., Geuken, M., van den Heuvel, F.A.J., et al., 2007. Decreased P-glycoprotein (P-gp/MDR1) expression in inflamed human intestinal epithelium is independent of PXR protein levels. Inflamm. Bowel Dis. 13, 710–720. http://dx.doi.org/10.1002/ibd.20088.

Blokzijl, H., van Steenpaal, A., Vander Borght, S., Bok, L.I.H., Libbrecht, L., Tamminga, M., et al., 2008. Up-regulation and cytoprotective role of epithelial multidrug resistance-associated protein 1 in inflammatory bowel disease. J. Biol. Chem. 283, 35630–35637. http://dx.doi.org/10.1074/jbc.M804374200.

Bonhomme-Faivre, L., Pelloquin, A., Tardivel, S., Urien, S., Mathieu, M.-C., Castagne, V., et al., 2002. Recombinant interleukin-2 treatment decreases P-glycoprotein activity and paclitaxel metabolism in mice. Anticancer Drugs 13, 51–57.

Borst, P., Evers, R., Kool, M., Wijnholds, J., 2000. A family of drug transporters: the multidrug resistance-associated proteins. J. Natl. Cancer Inst. 92, 1295–1302. http://dx.doi.org/10.1093/jnci/92.16.1295.

Brcakova, E., Fuksa, L., Cermanova, J., Kolouchova, G., Hroch, M., Hirsova, P., et al., 2009. Alteration of methotrexate biliary and renal elimination during extrahepatic and intrahepatic cholestasis in rats. Biol. Pharm. Bull. 32, 1978–1985.

Brechot, J.-M., Hurbain, I., Fajac, A., Daty, N., Bernaudin, J.-F., 1998. Different pattern of MRP localization in ciliated and basal cells from human bronchial epithelium. J. Histochem. Cytochem. 46, 513–517. http://dx.doi.org/10.1177/002215549804600411.

Burisch, J., Munkholm, P., 2015. The epidemiology of inflammatory bowel disease. Scand. J. Gastroenterol. 50, 942–951. http://dx.doi.org/10.3109/00365521.2015.1014407.

Buyse, M., Radeva, G., Bado, A., Farinotti, R., 2005. Intestinal inflammation induces adaptation of P-glycoprotein expression and activity. Biochem. Pharmacol. 69, 1745–1754. http://dx.doi.org/10.1016/j.bcp.2005.03.025.

Castagne, V., Bonhomme-Faivre, L., Urien, S., Ben Reguiga, M., Soursac, M., Gimenez, F., et al., 2004. Effect of recombinant interleukin-2 pretreatment on oral and intravenous digoxin pharmacokinetics and P-glycoprotein activity in mice. Drug Metab. Dispos. 32, 168–171. http://dx.doi.org/10.1124/dmd.32.2.168.

Cherrington, N.J., Slitt, A.L., Li, N., Klaassen, C.D., 2004. Lipopolysaccharide-mediated regulation of hepatic transporter mRNA levels in rats. Drug Metab. Dispos. 32, 734–741.

Cherrington, N.J., 2002. Organ distribution of multidrug resistance proteins 1, 2, and 3 (Mrp1, 2, and 3) mRNA and hepatic induction of Mrp3 by constitutive androstane receptor activators in rats. J. Pharmacol. Exp. Ther. 300, 97–104. http://dx.doi.org/10.1124/jpet.300.1.97.

Choy, E.H., Panayi, G.S., 2001. Cytokine pathways and joint inflammation in rheumatoid arthritis. N. Engl. J. Med. 344, 907–916. http://dx.doi.org/10.1056/NEJM200103223441207.

Collett, A., Higgs, N.B., Gironella, M., Zeef, L.A.H., Hayes, A., Salmo, E., et al., 2008. Early molecular and functional changes in colonic epithelium that precede increased gut permeability during colitis development in mdr1a(−/−) mice. Inflamm. Bowel Dis. 14, 620–631. http://dx.doi.org/10.1002/ibd.20375.

Copeland, S., Warren, H.S., Lowry, S.F., Calvano, S.E., Remick, D., 2005. Acute inflammatory response to endotoxin in mice and humans. Clin. Diagn. Lab. Immunol. 12, 60–67. http://dx.doi.org/10.1128/CDLI.12.1.60-67.2005.

Cray, C., Zaias, J., Altman, N.H., 2009. Acute phase response in animals: a review. Comp. Med. 59, 517–526.

Cressman, A.M., McDonald, C.R., Silver, K., Kain, K.C., Piquette-Miller, M., 2014. Malaria infection alters the expression of hepatobiliary and placental drug transporters in pregnant mice. Drug Metab. Dispos. 42, 603–610. http://dx.doi.org/10.1124/dmd.113.053983.

Cuperus, F.J.C., Claudel, T., Gautherot, J., Halilbasic, E., Trauner, M., 2014. The role of canalicular ABC transporters in cholestasis. Drug Metab. Dispos. 42, 546–560. http://dx.doi.org/10.1124/dmd.113.056358.

Dazert, P., Meissner, K., Vogelgesang, S., Heydrich, B., Eckel, L., Böhm, M., et al., 2003. Expression and localization of the multidrug resistance protein 5 (MRP5/ABCC5), a cellular export pump for cyclic nucleotides, in human heart. Am. J. Pathol. 163, 1567–1577. http://dx.doi.org/10.1016/S0002-9440(10)63513-4.

Diao, L., Li, N., Brayman, T.G., Hotz, K.J., Lai, Y., 2010. Regulation of MRP2/ABCC2 and BSEP/ABCB11 expression in sandwich cultured human and rat hepatocytes exposed to inflammatory cytokines TNF-{alpha}, IL-6, and IL-1 {beta}. J. Biol. Chem. 285, 31185–31192. http://dx.doi.org/10.1074/jbc.M110.107805.

Dipasquale, G., Welaj, P., Rassaert, C.L., 1974. Prolonged pentobarbital sleeping time in adjuvant-induced polyarthritic rats. Res. Commun. Chem. Pathol. Pharmacol. 9, 253–264.

Donner, M.G., Keppler, D., 2001. Up-regulation of basolateral multidrug resistance protein 3 (Mrp3) in cholestatic rat liver. Hepatology 34, 351–359. http://dx.doi.org/10.1053/jhep.2001.26213.

Donner, M.G., Warskulat, U., Saha, N., Häussinger, D., 2004. Enhanced expression of basolateral multidrug resistance protein isoforms Mrp3 and Mrp5 in rat liver by LPS. Biol. Chem. 385, 331–339. http://dx.doi.org/10.1515/BC.2004.029.

Elferink, M.G.L., Olinga, P., Draaisma, A.L., Merema, M.T., Faber, K.N., Slooff, M.J.H., et al., 2004. LPS-induced downregulation of MRP2 and BSEP in human liver is due to a posttranscriptional process. Am. J. Physiol. Gastrointest. Liver Physiol. 287, G1008–G1016. http://dx.doi.org/10.1152/ajpgi.00071.2004.

Englund, G., Rorsman, F., Rönnblom, A., Karlbom, U., Lazorova, L., Gråsjö, J., et al., 2006. Regional levels of drug transporters along the human intestinal tract: co-expression of ABC and SLC transporters and comparison with Caco-2 cells. Eur. J. Pharm. Sci. 29, 269–277. http://dx.doi.org/10.1016/j.ejps.2006.04.010.

Englund, G., Jacobson, A., Rorsman, F., Artursson, P., Kindmark, A., Rönnblom, A., 2007. Efflux transporters in ulcerative colitis: decreased expression of BCRP (ABCG2) and P-gp (ABCB1). Inflamm. Bowel Dis. 13, 291–297. http://dx.doi.org/10.1002/ibd.20030.

Erman, F., Tuzcu, M., Orhan, C., Sahin, N., Sahin, K., 2014. Effect of lycopene against cisplatin-induced acute renal injury in rats: organic anion and cation transporters evaluation. Biol. Trace Elem. Res. 158, 90–95. http://dx.doi.org/10.1007/s12011-014-9914-x.

Evseenko, D.A., Paxton, J.W., Keelan, J.A., 2007. Independent regulation of apical and basolateral drug transporter expression and function in placental trophoblasts by cytokines, steroids, and growth factors. Drug Metab. Dispos. 35, 595–601. http://dx.doi.org/10.1124/dmd.106.011478.

Fardel, O., Le Vée, M., 2009. Regulation of human hepatic drug transporter expression by pro-inflammatory cytokines. Expert Opin. Drug Metab. Toxicol. 5, 1469–1481. http://dx.doi.org/10.1517/17425250903304056.

Feghali, C.A., Wright, T.M., 1997. Cytokines in acute and chronic inflammation. Front Biosci. 2, d12–26.

Ferrari, L., Jouzeau, J.Y., Gillet, P., Herber, R., Fener, P., Batt, A.M., et al., 1993. Interleukin-1 beta differentially represses drug-metabolizing enzymes in arthritic female rats. J. Pharmacol. Exp. Ther. 264, 1012–1020.

Fortier, M.-E., Kent, S., Ashdown, H., Poole, S., Boksa, P., Luheshi, G.N., 2004. The viral mimic, polyinosinic:polycytidylic acid, induces fever in rats via an interleukin-1-dependent mechanism. Am. J. Physiol. Regul. Integr. Comp. Physiol. 287, R759–R766. http://dx.doi.org/10.1152/ajpregu.00293.2004.

Gabay, C., Kushner, I., 1999. Acute-phase proteins and other systemic responses to inflammation. N. Engl. J. Med. 340, 448–454. http://dx.doi.org/10.1056/NEJM199902113400607.

Gai, Z., Chu, L., Hiller, C., Arsenijevic, D., Penno, C.A., Montani, J.-P., et al., 2014. Effect of chronic renal failure on the hepatic, intestinal, and renal expression of bile acid transporters. Am. J. Physiol. Ren. Physiol. 306, F130–F137. http://dx.doi.org/10.1152/ajprenal.00114.2013.

Gandhi, R., Hayley, S., Gibb, J., Merali, Z., Anisman, H., 2007. Influence of poly I:C on sickness behaviors, plasma cytokines, corticosterone and central monoamine activity: moderation by social stressors. Brain Behav. Immun. 21, 477–489. http://dx.doi.org/10.1016/j.bbi.2006.12.005.

Gartung, C., Ananthanarayanan, M., Rahman, M.A., Schuele, S., Nundy, S., Soroka, C.J., et al., 1996. Down-regulation of expression and function of the rat liver Na^+/bile acid cotransporter in extrahepatic cholestasis. Gastroenterology 110, 199–209.

Geier, A., Dietrich, C.G., Voigt, S., Kim, S.-K., Gerloff, T., Kullak-Ublick, G.a, et al., 2003. Effects of proinflammatory cytokines on rat organic anion transporters during toxic liver injury and cholestasis. Hepatology 38, 345–354. http://dx.doi.org/10.1053/jhep.2003.50317.

Geier, A., Wagner, M., Dietrich, C.G., Trauner, M., 2007. Principles of hepatic organic anion transporter regulation during cholestasis, inflammation and liver regeneration. Biochim. Biophys. Acta 1773, 283–308. http://dx.doi.org/10.1016/j.bbamcr.2006.04.014.

Gibson, C.J., Hossain, M.M., Richardson, J.R., Aleksunes, L.M., 2012. Inflammatory regulation of ATP binding cassette efflux transporter expression and function in microglia. J. Pharmacol. Exp. Ther. 343, 650–660. http://dx.doi.org/10.1124/jpet.112.196543.

Goralski, K.B., Hartmann, G., Piquette-Miller, M., Renton, K.W., 2003. Downregulation of mdr1a expression in the brain and liver during CNS inflammation alters the in vivo disposition of digoxin. Br. J. Pharmacol. 139, 35–48. http://dx.doi.org/10.1038/sj.bjp.0705227.

Gruys, E., Toussaint, M.J.M., Niewold, T.A., Koopmans, S.J., 2005. Acute phase reaction and acute phase proteins. J. Zhejiang Univ. Sci. B 6, 1045–1056. http://dx.doi.org/10.1631/jzus.2005.B1045.

Guévin, C., Michaud, J., Naud, J., Leblond, F.A., Pichette, V., 2002. Down-regulation of hepatic cytochrome p450 in chronic renal failure: role of uremic mediators. Br. J. Pharmacol. 137, 1039–1046. http://dx.doi.org/10.1038/sj.bjp.0704951.

Gutmann, H., Hruz, P., Zimmermann, C., Straumann, A., Terracciano, L., Hammann, F., et al., 2008. Breast cancer resistance protein and P-glycoprotein expression in patients with newly diagnosed and therapy-refractory ulcerative colitis compared with healthy controls. Digestion 78, 154–162. http://dx.doi.org/10.1159/000179361.

Hagenbuch, B., Meier, P.J., 2003. The superfamily of organic anion transporting polypeptides. Biochim. Biophys. Acta 1609, 1–18.

Hagenbuch, B., Meier, P.J., 2004. Organic anion transporting polypeptides of the OATP/SLC21 family: phylogenetic classification as OATP/SLCO superfamily, new nomenclature and molecular/functional properties. Pflugers Arch. 447, 653–665. http://dx.doi.org/10.1007/s00424-003-1168-y.

Hanafy, S., El-Kadi, A.O.S., Jamali, F., 2012. Effect of inflammation on molecular targets and drug transporters. J. Pharm. Pharm. Sci. 15, 361–375.

Harati, R., Villégier, A.-S., Banks, W.A., Mabondzo, A., 2012. Susceptibility of juvenile and adult blood–brain barrier to endothelin-1: regulation of P-glycoprotein and breast cancer resistance protein expression and transport activity. J. Neuroinflammation 9, 273. http://dx.doi.org/10.1186/1742-2094-9-273.

Hartmann, G., Kim, H., Piquette-Miller, M., 2001. Regulation of the hepatic multidrug resistance gene expression by endotoxin and inflammatory cytokines in mice. Int. Immunopharmacol. 1, 189–199. http://dx.doi.org/10.1016/S0162-3109(00)00271-X.

Hartmann, G., Cheung, A.K.Y., Piquette-Miller, M., 2002. Inflammatory cytokines, but not bile acids, regulate expression of murine hepatic anion transporters in endotoxemia. J. Pharmacol. Exp. Ther. 303, 273–281. http://dx.doi.org/10.1124/jpet.102.039404.

Hartmann, G., Vassileva, V., Piquette-Miller, M., 2005. Impact of endotoxin-induced changes in P-glycoprotein expression on disposition of doxorubicin in mice. Drug Metab. Dispos. 33, 820–828. http://dx.doi.org/10.1124/dmd.104.002568.tion.

Haslett, C., 1992. Resolution of acute inflammation and the role of apoptosis in the tissue fate of granulocytes. Clin. Sci. 83, 639–648. http://dx.doi.org/10.1042/cs0830639.

Hayashi, H., Sugiyama, Y., 2013. Bile salt export pump (BSEP/ABCB11): trafficking and sorting disturbances. Curr. Mol. Pharmacol. 6, 95–103.

Hediger, M.A., Romero, M.F., Peng, J.-B., Rolfs, A., Takanaga, H., Bruford, E.A., 2004. The ABCs of solute carriers: physiological, pathological and therapeutic implications of human membrane transport proteinsIntroduction. Pflugers Arch. 447, 465–468. http://dx.doi.org/10.1007/s00424-003-1192-y.

Heemskerk, S., van Koppen, A., van den Broek, L., Poelen, G.J.M., Wouterse, A.C., Dijkman, H.B.P.M., et al., 2007. Nitric oxide differentially regulates renal ATP-binding cassette transporters during endotoxemia. Pflugers Arch. 454, 321–334. http://dx.doi.org/10.1007/s00424-007-0210-x.

Heemskerk, S., Peters, J.G.P., Louisse, J., Sagar, S., Russel, F.G.M., Masereeuw, R., 2010. Regulation of P-glycoprotein in renal proximal tubule epithelial cells by LPS and TNF-alpha. J. Biomed. Biotechnol. 2010, 525180. http://dx.doi.org/10.1155/2010/525180.

Helmick, C.G., Felson, D.T., Lawrence, R.C., Gabriel, S., Hirsch, R., Kwoh, C.K., et al., 2008. Estimates of the prevalence of arthritis and other rheumatic conditions in the United States. Part I. Arthritis Rheum. 58, 15–25. http://dx.doi.org/10.1002/art.23177.

Hidemura, K., Zhao, Y.L., Ito, K., Nakao, A., Tatsumi, Y., Kanazawa, H., et al., 2003. Shiga-like toxin II impairs hepatobiliary transport of doxorubicin in rats by down-regulation of hepatic P glycoprotein and multidrug resistance-associated protein Mrp2. Antimicrob. Agents Chemother. 47, 1636–1642.

Höcherl, K., Schmidt, C., Bucher, M., 2009. COX-2 inhibition attenuates endotoxin-induced downregulation of organic anion transporters in the rat renal cortex. Kidney Int. 75, 373–380. http://dx.doi.org/10.1038/ki.2008.557.

Hung, D.Y., Siebert, G.A., Chang, P., Whitehouse, M.W., Fletcher, L., Crawford, D.H.G., et al., 2006. Hepatic pharmacokinetics of propranolol in rats with adjuvant-induced systemic inflammation. Am. J. Physiol. Gastrointest. Liver Physiol. 290, G343–G351. http://dx.doi.org/10.1152/ajpgi.00155.2005.

Jahnel, J., Fickert, P., Langner, C., Högenauer, C., Silbert, D., Gumhold, J., et al., 2009. Impact of experimental colitis on hepatobiliary transporter expression and bile duct injury in mice. Liver Int. 29, 1316–1325. http://dx.doi.org/10.1111/j.1478-3231.2009.02044.x.

Jaisue, S., Gerber, J.P., Davey, a K., 2010. Pharmacokinetics of fexofenadine following LPS administration to rats. Xenobiotica 40, 743–750. http://dx.doi.org/10.3109/00498254.2010.506929.

Jansen, P.L., Müller, M., 2000. The molecular genetics of familial intrahepatic cholestasis. Gut 47, 1–5.

Jansen, P.L., Müller, M., Sturm, E., 2001. Genes and cholestasis. Hepatology 34, 1067–1074. http://dx.doi.org/10.1053/jhep.2001.29625.

Jessica Burch, P.B., Mary Onysko, P.B., 2012. Current Standards and Future Treatments of Rheumatoid Arthritis.

Ji, L., Masuda, S., Saito, H., Inui, K., 2002. Down-regulation of rat organic cation transporter rOCT2 by 5/6 nephrectomy. Kidney Int. 62, 514–524. http://dx.doi.org/10.1046/j.1523-1755.2002.00464.x.

Kalitsky-Szirtes, J., Shayeganpour, A., Brocks, D.R., Piquette-Miller, M., 2004. Suppression of drug-metabolizing enzymes and efflux transporters in the intestine of endotoxin-treated rats. Drug Metab. Dispos. 32, 20–27. http://dx.doi.org/10.1124/dmd.32.1.20.

Kawase, A., Tsunokuni, Y., Iwaki, M., 2007. Effects of alterations in CAR on bilirubin detoxification in mouse collagen-induced arthritis. Drug Metab. Dispos. 35, 256–261. http://dx.doi.org/10.1124/dmd.106.011536.

Kawase, A., Yoshida, I., Tsunokuni, Y., Iwaki, M., 2008. Decreased PXR and CAR inhibit transporter and CYP mRNA Levels in the liver and intestine of mice with collagen-induced arthritis. Xenobiotica 37 (4), 366–374.

Kawase, A., Wada, S., Iwaki, M., 2013. Changes in mRNA expression and activity of xenobiotic metabolizing enzymes in livers from adjuvant-induced arthritis rats. Pharmacol. Pharm. 04, 478–483. http://dx.doi.org/10.4236/pp.2013.46069.

Kawase, A., Norikane, S., Okada, A., Adachi, M., Kato, Y., Iwaki, M., 2014. Distinct alterations in ATP-binding cassette transporter expression in liver, kidney, small intestine, and brain in adjuvant-induced arthritic rats. J. Pharm. Sci. 103, 2556–2564. http://dx.doi.org/10.1002/jps.24043.

Kawauchi, S., Nakamura, T., Miki, I., Inoue, J., Hamaguchi, T., Tanahashi, T., et al., 2014. Downregulation of CYP3A and P-glycoprotein in the secondary inflammatory response of mice with dextran sulfate sodium-induced colitis and its contribution to cyclosporine A blood concentrations. J. Pharm. Sci. 124, 180–191.

Keitel, V., Burdelski, M., Warskulat, U., Kühlkamp, T., Keppler, D., Häussinger, D., et al., 2005. Expression and localization of hepatobiliary transport proteins in progressive familial intrahepatic cholestasis. Hepatology 41, 1160–1172. http://dx.doi.org/10.1002/hep.20682.

Kendall, M.J., Quarterman, C.P., Bishop, P.K., Schneider, R.E., 1979. Effects of inflammatory disease on plasma oxprenolol concentrations. Br. Med. J. 2, 465–468.

Keppler, D., 2011. Multidrug resistance proteins (MRPs, ABCCs): importance for pathophysiology and drug therapy. Handb. Exp. Pharmacol. 201, 299–323. http://dx.doi.org/10.1007/978-3-642-14541-4.

Kim, P.K., Chen, J., Andrejko, K.M., Deutschman, C.S., 2000. Intraabdominal sepsis down-regulates transcription of sodium taurocholate cotransporter and multidrug resistance-associated protein in rats. Shock 14, 176–181.

Klaassen, C.D., Aleksunes, L.M., 2010a. Xenobiotic, bile acid, and cholesterol transporters. Pharmacol. Rev. 62, 1–96. http://dx.doi.org/10.1124/pr.109.002014.1.

Klaassen, C.D., Aleksunes, L.M., 2010b. Xenobiotic, bile acid, and cholesterol transporters: function and regulation. Pharmacol. Rev. 62, 1–96. http://dx.doi.org/10.1124/pr.109.002014.

Koepsell, H., 1998. Organic cation transporters in intestine, kidney, liver, and brain. Annu. Rev. Physiol. 60, 243–266. http://dx.doi.org/10.1146/annurev.physiol.60.1.243.

Korolkova, O.Y., Myers, J.N., Pellom, S.T., Wang, L., M'Koma, A.E., 2015. Characterization of serum cytokine profile in predominantly colonic inflammatory bowel disease to delineate ulcerative and Crohn's colitides. Clin. Med. Insights Gastroenterol. 8, 29–44. http://dx.doi.org/10.4137/CGast.S20612.

Kosters, A., Karpen, S.J., 2008. Bile acid transporters in health and disease. Xenobiotica 38, 1043–1071. http://dx.doi.org/10.1080/00498250802040584.

Kosters, A., Karpen, S.J., 2010. The role of inflammation in cholestasis: clinical and basic aspects. Semin. Liver Dis. 30, 186–194. http://dx.doi.org/10.1055/s-0030-1253227.

Kozłowska-Rup, D., Czekaj, P., Plewka, D., Sikora, J., 2014. Immunolocalization of ABC drug transporters in human placenta from normal and gestational diabetic pregnancies. Ginekol Pol. 85, 410–419.

Kusuhara, H., Sugiyama, Y., 2005. Active efflux across the blood–brain barrier: role of the solute carrier family. NeuroRx 2, 73–85. http://dx.doi.org/10.1602/neurorx.2.1.73.

Langmann, T., Moehle, C., Mauerer, R., Scharl, M., Liebisch, G., Zahn, A., et al., 2004. Loss of detoxification in inflammatory bowel disease: dysregulation of pregnane X receptor target genes. Gastroenterology 127, 26–40.

Laouari, D., Yang, R., Veau, C., Blanke, I., Friedlander, G., 2001. Two apical multidrug transporters, P-gp and MRP2, are differently altered in chronic renal failure. Am. J. Physiol. Ren. Physiol. 280, F636–F645.

Lawrence, R.C., Felson, D.T., Helmick, C.G., Arnold, L.M., Choi, H., Deyo, R.A., et al., 2008. Estimates of the prevalence of arthritis and other rheumatic conditions in the United States. Part II. Arthritis Rheum. 58, 26–35. http://dx.doi.org/10.1002/art.23176.

Le Vee, M., Gripon, P., Stieger, B., Fardel, O., 2008. Down-regulation of organic anion transporter expression in human hepatocytes exposed to the proinflammatory cytokine interleukin 1beta. Drug Metab. Dispos. 36, 217–222. http://dx.doi.org/10.1124/dmd.107.016907.

Le Vee, M., Lecureur, V., Stieger, B., Fardel, O., 2009. Regulation of drug transporter expression in human hepatocytes exposed to the proinflammatory cytokines tumor necrosis factor-alpha or interleukin-6. Drug Metab. Dispos. 37, 685–693. http://dx.doi.org/10.1124/dmd.108.023630.pump.

Le Vee, M., Jouan, E., Moreau, A., Fardel, O., 2011a. Regulation of drug transporter mRNA expression by interferon-γ in primary human hepatocytes. Fundam. Clin. Pharmacol. 25, 99–103. http://dx.doi.org/10.1111/j.1472-8206.2010.00822.x.

Le Vee, M., Jouan, E., Stieger, B., Lecureur, V., Fardel, O., 2011b. Regulation of drug transporter expression by oncostatin M in human hepatocytes. Biochem. Pharmacol. 82, 304–311. http://dx.doi.org/10.1016/j.bcp.2011.04.017.

Leblond, F.A., Petrucci, M., Dubé, P., Bernier, G., Bonnardeaux, A., Pichette, V., 2002. Downregulation of intestinal cytochrome p450 in chronic renal failure. J. Am. Soc. Nephrol. 13, 1579–1585.

Lee, G., Piquette-Miller, M., 2001. Influence of IL-6 on MDR and MRP-mediated multidrug resistance in human hepatoma cells. Can. J. Physiol. Pharmacol. 79, 876–884.

Lee, P.Y., Li, Y., Kumagai, Y., Xu, Y., Weinstein, J.S., Kellner, E.S., et al., 2009. Type I interferon modulates monocyte recruitment and maturation in chronic inflammation. Am. J. Pathol. 175, 2023–2033. http://dx.doi.org/10.2353/ajpath.2009.090328.

Lemahieu, W., Maes, B., Verbeke, K., Rutgeerts, P., Geboes, K., Vanrenterghem, Y., 2005. Cytochrome P450 3A4 and P-glycoprotein activity and assimilation of tacrolimus in transplant patients with persistent diarrhea. Am. J. Transplant. 5, 1383–1391. http://dx.doi.org/10.1111/j.1600-6143.2005.00844.x.

Li, N.K.C., 2004. Role of liver-enriched transcription factors in the down-regulation of organic anion transporting polypeptide 4 (oatp4; oatplb2; slc21a10) by lipopolysaccharide. Mol. Pharmacol. 66, 694–701.

Lickteig, A.J., Slitt, A.L., Arkan, M.C., Karin, M., Cherrington, N.J., 2007. Differential regulation of hepatic transporters in the absence of tumor necrosis factor-alpha, interleukin-1beta, interleukin-6, and nuclear factor-kappaB in two models of cholestasis. Drug Metab. Dispos. 35, 402–409. http://dx.doi.org/10.1124/dmd.106.012138.

Ling, S., Jamali, F., 2005. Effect of early phase adjuvant arthritis on hepatic P450 enzymes and pharmacokinetics of verapamil: an alternative approach to the use of an animal model of inflammation for pharmacokinetic studies. Drug Metab. Dispos. 33, 579–586. http://dx.doi.org/10.1124/dmd.104.002360.

Liu, Z., Liu, K., 2016. Application of model-based approaches to evaluate hepatic transporter-mediated drug clearance: in vitro, in vivo, and in vitro-in vivo extrapolation. Curr. Drug Metab. 17 (5), 456–468.

Lye, P., Bloise, E., Javam, M., Gibb, W., Lye, S.J., Matthews, S.G., 2015. Impact of bacterial and viral challenge on multidrug resistance in first- and third-trimester human placenta. Am. J. Pathol. 185, 1666–1675. http://dx.doi.org/10.1016/j.ajpath.2015.02.013.

Mason, C.W., Buhimschi, I.A., Buhimschi, C.S., Dong, Y., Weiner, C.P., Swaan, P.W., 2011. ATP-binding cassette transporter expression in human placenta as a function of pregnancy condition. Drug Metab. Dispos. 39, 1000–1007. http://dx.doi.org/10.1124/dmd.111.038166.

Matsuzaki, T., Morisaki, T., Sugimoto, W., Yokoo, K., Sato, D., Nonoguchi, H., et al., 2008. Altered pharmacokinetics of cationic drugs caused by down-regulation of renal rat organic cation transporter 2 (Slc22a2) and rat multidrug and toxin extrusion 1 (Slc47a1) in ischemia/reperfusion-induced acute kidney injury. Drug Metab. Dispos. 36, 649–654. http://dx.doi.org/10.1124/dmd.107.019869.

Mayo, P.R., Skeith, K., Russell, A.S., Jamali, F., 2000. Decreased dromotropic response to verapamil despite pronounced increased drug concentration in rheumatoid arthritis. Br. J. Clin. Pharmacol. 50, 605–613.

Meier, Y., Eloranta, J.J., Darimont, J., Ismair, M.G., Hiller, C., Fried, M., et al., 2007. Regional distribution of solute carrier mRNA expression along the human intestinal tract. Drug Metab. Dispos. 35, 590–594. http://dx.doi.org/10.1124/dmd.106.013342.

Merrell, M.D., Nyagode, B.A., Clarke, J.D., Cherrington, N.J., Morgan, E.T., 2014. Selective and cytokine-dependent regulation of hepatic transporters and bile acid homeostasis during infectious colitis in mice. Drug Metab. Dispos. 42, 596–602. http://dx.doi.org/10.1124/dmd.113.055525.

Meunier, C.J., Verbeeck, R.K., 1999. Glucuronidation of R- and S-ketoprofen, acetaminophen, and diflunisal by liver microsomes of adjuvant-induced arthritic rats. Drug Metab. Dispos. 27, 26–31.

Mizoguchi, A., 2012. Animal models of inflammatory bowel disease. Prog. Mol. Biol. Transl. Sci. 105, 263–320. http://dx.doi.org/10.1016/B978-0-12-394596-9.00009-3.

Molodecky, N.A., Soon, I.S., Rabi, D.M., Ghali, W.A., Ferris, M., Chernoff, G., et al., 2012. Increasing incidence and prevalence of the inflammatory bowel diseases with time, based on systematic review. Gastroenterology 142, 46–54. http://dx.doi.org/10.1053/j.gastro.2011.10.001 e42; quiz e30.

Nakamura, J., Nishida, T., Hayashi, K., Kawada, N., Ueshima, S., Sugiyama, Y., et al., 1999. Kupffer cell-mediated down regulation of rat hepatic CMOAT/MRP2 gene expression. Biochem. Biophys. Res. Commun. 255, 143–149.

Naud, J., Michaud, J., Boisvert, C., Desbiens, K., Leblond, F.A., Mitchell, A., et al., 2007. Down-regulation of intestinal drug transporters in chronic renal failure in rats. J. Pharmacol. Exp. Ther. 320, 978–985. http://dx.doi.org/10.1124/jpet.106.112631.

Naud, J., Michaud, J., Leblond, F.A., Lefrancois, S., Bonnardeaux, A., Pichette, V., 2008. Effects of chronic renal failure on liver drug transporters. Drug Metab. Dispos. 36, 124–128. http://dx.doi.org/10.1124/dmd.107.018192.

Naud, J., Michaud, J., Beauchemin, S., Hébert, M.-J., Roger, M., Lefrancois, S., et al., 2011. Effects of chronic renal failure on kidney drug transporters and cytochrome P450 in rats. Drug Metab. Dispos. 39, 1363–1369. http://dx.doi.org/10.1124/dmd.111.039115.

Naud, J., Laurin, L.-P., Michaud, J., Beauchemin, S., Leblond, F.A., Pichette, V., 2012. Effects of chronic renal failure on brain drug transporters in rats. Drug Metab. Dispos. 40, 39–46. http://dx.doi.org/10.1124/dmd.111.041145.

Ni, Z., Bikadi, Z., Rosenberg, M.F., Mao, Q., 2010. Structure and function of the human breast cancer resistance protein (BCRP/ABCG2). Curr. Drug Metab. 11, 603–617.

Nies, A.T., Koepsell, H., Damme, K., Schwab, M., 2011. Organic cation transporters (OCTs, MATEs), in vitro and in vivo evidence for the importance in drug therapy. Handb. Exp. Pharmacol. 105–167. http://dx.doi.org/10.1007/978-3-642-14541-4_3.

Nishimura, M., Naito, S., 2005. Tissue-specific mRNA expression profiles of human ATP-binding cassette and solute carrier transporter superfamilies. Drug Metab. Pharmacokinet. 20, 452–477.

Nolin, T.D., Naud, J., Leblond, F.a, Pichette, V., 2008. Emerging evidence of the impact of kidney disease on drug metabolism and transport. Clin. Pharmacol. Ther. 83, 898–903. http://dx.doi.org/10.1038/clpt.2008.59.

Nones, K., Knoch, B., Dommels, Y.E.M., Paturi, G., Butts, C., McNabb, W.C., et al., 2009. Multidrug resistance gene deficient (mdr1a-/-) mice have an altered caecal microbiota that precedes the onset of intestinal inflammation. J. Appl. Microbiol. 107, 557–566. http://dx.doi.org/10.1111/j.1365-2672.2009.04225.x.

Oswald, S., Gröer, C., Drozdzik, M., Siegmund, W., 2013. Mass spectrometry-based targeted proteomics as a tool to elucidate the expression and function of intestinal drug transporters. AAPS J. 15, 1128–1140. http://dx.doi.org/10.1208/s12248-013-9521-3.

Panwala, C.M., Jones, J.C., Viney, J.L., 1998. A novel model of inflammatory bowel disease: mice deficient for the multiple drug resistance gene, mdr1a, spontaneously develop colitis. J. Immunol. 161, 5733–5744.

Pauli-Magnus, C., von Richter, O., Burk, O., Ziegler, A., Mettang, T., Eichelbaum, M., et al., 2000. Characterization of the major metabolites of verapamil as substrates and inhibitors of P-glycoprotein. J. Pharmacol. Exp. Ther. 293, 376–382.

Petrovic, V., Piquette-Miller, M., 2010. Impact of polyinosinic/polycytidylic acid on placental and hepatobiliary drug transporters in pregnant rats. Drug Metab. Dispos. 38, 1760–1766. http://dx.doi.org/10.1124/dmd.110.034470.

Petrovic, V., Teng, S., Piquette-Miller, M., 2007. Regulation of drug transporters during infection and inflammation. Mol. Interv. 7, 99–111. http://dx.doi.org/10.1124/mi.7.2.10.

Petrovic, V., Wang, J.-H., Piquette-Miller, M., 2008. Effect of endotoxin on the expression of placental drug transporters and glyburide disposition in pregnant rats. Drug Metab. Dispos. 36, 1944–1950. http://dx.doi.org/10.1124/dmd.107.019851.very.

Petrovic, V., Kojovic, D., Cressman, A., Piquette-Miller, M., 2015. Maternal bacterial infections impact expression of drug transporters in human placenta. Int. Immunopharmacol. 26, 349–356. http://dx.doi.org/10.1016/j.intimp.2015.04.020.

Pichette, V., Leblond, F.A., 2003. Drug metabolism in chronic renal failure. Curr. Drug Metab. 4, 91–103.

Piquette-Miller, M., Jamali, F., 1992. Effect of adjuvant arthritis on the disposition of acebutolol enantiomers in rats. Agents Actions 37, 290–296.

Piquette-Miller, M., Jamali, F., 1993. Selective effect of adjuvant arthritis on the disposition of propranolol enantiomers in rats detected using a stereospecific HPLC assay. Pharm. Res. 10, 294–299.

Piquette-Miller, M., Pak, A., Kim, H., Anari, R., Shahzamani, A., 1998. Decreased expression and activity of P-glycoprotein in rat liver during acute inflammation. Pharm. Res. 15, 706–711.

Poller, B., Drewe, J., Krähenbühl, S., Huwyler, J., Gutmann, H., 2010. Regulation of BCRP (ABCG2) and P-glycoprotein (ABCB1) by cytokines in a model of the human blood–brain barrier. Cell Mol. Neurobiol. 30, 63–70. http://dx.doi.org/10.1007/s10571-009-9431-1.

Poloyac, S.M., Tosheva, R.T., Gardner, B.M., Shedlofsky, S.I., Blouin, R.A., 1999. The effect of endotoxin administration on the pharmacokinetics of chlorzoxazone in humans. Clin. Pharmacol. Ther. 66, 554–562. http://dx.doi.org/10.1053/cp.1999.v66.103172001.

Raddatz, D., Bockemühl, M., Ramadori, G., 2005. Quantitative measurement of cytokine mRNA in inflammatory bowel disease: relation to clinical and endoscopic activity and outcome. Eur. J. Gastroenterol. Hepatol. 17, 547–557.

Roe, A.L., Warren, G., Hou, G., Howard, G., Shedlofsky, S.I., Blouin, R.A., 1998. The effect of high dose endotoxin on CYP3A2 expression in the rat. Pharm. Res. 15, 1603–1608.

Ronaldson, P.T., Bendayan, R., 2006. HIV-1 viral envelope glycoprotein gp120 triggers an inflammatory response in cultured rat astrocytes and regulates the functional expression of P-glycoprotein. Mol. Pharmacol. 70, 1087–1098. http://dx.doi.org/10.1124/mol.106.025973.

Roth, M., Obaidat, A., Hagenbuch, B., 2012. OATPs, OATs and OCTs: the organic anion and cation transporters of the SLCO and SLC22A gene superfamilies. Br. J. Pharmacol. 165, 1260–1287. http://dx.doi.org/10.1111/j.1476-5381.2011.01724.x.

Sacks, J.J., Luo, Y.-H., Helmick, C.G., 2010. Prevalence of specific types of arthritis and other rheumatic conditions in the ambulatory health care system in the United States, 2001–2005. Arthritis Care Res. (Hoboken) 62, 460–464. http://dx.doi.org/10.1002/acr.20041.

Sanada, H., Sekimoto, M., Kamoshita, A., Degawa, M., 2011. Changes in expression of hepatic cytochrome P450 subfamily enzymes during development of adjuvant-induced arthritis in rats. J. Toxicol. Sci. 36, 181–190.

Schneider, R.E., Babb, J., Bishop, H., Mitchard, M., Hoare, A.M., 1976. Plasma levels of propranolol in treated patients with coeliac disease and patients with Crohn's disease. Br. Med. J. 2, 794–795.

Schneider, R., Sauvant, C., Betz, B., Otremba, M., Fischer, D., Holzinger, H., et al., 2007. Downregulation of organic anion transporters OAT1 and OAT3 correlates with impaired secretion of para-aminohippurate after ischemic acute renal failure in rats. Am. J. Physiol. Ren. Physiol. 292, F1599–F1605. http://dx.doi.org/10.1152/ajprenal.00473.2006.

Schuetz, E.G., Strom, S., Yasuda, K., Lecureur, V., Assem, M., Brimer, C., et al., 2001. Disrupted bile acid homeostasis reveals an unexpected interaction among nuclear hormone receptors, transporters, and cytochrome P450. J. Biol. Chem. 276, 39411–39418. http://dx.doi.org/10.1074/jbc.M106340200.

Siewert, E., Dietrich, C.G., Lammert, F., Heinrich, P.C., Matern, S., Gartung, C., et al., 2004. Interleukin-6 regulates hepatic transporters during acute-phase response. Biochem. Biophys. Res. Commun. 322, 232–238. http://dx.doi.org/10.1016/j.bbrc.2004.07.102.

Smolen, J.S., Steiner, G., 2003. Therapeutic strategies for rheumatoid arthritis. Nat. Rev. Drug Discov. 2, 473–488. http://dx.doi.org/10.1038/nrd1109.

Staley, E.M., Dimmitt, R.A., Schoeb, T.R., Tanner, S.M., Lorenz, R.G., 2011. Critical role for P-glycoprotein expression in hematopoietic cells in the FVB.Mdr1a(−/−) model of colitis. J. Pediatr. Gastroenterol. Nutr. 53, 666–673. http://dx.doi.org/10.1097/MPG.0b013e31822860f1.

Stephens, R.H., O'Neill, C.A., Bennett, J., Humphrey, M., Henry, B., Rowland, M., et al., 2002a. Resolution of P-glycoprotein and non-P-glycoprotein effects on drug permeability using intestinal tissues from mdr1a (−/−) mice. Br. J. Pharmacol. 135, 2038–2046. http://dx.doi.org/10.1038/sj.bjp.0704668.

Stephens, R.H., Tanianis-Hughes, J., Higgs, N.B., Humphrey, M., Warhurst, G., 2002b. Region-dependent modulation of intestinal permeability by drug efflux transporters: in vitro studies in mdr1a(−/−) mouse intestine. J. Pharmacol. Exp. Ther. 303, 1095–1101. http://dx.doi.org/10.1124/jpet.102.041236.

Su, Y., Zhang, Y., Chen, M., Jiang, Z., Sun, L., Wang, T., et al., 2014. Lipopolysaccharide exposure augments isoniazide-induced liver injury. J. Appl. Toxicol. 34, 1436–1442. http://dx.doi.org/10.1002/jat.2979.

Sukhai, M., Yong, A., Kalitsky, J., Piquette-Miller, M., 2000. Inflammation and interleukin-6 mediate reductions in the hepatic expression and transcription of the mdr1a and mdr1b Genes. Mol. Cell Biol. Res. Commun. 4, 248–256. http://dx.doi.org/10.1006/mcbr.2001.0288.

Sukhai, M., Yong, A., Pak, A., Piquette-Miller, M., 2001. Decreased expression of P-glycoprotein in interleukin-1β and interleukin-6 treated rat hepatocytes. Inflamm. Res. 50, 362–370. http://dx.doi.org/10.1007/PL00000257.

Sun, H., Frassetto, L., Benet, L.Z., 2006. Effects of renal failure on drug transport and metabolism. Pharmacol. Ther. 109, 1–11. http://dx.doi.org/10.1016/j.pharmthera.2005.05.010.

Takeda, M., Khamdang, S., Narikawa, S., Kimura, H., Hosoyamada, M., Cha, S.H., et al., 2002. Characterization of methotrexate transport and its drug interactions with human organic anion transporters. J. Pharmacol. Exp. Ther. 302, 666–671. http://dx.doi.org/10.1124/jpet.102.034330.

Tang, W., Yi, C., Kalitsky, J., Piquette-Miller, M., 2000. Endotoxin downregulates hepatic expression of P-glycoprotein and MRP2 in 2-acetylaminofluorene-treated rats. Mol. Cell Biol. Res. Commun. 4, 90–97. http://dx.doi.org/10.1006/mcbr.2000.0264.

Trauner, M., Boyer, J.L., 2003. Bile salt transporters: molecular characterization, function, and regulation. Physiol. Rev. 633–671.

Trauner, M., Arrese, M., Lee, H., Boyer, J.L., Karpen, S.J., 1998. Endotoxin downregulates rat hepatic ntcp gene expression via decreased activity of critical transcription factors. J. Clin. Invest. 101, 2092–2100. http://dx.doi.org/10.1172/JCI1680.

Ufer, M., Häsler, R., Jacobs, G., Haenisch, S., Lächelt, S., Faltraco, F., et al., 2009. Decreased sigmoidal ABCB1 (P-glycoprotein) expression in ulcerative colitis is associated with disease activity. Pharmacogenomics 10, 1941–1953. http://dx.doi.org/10.2217/pgs.09.128.

Uno, S., Uraki, M., Ito, A., Shinozaki, Y., Yamada, A., Kawase, A., et al., 2009. Changes in mRNA expression of ABC and SLC transporters in liver and intestines of the adjuvant-induced arthritis rat. Biopharm. Drug Dispos. 30, 49–54. http://dx.doi.org/10.1002/bdd.639.

van Herwaarden, A.E., Jonker, J.W., Wagenaar, E., Brinkhuis, R.F., Schellens, J.H.M., Beijnen, J.H., et al., 2003. The breast cancer resistance protein (Bcrp1/Abcg2) restricts exposure to the dietary carcinogen 2-amino-1-methyl-6-phenylimidazo[4,5-b]pyridine. Cancer Res. 63, 6447–6452.

van Herwaarden, A.E., Wagenaar, E., Karnekamp, B., Merino, G., Jonker, J.W., Schinkel, A.H., 2006. Breast cancer resistance protein (Bcrp1/Abcg2) reduces systemic exposure of the dietary carcinogens aflatoxin B1, IQ and Trp-P-1 but also mediates their secretion into breast milk. Carcinogenesis 27, 123–130. http://dx.doi.org/10.1093/carcin/bgi176.

Veau, C., Faivre, L., Tardivel, S., Soursac, M., Banide, H., Lacour, B., et al., 2002. Effect of interleukin-2 on intestinal P-glycoprotein expression and functionality in mice. J. Pharmacol. Exp. Ther. 302, 742–750.

Vlaming, M.L.H., Teunissen, S.F., van de Steeg, E., van Esch, A., Wagenaar, E., Brunsveld, L., et al., 2014. Bcrp1;Mdr1a/b;Mrp2 combination knockout mice: altered disposition of the dietary carcinogen PhIP (2-amino-1-methyl-6-phenylimidazo[4,5-b]pyridine) and its genotoxic metabolites. Mol. Pharmacol. 85, 520–530. http://dx.doi.org/10.1124/mol.113.088823.

von Wedel-Parlow, M., Wölte, P., Galla, H.-J., 2009. Regulation of major efflux transporters under inflammatory conditions at the blood—brain barrier in vitro. J. Neurochem. 111, 111—118. http://dx.doi.org/10.1111/j.1471-4159.2009.06305.x.

Vos, T.A., Hooiveld, G.J., Koning, H., Childs, S., Meijer, D.K., Moshage, H., et al., 1998. Up-regulation of the multidrug resistance genes, Mrp1 and Mdr1b, and down-regulation of the organic anion transporter, Mrp2, and the bile salt transporter, SP-gp, in endotoxemic rat liver. Hepatology 28, 1637—1644. http://dx.doi.org/10.1002/hep.510280625.

Wagner, M., Fickert, P., Zollner, G., Fuchsbichler, A., Silbert, D., Tsybrovskyy, O., et al., 2003. Role of farnesoid X receptor in determining hepatic ABC transporter expression and liver injury in bile duct-ligated mice. Gastroenterology 125, 825—838.

Wahba, M.G.F., Messiha, B.A.S., Abo-Saif, A.A., 2015. Protective effects of fenofibrate and resveratrol in an aggressive model of rheumatoid arthritis in rats. Pharm. Biol. 1—11. http://dx.doi.org/10.3109/13880209.2015.1125931.

Wang, J., Scollard, D., Teng, S., Reilly, R., Piquette-Miller, M., 2005. Detection of P-glycoprotein activity in endotoxemic rats by 99mTc-sestamibi imaging. J. Nucl. Med. 46, 1537—1545.

Wang, Y., Fang, Y., Huang, W., Zhou, X., Wang, M., Zhong, B., et al., 2005. Effect of sinomenine on cytokine expression of macrophages and synoviocytes in adjuvant arthritis rats. J. Ethnopharmacol. 98, 37—43. http://dx.doi.org/10.1016/j.jep.2004.12.022.

Whitehouse, M.W., Beck, F.J., 1973. Impaired drug metabolism in rats with adjuvant-induced arthritis: a brief review. Drug Metab. Dispos. 1, 251—255.

Wojtal, K.A., Eloranta, J.J., Hruz, P., Gutmann, H., Drewe, J., Staumann, A., et al., 2009. Changes in mRNA expression levels of solute carrier transporters in inflammatory bowel disease patients. Drug Metab. Dispos. 37, 1871—1877. http://dx.doi.org/10.1124/dmd.109.027367.

Wright, S.R., Boag, A.H., Valdimarsson, G., Hipfner, D.R., Campling, B.G., Cole, S.P., et al., 1998. Immunohistochemical detection of multidrug resistance protein in human lung cancer and normal lung. Clin. Cancer Res. 4, 2279—2289.

Xavier, R.J., Podolsky, D.K., 2007. Unravelling the pathogenesis of inflammatory bowel disease. Nature 448, 427—434. http://dx.doi.org/10.1038/nature06005.

Yang, H., Lisman, T., Gouw, A.S.H., Porte, R.J., Verkade, H.J., Jan, B., et al., 2009. Inflammation mediated downregulation of hepatobiliary transporters contributes to intrahepatic cholestasis and liver damage in murine biliary atresia. Pediatr. Res. http://dx.doi.org/10.1203/PDR.0b013e3181b454a4.

Zhao, Y.L., Du, J., Kanazawa, H., Sugawara, A., Takagi, K., Kitaichi, K., et al., 2002a. Effect of endotoxin on doxorubicin transport across blood—brain barrier and P-glycoprotein function in mice. Eur. J. Pharmacol. 445, 115—123.

Zhao, Y.L., Du, J., Kanazawa, H., Cen, X.B., Takagi, K., Kitaichi, K., et al., 2002b. Shiga-like toxin II modifies brain distribution of a P-glycoprotein substrate, doxorubicin, and P-glycoprotein expression in mice. Brain Res. 956, 246—253.

Zollner, G., Fickert, P., Zenz, R., Fuchsbichler, A., Stumptner, C., Kenner, L., et al., 2001. Hepatobiliary transporter expression in percutaneous liver biopsies of patients with cholestatic liver diseases. Hepatology 33, 633—646. http://dx.doi.org/10.1053/jhep.2001.22646.

Zollner, G., Fickert, P., Silbert, D., Fuchsbichler, A., Marschall, H.U., Zatloukal, K., et al., 2003. Adaptive changes in hepatobiliary transporter expression in primary biliary cirrhosis. J. Hepatol. 38, 717—727.

Zollner, G., Wagner, M., Moustafa, T., Fickert, P., Silbert, D., Gumhold, J., et al., 2006. Coordinated induction of bile acid detoxification and alternative elimination in mice: role of FXR-regulated organic solute transporter-alpha/beta in the adaptive response to bile acids. Am. J. Physiol. Gastrointest. Liver Physiol. 290, G923—G932. http://dx.doi.org/10.1152/ajpgi.00490.2005.

4

Drug Metabolism in Kidney Disease

T.D. Nolin

University of Pittsburgh, Pittsburgh, PA, United States

OUTLINE

Conventional Drug-Dosing Paradigm in
Kidney Disease   92

Nonrenal Clearance   93

Influence of Experimental Kidney
Disease on Drug Metabolism   94
   Metabolism in Experimental Models of
     Chronic Kidney Disease   95
   Metabolism in Experimental Models of
     Acute Kidney Injury
     (Acute Renal Failure)   97

Influence of Kidney Disease on Drug
Metabolism in Humans   99

Altered Nonrenal Clearance   99
Phenotypic Assessments of Metabolic
   Pathways in Kidney Disease   102

Mechanisms of Altered Drug
Metabolism in Kidney Disease   105
   Modified Gene or Protein Expression   105
   Posttranslational Modifications (Direct
     Competitive Inhibition)   106

Summary   107

References   107

Chronic kidney disease (CKD) is a significant global public health problem, affecting over 10% of the world's population (Levey et al., 2015). Moreover, an estimated 14% of US adults are afflicted with CKD, and the number of patients with end-stage renal disease (ESRD) alone was approximately 662,000 at the end of 2013, representing 2034 prevalent cases per million in the US population (United States Renal Data System, 2015). Notably, the number of ESRD prevalent cases continues to rise by about 21,000 cases per year, primarily due to the steady incidence rate and a simultaneous decline in mortality rate among patients with ESRD. Despite the decline, however, the all-cause mortality rate for Medicare patients aged 66 years and older with CKD is 117.5 per 1000 patient-years (after adjusting for age, sex, and race), which is more than double the mortality rate observed in patients without CKD of 47.2

per 1000 patient-years (United States Renal Data System, 2015). The precise reasons for this are unknown, but a high burden of serious comorbidities in patients with CKD, such as diabetes, hypertension, and cardiovascular disease likely contributes.

Patients with CKD are prescribed a disproportionately high number of medications compared with patients without kidney disease due to the presence of numerous underlying comorbidities. In particular, patients with ESRD receiving chronic hemodialysis treatment have been reported to take an average of 12 medications (prescribed and over the counter) with a median pill burden of 19 per day (Chiu et al., 2009; St Peter, 2015). Consequently, patients with CKD are at high risk for developing medication-related problems, including adverse drug effects and drug interactions, leading to suboptimal therapeutic outcomes. A better understanding of the effects of kidney disease on drug disposition, including nonrenal drug clearance mediated by metabolizing enzymes, will facilitate improved drug selection and dosing in these patients who comprise a considerable proportion of the US population.

CONVENTIONAL DRUG-DOSING PARADIGM IN KIDNEY DISEASE

The pharmacokinetics (PK) of many drugs are altered in patients with kidney disease. Early investigations characterizing PK in the setting of CKD focused on the decrease in renal drug clearance, leading to pioneering clinically relevant dosing recommendations for renally cleared drugs (Kunin, 1967; Bennett et al., 1970; Dettli et al., 1970) as well as the establishment of a drug-dosing paradigm that persisted for more than 40 years, namely that one of two strategies be used when prescribing drugs for patients with impaired kidney function in an effort to optimize systemic exposure and minimize toxicity: (1) use medications that are not cleared by the kidney or (2) use nomograms, guidelines, recommendations, or prospective PK calculations to adjust the dose of medications that are predominantly renally eliminated (Matzke et al., 1984; Bennett, 1988; Talbert, 1994). The latter is based on the premise that total body or systemic clearance (CL_T), which reflects renal clearance (CL_R) of these drugs, and corresponding systemic exposure are proportional to the level of kidney function (Dettli, 1973, 1974). This is often referred to as the Dettli method of drug dosing, named after Dr. Luzius Dettli, who championed the approach to individualizing therapy in patients with impaired kidney function by using creatinine clearance to estimate appropriate drug doses a priori (Dettli, 1976).

Despite the implementation and routine use of these strategies for decades, variability in response and the frequency of adverse drug events appear to be greater in patients with kidney disease than in those with normal kidney function (Zaidenstein et al., 2002; Bates et al., 1999; Hug et al., 2009). Numerous studies indicate that changes in systemic exposure of drugs that undergo nonrenal clearance (CL_{NR}) (e.g., hepatic and extrahepatic metabolism) are altered in patients with kidney disease (Nolin, 2008; Nolin et al., 2008; Momper et al., 2010; Yeung et al., 2014; Velenosi and Urquhart, 2014), likely leading to drug concentrations at the site of action that are disproportionate to the dose. These studies draw attention to a fundamentally important and flawed assumption of the Dettli method—that nonrenal drug clearance is constant, i.e., does not change as kidney function declines (Fig. 4.1) (Atkinson Jr. and Huang, 2009). In fact, extensive data derived from experimental models and clinical studies

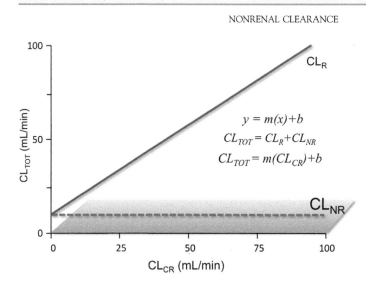

FIGURE 4.1 The Dettli method of drug dosing, depicting the relationship between total systemic drug clearance (CL_{TOT}) and creatinine clearance (CL_{CR}). CL_R, renal clearance; CL_{NR}, nonrenal clearance. *Adapted from Dettli, L., 1974. Individualization of drug dosage in patients with renal disease. Med. Clin. North Am. 58, 977–985.*

now clearly indicate that kidney disease has differential effects on drug-metabolizing enzymes that may lead to alterations in CL_{NR} (Zhang et al., 2009; Huang et al., 2009).

NONRENAL CLEARANCE

Nonrenal clearance encompasses all routes of drug elimination, excluding renal excretion of unchanged drug. It largely comprises hepatic and extrahepatic metabolism (together called metabolic clearance) and drug transport. The concept that kidney disease affects metabolic drug clearance is not new. Several historical reviews of the subject tabulated alterations in CL, CL_R, and CL_{NR} in humans derived from clinical PK studies, with little or no description of effects on specific drug-metabolizing enzymes (Balant et al., 1983; Gibson, 1986; Touchette and Slaughter, 1991; Elston et al., 1993). For example, the effect of CKD on cytochrome P450 (CYP) activity has been described semiquantitatively (i.e., inhibition, induction, or no change) based on the changes in CL or CL_{NR} of known CYP substrates (Elston et al., 1993). These findings must be interpreted within the context of their limitations, however, including use of nonspecific CYP substrates as phenotypic probe drugs, lack of information regarding CYP genetic data, and poor control of environmental factors (e.g., smoking, diet) known to lack impact on enzyme function. Lastly, lack of information regarding transporter function is an important limitation because of the substantial overlap in substrate specificity between metabolizing enzymes and transporters (Kim et al., 1999; Benet et al., 2003, 2004). If not taken into consideration, changes in transporter function could lead to inaccurate conclusions regarding enzyme function based on PK changes of substrates with overlapping specificity. The emergence of more specific phenotypic probe drugs and robust experimental models of CKD and acute kidney injury (AKI) have enabled investigators to more clearly elucidate the effects of kidney disease on drug metabolism.

INFLUENCE OF EXPERIMENTAL KIDNEY DISEASE ON DRUG METABOLISM

Several early reports of reduced hepatic microsomal CYP content and/or activity in various animal models of chronic renal failure (CRF) were published prior to 1990 (Leber and Schutterle, 1972; Van Peer and Belpaire, 1977; Leber et al., 1978; Patterson and Cohn, 1984). These early investigations are limited because they included the use of nonspecific substrates (e.g., aniline, antipyrine, aminopyrine, and acetanilide), and there is an absence of data concerning the in vivo relevance of the changes noted. Although subsequent studies of animals with experimental renal failure indicate that expression of several CYP isoforms is dramatically and differentially altered (Ikemoto et al., 1992; Ohishi et al., 1994; Uchida et al., 1995; Rege et al., 2003; Chung et al., 2002), disparate results led to skepticism regarding effects observed. As presented in Table 4.1, possible sources of variability in results stem from the use of different models of renal failure, including models that more closely mimic CRF (e.g., surgical nephrectomy) and others that reflect AKI (e.g., chemically induced). For example, Uchida et al. (1995) used a surgical nephrectomy rat model and demonstrated an increase in expression of CYP1A2, and a decrease in the levels of CYP2C6, 2C11, and 3A2 protein expression, with no change in CYP2E1. A relationship between blood urea nitrogen concentration and CYP content ($r^2 = 0.73$; $p < .0007$) and aminopyrine N-demethylase activity ($r^2 = 0.77$; $p < .002$) was also observed. Conversely, others used a chemically induced (*cis*-diamminedichloroplatinum) nephrotoxicity model and reported nearly opposite effects. Specifically, a decrease in expression of CYPs 1A2, 2C11, and 3A2 was found, along with increased levels of CYP2C6 and CYP2E1 (Table 4.1) (Ohishi et al., 1994).

TABLE 4.1   Disparate Hepatic CYP Expression Findings in Various Rat Models of Renal Failure

1A2	2C6	2C11	2D1	2E1	3A1	3A2	Exp. Method	Model	Duration	References
na	+14	−64[a]	na	+23	na	−67[a]	WB	SN	35	Ikemoto et al. (1992)
−25	+31	−52[a]	na	+76[b]	na	−77[a]	WB	CDDP	7	Ohishi et al. (1994)
↑	↓	↓	na	↔	na	↓	WB	SN	21	Uchida et al. (1995)
na	na	na	↔	na	↔	↓[c]	PCR	SN	35	Rege et al. (2003)
na	na	na	na	↑[d]	na	na	WB	UN	5	Chung et al. (2002)
↔	na	↓	na	↑[e]	na	na	NB	UN	5	Chung et al. (2002)

Expressed as percentage increase (+) or decrease (−) in expression compared with control where indicated. Otherwise relative increase (↑), decrease (↓), or no change (↔) compared with control is noted.
CDDP, *cis*-diamminedichloroplatinum; *CYP*, cytochrome P450; *Duration*, duration of renal failure at time of sacrifice (days); *Exp. method*, method of determining expression level; *na*, not assessed; *NB*, Northern blot; *PCR*, semiquantitative reverse-transcriptase polymerase chain reaction; *SN*, surgical nephrectomy; *UN*, uranyl nitrate; *WB*, Western blot.
[a]$p < .01$, significant as compared with control; [b]$p < .05$, significant as compared with control; [c]$p < .01$, significant as compared with control; [d]More than twofold increase reported; [e]More than fourfold increase reported.

TABLE 4.2 Alterations in Phase I and II Metabolic Enzymes Observed in the Five-Sixth Nephrectomy Rat Model of CRF

Phase	Enzyme	Intestine (Leblond et al., 2002)				Liver (Leblond et al., 2001, 2000; Simard et al., 2008; Yu et al., 2006; Alshogran et al., 2015a)			
		Protein	RNA	Activity	F	Protein	RNA	Activity	Effect
I	CYP1A1	↓ 43%	↓ 32%	↓ 25%	↑	↔	↔	↔	↔ metabolic CL
I	CYP2B1	↔	↔	na	↔	na	na	na	na
I	CYP2C6	↔	↔	na	↔	na	na	na	na
I	CYP2C11	↔	↔	na	↔	↓ 45%	↓	↓ 35%	↓ metabolic CL
I	CYP2D	na	na	na	na	↔	↔	na	↔ metabolic CL
I	CYP3A1	na	na	na	na	↓ 85%	↓	↓ 35%	↓ metabolic CL
I	CYP3A2	↓ 71%	↓ 36%	↓ 25%	↑	↓ 65%	↓	↓ 35%	↓ metabolic CL
I	CBR1	na	na	na	na	↓ 43%	↓ 34%	↓	↓ metabolic CL
I	AKR1C3/18	na	na	na	na	↓ 76%	↓ 93%	↓	↓ metabolic CL
I	11β-HSD1	na	na	na	na	↓ 70%	↓ 35%	↓	↓ metabolic CL
II	NAT1	na	na	na	na	↓ 33%	na	↓ 45%	↓ metabolic CL
II	NAT2	na	na	na	na	↓ 50%	↓ 35%	↓ 50%	↓ metabolic CL
II	UGT1a	na	na	na	na	↔	↔	↔	↔ metabolic CL
II	UGT2b	na	na	na	na	↔	↔	↔	↔ metabolic CL

Increase (↑), decrease (↓), or no change (↔) compared with control is noted.
AKR, aldo-keto reductase; *CBR*, carbonyl reductase; *CL*, clearance; *CRF*, chronic renal failure; *CYP*, cytochrome P450; *F*, bioavailability; *HSD*, hydroxysteroid dehydrogenase; *na*, not assessed; *NAT*, N-acetyltransferase; *UGT*, uridine diphosphate-glucuronosyltransferase.

Metabolism in Experimental Models of Chronic Kidney Disease

The most consistent and reproducible mechanistic insight and evidence to date that phases I and II metabolic pathways are differentially altered in CKD are provided by the extensive body of work by Leblond et al. (Table 4.2) (Leblond et al., 2001, 2000, 2002; Guevin et al., 2002; Michaud et al., 2005, 2006; Naud et al., 2007; Simard et al., 2008; Yu et al., 2006; Alshogran et al., 2015a). Over nearly two decades, they have systematically evaluated the effect of experimental CKD (induced via two-stage five-sixth nephrectomy) on multiple metabolic enzymes and transporters in intestine and liver, as well as in vivo hepatic metabolism in rats. Total microsomal CYP activity, which correlated negatively with creatinine clearance ($r^2 = 0.7$; $p < .001$), was reduced by up to 47% compared with control paired-fed animals ($p < .01$) (Leblond et al., 2000, 2001). Moreover, protein expression (determined by Western blot analysis) of CYP2C11, CYP3A1 (CYP3A23), and CYP3A2 in CKD rats was reduced by 45%, 85%, and 65%, respectively, compared with controls ($p < .001$). The expression of CYPs 1A1 and 2D was unchanged (Table 4.2). This group then evaluated the in vivo relevance of reduced

CYP protein expression using enzyme-specific breath tests (Leblond et al., 2000). The amino-pyrine and erythromycin breath tests (EBTs), probes of hepatic CYP2C11 and CYP3A activity, respectively, were reduced by 35% ($p < .001$), whereas the caffeine breath test (a CYP1A1 probe) was unchanged compared with control animals. Significant correlations existed between breath test results and both creatinine clearance and protein expression. Northern blotting confirmed and was consistent with Western blot results, demonstrating that hepatic CYP2C11, CYP3A1 (CYP3A23), and CYP3A2 mRNA expression was decreased in CKD animals (Leblond et al., 2001). Interestingly, for the first time, Velenosi et al. (2012) demonstrated that surgically induced moderate CKD results in decreased CYP3A2 and CYP2C11 expression, and a corresponding decrease in the activity of each enzyme of more than 60% when compared with controls.

The effects of CKD on intestinal CYP have also been explored (Leblond et al., 2002). Total intestinal CYP activity was correlated with creatinine clearance ($r^2 = 0.9$; $p < .001$) and was reduced by 32% in CKD animals compared with control ($p < .001$). Protein expression of CYP1A1 and CYP3A2 was reduced by 43% and 71%, respectively ($p < .001$), and corresponding mRNA levels were decreased by 32% and 36%, respectively ($p < .001$). Expression of CYP2B1, CYP2C6, and CYP2C11 did not change (Table 4.2). Microsomal activities of CYP3A and CYP1A were also reduced by 25% (Leblond et al., 2002). These studies demonstrated for the first time that the selective modulation of hepatic and intestinal CYP enzyme activity observed in kidney disease is likely due to reduced mRNA expression, indicating transcriptionally mediated downregulation of CYP genes.

The effect of experimental CKD on CYP inducibility has also been investigated using dexamethasone and phenobarbital. The drugs were administered to five-sixth nephrectomy rats in an effort to induce hepatic CYP3A1 (CYP3A23) and CYP3A2 (Leblond et al., 2001). Both drugs enhanced hepatic protein and mRNA expression. Dexamethasone also maintained its ability to induce intestinal CYP3A2 (Leblond et al., 2002). These data are consistent with findings in patients with ESRD, in whom rifampin was successfully used to induce CYP3A activity (Dowling et al., 2003). This suggests that, despite initial reductions in CYP expression, inducibility is maintained. The implications of this are that CYP-mediated drug, diet, and environmental interactions are still legitimate possibilities in patients with CKD.

Evidence suggests that drug reduction, another important phase I metabolic pathway, may be impacted by kidney disease (Table 4.2). For example, the reductase substrate warfarin was used to show that hepatic drug reduction is selectively impaired in the five-sixth nephrectomy rat model of CKD (Alshogran et al., 2015a). Warfarin is a highly metabolized drug that undergoes phase I oxidation mediated by CYP450 enzymes, as well as reduction. The acetonyl side-chain reduction of warfarin by hepatic reductases generates warfarin alcohols. Warfarin reduction results in creation of second chiral center, thus two diastereoisomers of warfarin alcohols are produced: alcohol 1 (*RS/SR*) and alcohol 2 (*RR/SS*) (Chan et al., 1972). The decrease in reductase activity in kidney disease was demonstrated by reduced formation of warfarin alcohol 1 by 39% in cytosol and 43% in microsomes of nephrectomized versus control rats ($n = 10$ per group) (Alshogran et al., 2015a). This study also showed decreased mRNA expression of cytosolic carbonyl reductase 1 (CBR1), aldo-keto reductase 1C3 (AKR1C3), and microsomal 11β-hydroxysteroid dehydrogenase 1 (HSD1) by 34%, 93%, and 35%, respectively, in CKD rats. Additionally, downregulation in protein expression of CBR1, AKR1C18 (encoded by AKR1C3), and 11β-HSD1 by 43%, 76%, and 70%, respectively, was observed in CKD rats (Alshogran et al., 2015a). More recently, human reductase activity and expression was assessed in livers of deceased patients with ESRD ($n = 10$) and control patients without kidney disease ($n = 11$). A 65% decrease in CBR1 protein expression, as well as a trend toward a selective decrease in reductase mRNA expression and activity (using warfarin as a probe substrate), was observed in ESRD livers versus controls (Alshogran et al., 2015b). Together, these findings suggest that kidney disease may selectively impair hepatic reductase function and expression.

Phase II drug metabolism pathways are also vital for the elimination of drugs. Uridine diphosphate-glucuronosyltransferase (UGT)-mediated glucuronidation and N-acetyltransferase (NAT)-mediated acetylation are among the most important phase II metabolic pathways and have been evaluated in the five-sixth nephrectomy rat model of CKD. Although hepatic UGTs have been shown to be unaffected in this model (Yu et al., 2006), decreases of more than 30% in hepatic protein and mRNA expression of NAT1 and NAT2 have been demonstrated (Table 4.2) (Simard et al., 2008). A 50% decrease in N-acetylation of p-aminobenzoic acid by NAT2 was also observed in vitro. The purported uremic toxin parathyroid hormone may be involved in the mechanism of the enzyme inhibition since parathyroidectomy prevented the decreases in NAT functional expression (Simard et al., 2008).

Metabolism in Experimental Models of Acute Kidney Injury (Acute Renal Failure)

In contrast to the commonly used five-sixth nephrectomy rat model of CKD described earlier, several models of AKI (formerly known as acute renal failure) have been used and striking differences in results have been reported (Table 4.3) (Lane et al., 2013). Numerous investigations employing many different phenotypic probe drugs and animals (e.g., rats, dogs, and rabbits) illustrate this point (Gurley et al., 1997; Lee et al., 1992; Choi et al., 2001). For instance, the PK of the macrolide antibiotics clarithromycin and telithromycin were assessed in rats with uranyl nitrate−induced AKI, and no change in CL_{NR} was observed, suggesting that CYP3A metabolism was unchanged (Lee et al., 2004; Lee and Lee, 2007). Similar findings of unaltered CYP3A activity were reported in a gentamicin-induced AKI model using cyclosporine as a phenotypic probe drug (Shibata et al., 2004). On the other hand, others have reported altered metabolic clearance, presumably via CYP3A, of etoposide and losartan in rats with uranyl nitrate−induced AKI (Venkatesh et al., 2007; Yoshitani et al., 2002). Decreased CYP3A activity was also reported following cisplatin-induced AKI in rats, based on decreased clearance of tacrolimus and quinidine (Okabe et al., 2002; Izuwa et al., 2009), following folate-induced AKI in rabbits (Choi et al., 2001), and following renal ischemia−reperfusion injury in rabbits based on altered cyclosporine clearance (Table 4.3) (Karim et al., 1990).

Using the bilateral renal ischemia−reperfusion AKI model in rats, DNA microarray technology, and reverse transcription polymerase chain reaction, Yoshida et al. (2002) demonstrated a rapid and significant reduction in CYP2D expression. Expression declined to 20% of that observed in sham controls within 24 h, then gradually increased as kidney function improved to approximately 70% of control by day four. Conversely, AKI induced by bilateral ureteric ligation or by glycerol did not result in altered CYP2D6-mediated metabolism of

TABLE 4.3   Alterations in CYPs Observed in Various Experimental Models of AKI

Substrate	CYP(s) Assessed	Animal	Model	Effect on Metabolism	References
Antipyrine	1A, 2B, 2C8, 2C9, 2C18, 3A	Dog	IRI	Decreased	Gurley et al. (1997)
Clarithromycin	3A	Rat	UN	No change	Lee et al. (2004)
Cyclosporine	3A	Rat	Gent	No change	Shibata et al. (2004)
Cyclosporine	3A	Rabbit	IRI	Decreased	Karim et al. (1990)
Diltiazem	3A	Rat	UN	Decreased	Lee et al. (1992)
Diltiazem	3A	Rabbit	Folate	Decreased	Choi et al. (2001)
Etoposide	3A	Rat	UN	Decreased	Venkatesh et al. (2007)
Losartan	2C9, 3A	Rat	UN, BUL	Decreased	Yoshitani et al. (2002)
Metoprolol	2D	Rat	BUL	No change	Okabe et al. (2004)
Metoprolol	2D	Rat	Glycerol	No change	Tanabe et al. (2007)
Mirodenafil	1A, 2B, 2D, 3A	Rat	UN	Increased	Choi et al. (2009)
Propranolol	2D	Rat	Cisplatin	No change	Okabe et al. (2003)
Propranolol	2D	Rat	BUL	Decreased	Okabe et al. (2004)
Quinidine	3A	Rat	Cisplatin, Glycerol	Decreased	Izuwa et al. (2009)
Tacrolimus	3A	Rat	Cisplatin	Decreased	Okabe et al. (2002)
Telithromycin	3A	Rat	UN	No change	Lee and Lee (2007)
Theophylline	2E1	Rat	UN	Increased	Yu (2002)

AKI, acute kidney injury; *BUL*, bilateral ureteral ligation; *CYP*, cytochrome P450; *Gent*, gentamicin; *IRI*, ischemia reperfusion injury; *UN*, uranyl nitrate.
Adapted from Lane, K., Dixon J.J., MacPhee, I.A., Philips, B.J., 2013. Renohepatic crosstalk: does acute kidney injury cause liver dysfunction? Nephrol. Dial. Transplant. 28, 1634–1647.

metoprolol (Tanabe et al., 2007; Okabe et al., 2004), and cisplatin-induced AKI had no effect on CYP2D6-mediated metabolism of propranolol (Okabe et al., 2003). However, increased propranolol concentrations were observed when AKI was induced by bilateral ureteric ligation in rats, suggesting that CYP2D6 activity was decreased (Okabe et al., 2003). Lastly, uranyl nitrate–induced AKI reportedly led to increased metabolic clearance of mirodenafil (Choi et al., 2009), a substrate of several CYPs, as well as theophylline, presumably by CYP2E1 (Yu, 2002). Interestingly, CYP2E1 expression is increased up to fourfold in rats with uranyl nitrate–induced AKI (Chung et al., 2002). Collectively, these findings suggest that drug metabolism is altered in the setting of experimental AKI, but disparate results indicate that AKI model–specific differences exist.

INFLUENCE OF KIDNEY DISEASE ON DRUG METABOLISM IN HUMANS

The assessment of drug metabolism in humans with kidney disease is limited to determination of PK parameters in patients with impaired kidney function when compared with healthy control subjects. When highly hepatically metabolized compounds (i.e., fraction of drug excreted unchanged in the urine $<5-10\%$) exhibit altered CL_T (in the absence of blood flow or protein binding changes), one may assume that it is due to a change in CL_{NR}, and in fact, a change in intrinsic metabolic activity in the liver (CL_{INT}). When drugs are eliminated by more than one CL_{NR} pathway, then only general conclusions can be drawn regarding those pathways. Conversely, direct phenotypic assessments of metabolic pathways are possible using specific probe drugs (Tucker et al., 2001). In either scenario, the assessment and interpretation of CL_{NR} changes in kidney disease within the context of drug metabolism requires knowledge of the specificity of the substrate for individual CL_{NR} pathways. Fortunately, the last decade has witnessed an enormous increase in our understanding of CL_{NR} pathways and the impact of overlapping substrate specificity on the interpretation of PK findings (Benet, 2009). In turn, this has enabled investigators to elucidate the effects of disease states on specific pathways.

Altered Nonrenal Clearance

Numerous drugs that exhibit altered CL_{NR} in patients with impaired kidney function are listed in Table 4.4. For many of these drugs, CL_{NR} decreases as kidney function declines, i.e., as kidney disease progresses. Also, for many of the drugs that undergo first-pass metabolism in the intestine and/or liver (e.g., erythromycin and nicardipine), an increase in oral bioavailability has been reported. The pathways responsible for the CL_{NR} of some drugs are unclear, so one cannot readily extrapolate these observations to other structurally similar compounds. Additionally, CL_{NR} may decline over time in patients with AKI as the duration of AKI is prolonged. For example, the CL_{NR} of imipenem and vancomycin is higher in subjects with AKI than in those with CKD but declines over time and may eventually approach values similar to those seen in patients with CKD (Macias et al., 1991; Mueller et al., 1993).

Reports of altered PK of known CYP substrates illustrate the influence of CKD on oxidative metabolism. CYP3A is highly expressed in human liver and metabolizes a large percentage of drugs in current clinical use, so it is not surprising that CYP3A substrates have extensively been studied (Zhang et al., 2009). The hypoglycemic agent repaglinide is predominantly metabolized by CYP2C8 and CYP3A4 followed by biliary excretion in normal volunteers, with $<0.1\%$ of parent drug excreted unchanged in the urine (van Heiningen et al., 1999; Niemi et al., 2001, 2003; Guay, 1998). Although PK parameters are similar in the presence of mild-to-moderate CKD to those observed in subjects with normal kidney function, the mean $t_{1/2}$ increased nearly fourfold after a week of treatment in patients with severe CKD, and the area under the plasma-concentration time curve (AUC) was significantly higher after both single and multiple dosing (Marbury et al., 2000; Schumacher et al., 2001). No differences in the maximal serum concentrations were observed, suggesting that oral bioavailability

TABLE 4.4   Selected Drugs Exhibiting Decreased Nonrenal Clearance and/or Increased Bioavailability in Patients With Impaired Kidney Function

Acyclovir	Cilastatin	Ketoprofen	Propranolol
Alfuzosin	Cimetidine	Ketorolac	Quinapril
Aliskiren	Ciprofloxacin	Lanthanum	Raloxifene
Aprepitant	Cyclophosphamide	Lidocaine	Ranolazine
Aztreonam	Darifenacin	Lomefloxacin	Reboxetine
Bufurolol	Desmethyldiazepam	Losartan	Repaglinide
Bupropion	Diacerein	Lovastatin	Rosuvastatin
Captopril	Didanosine	Metoclopromide	Roxithromycin
Carvedilol	Dihydrocodeine	Minoxidil	Sildenafil
Caspofungin	Doxorubicin	Morphine	Simvastatin
Cefepime	Duloxetine	Moxalactam	Solifenacin
Cefmenoxime	Encainide	Naltrexone	Sparfloxacin
Cefmetazole	Eprosartan	Nefopam	Tacrolimus
Cefonicid	Erythromycin	Nicardipine	Tadalafil
Cefotaxime	Felbamate	Nimodipine	Telithromycin
Cefsulodin	Fexofenadine	Nitrendipine	Valsartan
Ceftibuten	Fluorouracil	Nortriptyline	Vancomycin
Ceftizoxime	Guanadrel	Oxcarbazepine	Vardenafil
Ceftriaxone	Idarubicin	Oxprenolol	Verapamil
Cerivastatin	Imipenem	Procainamide	Warfarin
Cibenzoline	Isoniazid	Propoxyphene	Zidovudine

Adapted in part from Nolin, T.D., 2008. Altered nonrenal drug clearance in ESRD. Curr. Opin. Nephrol. Hypertens. 17, 555–559, Momper, J.D., Venkataramanan, R., Nolin, T.D., 2010. Nonrenal drug clearance in CKD: searching for the path less traveled. Adv. Chronic Kidney Dis. 17, 384–391, and Yeung, C.K., Shen, D.D., Thummel, K.E., Himmelfarb, J., 2014. Effects of chronic kidney disease and uremia on hepatic drug metabolism and transport. Kidney Int. 85, 522–528.

was also not different. These data suggest that intrinsic hepatic clearance of repaglinide mediated by CYP2C8 and/or CYP3A4 is decreased in subjects with severe CKD.

Reboxetine is a selective norepinephrine reuptake inhibitor that is eliminated via CYP3A4-mediated metabolism (Wienkers et al., 1999), with only 9% of the parent drug excreted unchanged in the urine (Edwards et al., 1995). Like repaglinide, it also exhibits decreased CL_{NR} in patients with severe CKD (Coulomb et al., 2000). The AUC and $t_{1/2}$ values observed in subjects with severe CKD (creatinine clearance 10–20 mL/min) after a single 4-mg dose were more than twice those previously demonstrated in healthy subjects

(Edwards et al., 1995; Coulomb et al., 2000). Furthermore, CL_{NR} was decreased by 67% compared with healthy subjects. The phosphodiesterase type 5 enzyme inhibitor tadalafil, which is predominantly metabolized by CYP3A4, exhibits even more pronounced changes with up to fourfold higher AUCs in patients with ESRD compared with healthy subjects (Zhang et al., 2009). Overall, data from the above-mentioned and other clinical studies suggest the most likely explanation for increased exposure and decreased systemic clearance of nonspecific CYP3A substrates in subjects with advanced CKD is decreased metabolic clearance. Together with numerous reports of decreased expression and activity of hepatic CYP3A in experimental models of CKD and AKI, the logical and frequent conclusion has been that hepatic CYP3A function is altered in patients with impaired kidney function (Momper et al., 2010).

Altered PK of multiple reductase drug substrates have also been demonstrated in patients with impaired kidney function. For example, idarubicin is an anthracycline anticancer drug that undergoes reduction to produce idarubicinol. The drug is extensively metabolized by reductase enzymes, specifically AKR and CBR (Kang and Weiss, 2003), with 3–5% of the parent drug excreted unchanged in the urine (Tamassia et al., 1987; Robert, 1993). The PK of idarubicin were investigated in patients with cancer with varying levels of kidney function after a rapid single-dose intravenous infusion of $12 \, mg/m^2$ (Camaggi et al., 1992). A 30% decrease in the total clearance was reported in patients with creatinine clearance of <60 mL/min compared with subjects with normal kidney function. A corresponding 38% increase in idarubicin exposure (AUC) was also observed in patients with kidney disease. These findings strongly suggest that hepatic reduction of idarubicin is impaired in the setting of kidney disease.

Similarly, the PK of the anthracycline agent doxorubicin were evaluated in hemodialysis patients and control subjects after intravenous infusion of 40–60 mg (Yoshida et al., 1994). A 71% increase in AUC and a 41% decrease in the total clearance of doxorubicin were observed in hemodialysis patients compared with the control group. The compartmental analysis of the data indicated that increased doxorubicin exposure in patients with HD resulted from decreased formation of the alcohol metabolite (doxorubicinol) (Yoshida et al., 1994). Metabolic reduction of doxorubicin is primarily mediated by CBR1 and AKR1C3 (Kassner et al., 2008). Therefore, changes in doxorubicin PK in CKD may be attributed to altered metabolic clearance by these isoforms.

Several other hepatic reductase drug substrates, including bupropion, dolasetron, ketoprofen, naltrexone, and oxcarbazepine, have been reported to exhibit significant PK changes in patients with impaired kidney function. Given the contribution of reductases to elimination of these drugs (Malatkova and Wsol, 2014; Barski et al., 2008), the alterations in their disposition suggest that metabolic reduction may be modulated in kidney disease. For example, PK studies of bupropion suggest that its metabolic clearance is decreased in patients with kidney disease. Bupropion is a highly metabolized drug that undergoes phase I oxidation and reduction, with <0.5% of parent drug excreted unchanged in urine (Lai and Schroeder, 1983). Oxidation is primarily mediated by CYP2B6 (Faucette et al., 2000), and reduction is catalyzed by multiple reductase isoforms including AKR1C1 and 11β-HSD1 (Skarydova et al., 2014; Molnari and Myers, 2012). Bupropion AUC and maximal plasma concentrations were 126% and 86% higher, respectively, and the apparent oral clearance was 63% lower in patients with kidney disease (mean GFR 31 mL/min) compared with healthy control subjects after single-dose oral administration (Turpeinen et al., 2007). CYP2B6 genotype did not account for the differences observed. Reduced bupropion clearance has also been reported in patients with glomerular kidney disease with preserved kidney function (mean creatinine clearance 102 mL/min) (Joy et al., 2010), suggesting that altered metabolic capacity may not be restricted to uremic patients with advanced kidney disease. Overall, these findings likely suggest that bupropion metabolic clearance mediated by CYP2B6, AKR1C1, and/or 11β-HSD1 is decreased in patients with kidney disease.

Decreases in CL_{NR} of some drugs that undergo conjugative metabolism have also been described (Debord et al., 1994; Kim et al., 1993; Osborne et al., 1993). The PK of isoniazid, a NAT2 substrate, were evaluated in patients with ESRD before and after kidney transplantation (Kim et al., 1993). Isoniazid CL_{NR} was increased more than 50% and 225% posttransplant in rapid and slow acetylators, respectively. This suggests that NAT activity is decreased in ESRD and may indicate that NAT function is impacted to a greater extent in patients with CKD exhibiting the slow acetylator phenotype. Moreover, clearance of isoniazid and procainamide (also a NAT substrate) in patients with CKD is significantly decreased compared with healthy subjects after stratifying both groups into rapid and slow acetylators (Kim et al., 1993; Gibson et al., 1977).

Decreased metabolism has been implicated in the significant increase in AUC and decrease in clearance of morphine in patients with CKD compared with normal volunteers (Osborne et al., 1993). Morphine is primarily glucuronidated by UGT2B7 and UGT1A3, suggesting that UGT-mediated metabolic clearance is decreased in kidney disease. Similarly, CL_{NR} of the nonsteroidal antiinflammatory agent diacerein, which is primarily hepatically metabolized, undergoing 60% glucuronidation and 20% sulfation (Nicolas et al., 1998), is decreased by nearly 40% in subjects with CKD compared with those with normal kidney function (Debord et al., 1994). Lastly, glucuronidation of zidovudine is also changed in CKD subjects compared with healthy subjects, with significant decreases in its apparent oral clearance and CL_{NR} of 52% and 48%, respectively (Singlas et al., 1989).

Phenotypic Assessments of Metabolic Pathways in Kidney Disease

Direct assessments of CYP activity in vivo, including patients with kidney disease, has been facilitated by recognition and use of isoform-specific probe drugs (Streetman et al., 2000). This has minimized, if not overcome, well-known limitations of nonselective CYP probes, which have generated conflicting results (Teunissen et al., 1985; Lanchote et al., 1996), and has provided a clearer phenotypic picture of drug metabolism in kidney disease. The activities of CYPs 2E1, 2D6, and 2C19 have been assessed in patients with CKD using the probes chlorzoxazone (CZ) (Nolin et al., 2003), mephenytoin (MP) (Nolin et al., 2007), and sparteine (Kevorkian et al., 1996), respectively.

CZ, a centrally acting skeletal muscle relaxant, is used extensively as a phenotypic probe because of its relative safety and selectivity (Lucas et al., 1999). The drug is extensively hydroxylated by CYP2E1 to form 6-hydroxychlorzoxazone (6-HCZ), and the formation clearance of 6-HCZ (i.e., CYP2E1-mediated metabolic clearance of CZ to 6-HCZ) is a commonly used phenotypic index of CYP2E1 activity. No relationship between 6-HCZ formation clearance and kidney function was observed in patients with varying levels of kidney function, and CZ PK parameters were similar to those previously reported in subjects with normal kidney function, indicating that kidney disease does not affect CYP2E1 activity (Nolin et al., 2003).

The anticonvulsant agent MP is a racemic mixture of optical enantiomers, R-mephenytoin (R-MP) and S-mephenytoin (S-MP), that exhibit stereoselective metabolism (Wilkinson et al., 1989). S-MP undergoes rapid hydroxylation via CYP2C19 to form 4'-hydroxymephenytoin (HMP), whereas R-MP is slowly demethylated (Goldstein et al., 1994). As such, MP has been used as a phenotypic probe, with HMP formation clearance reflecting CYP2C19 activity. After single-dose administration to patients with varying levels of kidney function, PK analysis revealed that the AUC of S-MP and HMP formation clearance was not affected by kidney disease. Specifically, no relationship between kidney function and S-MP AUC or HMP formation clearance was observed, indicating that CYP2C19 activity is not changed in patients with CKD (Nolin et al., 2007).

Sparteine, a class 1A antiarrhythmic agent, is a prototypical CYP2D6 substrate and phenotypic probe (Streetman et al., 2000). It is rapidly metabolized by CYP2D6 to form 5- and 2-dehydrosparteine. A PK study of sparteine in patients with CKD demonstrated a 49% decrease in dehydrosparteine formation clearance compared with controls (Kevorkian et al., 1996). These data suggest that CYP2D6 activity declines in the setting of impaired kidney function (Rostami-Hodjegan et al., 1999). A systematic and quantitative analysis of CYP2D6 substrates by investigators at the Food and Drug Administration (FDA) corroborates these findings (Yoshida et al., 2016). Specifically, PK data generated from dedicated CKD studies were available for 13 CYP2D6 drug substrates. Analysis of these data indicated that CYP2D6-mediated clearance is generally decreased in parallel with the severity of CKD (Yoshida et al., 2016).

CYP2C9 activity has been assessed in patients with ESRD utilizing warfarin (Dreisbach et al., 2003). The S-enantiomer of warfarin is primarily metabolized by CYP2C9, whereas R-warfarin is metabolized by multiple CYPs. The plasma S/R warfarin ratio has been used as a measure of CYP2C9 activity in vivo. The ratio was increased by 51% in patients with ESRD compared with control individuals ($p < .02$), suggesting a decrease in CYP2C9 activity in ESRD (Dreisbach et al., 2003).

As described previously, numerous reports of decreased CYP3A functional expression in experimental models of CKD and AKI, along with PK data from extensive clinical studies of nonspecific CYP3A substrates, have led many to conclude that hepatic CYP3A function is altered in patients with impaired kidney function. However, studies that take into consideration enzyme—transporter interplay and overlapping substrate specificity have employed more specific phenotypic probes to interrogate CL_{NR} pathways in humans, showing inconsistent results and suggesting that CYP3A is probably not significantly impacted by CKD (Yoshida et al., 2016; Nolin et al., 2009; Thomson et al., 2015). Studies using erythromycin versus midazolam and fexofenadine as phenotypic probes illustrate this point.

Hepatic metabolism has been assessed in patients with ESRD utilizing various formulations of erythromycin (Dowling et al., 2003; Nolin et al., 2006; Frassetto et al., 2007; Sun et al., 2010), which was long considered an excellent phenotypic probe of CYP3A4. In particular, the ^{14}C-EBT was commonly used for this purpose (Rivory et al., 2001). It is based on the principle that erythromycin is N-demethylated by CYP3A4 and the demethylated carbon rapidly appears in the breath as carbon dioxide. Thus, when the erythromycin

N-methyl carbon is labeled with ^{14}C, activity of CYP3A4 may be estimated from changes in the rate of production of radiolabeled carbon dioxide ($^{14}CO_2$) in the breath (Rivory and Watkins, 2001). According to the standard interpretation, a decrease in excretion of $^{14}CO_2$ translated into a reduction in CYP3A4 activity, and an increase in excretion of $^{14}CO_2$ translated into an increase in CYP3A4 activity. Previous studies showed that $^{14}CO_2$ excretion was decreased by 28% in patients with ESRD compared with individuals with normal kidney function (Dowling et al., 2003) and that hemodialysis significantly improves $^{14}CO_2$ excretion by 27%, indicating that erythromycin clearance is increased postdialysis (Nolin et al., 2006). Again, based on the standard interpretation, these results suggest that hemodialysis acutely improves altered hepatic CYP3A4 activity in ESRD. However, it is now known that erythromycin also undergoes organic anion transporting polypeptide (OATP) uptake and P-glycoprotein (P-gp) efflux in the liver (Frassetto et al., 2007; Kurnik et al., 2006) and that alterations in transporters but not CYP3A4, per se, may result in significant changes in the PK of CYP3A4 substrates like erythromycin (Frassetto et al., 2007; Sun et al., 2010; Lam et al., 2006; Lau et al., 2007). In fact, improved excretion of $^{14}CO_2$ postdialysis may indicate that OATP-mediated hepatic uptake of erythromycin is increased, which then increases the amount of intracellular substrate available for CYP3A4 metabolism, resulting in increased $^{14}CO_2$ excretion (Nolin et al., 2006). Since the PK of midazolam, a selective phenotypic probe of CYP3A, which is neither a P-gp nor an OATP transporter substrate, and its 1-hydroxymidazolam metabolite are not altered in patients with ESRD, it is unlikely that hepatic CYP3A function is affected (Nolin et al., 2009). This is mechanistically corroborated by studies showing that the apparent oral clearance of the OATP substrate fexofenadine is decreased in patients with CKD with and without ESRD (Nolin et al., 2009; Thomson et al., 2015) and that OATP-mediated uptake of erythromycin is directly inhibited by the uremic toxin 3-carboxy-4-methyl-5-propyl-2-furanpropanoic acid (Sun et al., 2004), suggesting that this may be a mechanism by which the hepatic clearance of erythromycin is decreased in kidney disease. A clinical PK study of orally and intravenously administered erythromycin in patients with ESRD demonstrated that hepatic clearance but not oral absorption is significantly reduced (Sun et al., 2010), further supporting the concept that hepatic OATP uptake is decreased in ESRD. Conflicting results have been reported, however, with studies reporting that midazolam clearance was significantly decreased in patients with ESRD (Thomson et al., 2015) and AKI (Kirwan et al., 2012). Systematic analyses by FDA investigators of PK data generated from dedicated CKD studies further demonstrates inconsistent effects of kidney disease on CYP3A (Zhang et al., 2009; Yoshida et al., 2016). Analysis of PK data for 18 CYP3A4/5 drug substrates revealed no apparent relationship between the severity of CKD and metabolic drug clearance, suggesting that CYP3A4/5 is probably not significantly impacted by CKD (Yoshida et al., 2016). Collectively, inconsistent findings surrounding the effect of kidney disease on CYP3A metabolic function likely indicate a small to negligible effect and may indicate that altered drug disposition in CKD previously thought to be due to a reduction in CYP3A-mediated hepatic metabolism may in fact be a manifestation of altered drug transport pathways. Clearly, further mechanistically focused research is required to elucidate the effect of kidney disease on CYP3A function in humans.

MECHANISMS OF ALTERED DRUG METABOLISM IN KIDNEY DISEASE

The underlying mechanism of the changes in drug-metabolizing enzyme activity and expression observed in kidney disease is unclear. The most commonly proposed explanation is that substances that are normally excreted by the kidneys, also known as "uremic toxins," (e.g., urea, parathyroid hormone, indoxyl sulfate, *p*-cresol, cytokines) are responsible for either (1) transcriptional or translational modifications or (2) direct competitive inhibition of the metabolic enzyme (Nolin et al., 2008).

Modified Gene or Protein Expression

As presented in Table 4.2, numerous preclinical studies utilizing the five-sixth nephrectomy rat model of CRF have demonstrated broad changes in the expression of phase I and II metabolic enzymes. Decreased expression of mRNA and protein have been demonstrated in the intestine and liver with corresponding changes in enzyme function (Leblond et al., 2001, 2000, 2002; Simard et al., 2008; Yu et al., 2006; Alshogran et al., 2015a). Although the precise mechanism is unknown, uremic toxins may exert effects on gene transcription (Toell et al., 1999; Beigneux et al., 2002). For instance, uremic plasma ultrafiltrate and peritoneal dialyzate have been shown to inhibit vitamin D receptor (VDR)-retinoid X receptor (RXR) heterodimerization and attenuate activation of vitamin D responsive genes, including CYP3A4 (Toell et al., 1999; Schmiedlin-Ren et al., 2001). Proinflammatory cytokines and mediators of the acute phase response (e.g., interleukin-1, interleukin-6, interferon, tumor necrosis factor-α), which are well-known uremic toxins (Neirynck et al., 2013), are associated with downregulation of CYPs (see Chapter 2) (Morgan et al., 2008). It is known that pregnane X receptor (PXR), constitutive androstane receptor, and RXR mRNA expression are downregulated during the acute phase response (Beigneux et al., 2002), and PXR and RXR are involved in the regulation of CYP3A (Liddle and Goodwin, 2002). CKD is a chronic inflammatory state, and these patients are subject to increased levels of oxidative stress (Akchurin and Kaskel, 2015), so it is possible that PXR and/or RXR are chronically downregulated leading to alterations in drug metabolism. Furthermore, decreased PXR and hepatocyte nuclear factor-4α binding to the promoters of CYP2C11 and CYP3A2 may decrease transcription in CKD (Velenosi et al., 2014). AKI may impact metabolic pathways in a similar fashion, as the mRNA expression of peroxisome proliferator-activated receptor (PPAR)α and PPARγ is downregulated in animal models of AKI (Yoshida et al., 2002; Portilla et al., 2002). Moreover, a study in critically ill patients with AKI demonstrated not only that the metabolic clearance of the CYP3A4/5 probe midazolam was decreased, but also that the magnitude of the decrease associated with the severity and duration of AKI (Kirwan et al., 2012). This may support the idea that altered gene transcription and/or protein translation are responsible.

Transcriptionally mediated alterations in drug-metabolizing enzymes have also been shown in several experiments utilizing primary cultures of rat hepatocytes (Guevin et al., 2002; Michaud et al., 2005, 2006, 2008). For example, after incubating normal rat hepatocytes with uremic serum obtained from five-sixth nephrectomized rats, the expression of CYPs 2C6, 2C11, 3A1 (3A23), and 3A2 protein was decreased up to 57% (Guevin et al., 2002).

In addition, CYP2C11 and CYP3A2 mRNA expression was decreased 27% and 36%, respectively. The impact of varying molecular weight fractions of uremic serum was also studied by incubating normal hepatocytes with one of three subfractions: <10, 10–30, and >30 kDa CYP3A2 expression was reduced by 40% when in the presence of the 10–30 kDa uremic subfraction compared with control (Guevin et al., 2002). Subsequent work that investigated the effects of incubating hepatocytes with human sera obtained from patients with ESRD showed similar results (Michaud et al., 2008). Specifically, serum drawn immediately prehemodialysis (presumably maximally uremic), resulted in significant reductions in CYPs 1A (44%), 2C (27%), and 3A (35%) protein expression compared with control serum, whereas dialyzed serum (obtained immediately posthemodialysis) had no effect. Moreover, mRNA expression of CYPs 1A2, 2C11, and 3A2 were similarly impacted by uremic serum and were improved to >80% of control values after incubation with dialyzed serum. Interestingly, nuclear factor-κB (NF-κB) inhibition nearly eliminated the effect of prehemodialysis serum on CYP expression, suggesting that NF-κB is a key transcriptional factor in CYP downregulation observed in uremia (Michaud et al., 2008). Parathyroid hormone acts via the NF-κB signaling pathway and has been implicated as a potential uremic mediator of drug metabolism (Michaud et al., 2006).

Posttranslational Modifications (Direct Competitive Inhibition)

In addition to modified gene and protein expression, kidney disease also appears to elicit acute, posttranslational modifications in drug-metabolizing enzymes. Uremic blood and plasma are capable of inducing acute changes in CYP activity when placed in contact with normal hepatic tissue for short periods of time (i.e., minutes), presumably caused by circulating uremic toxins that act as competitive inhibitors (Taburet et al., 1996). Classic isolated rat liver cross-perfusion experiments explored this phenomenon by assessing the hepatic extraction, reflecting primarily intrinsic metabolic clearance, of the CYP2D6 substrate propranolol (Terao and Shen, 1985). Perfusion of normal rat livers with uremic blood obtained from rats with uranyl nitrate–induced AKI resulted in more than a 50% decrease in the hepatic extraction of propranolol compared with control (normal liver perfused with normal blood); the reduced clearance was nearly identical to that observed when uremic livers from AKI rats were perfused with uremic blood. Furthermore, perfusion of uremic liver with normal blood increased the clearance of propranolol to values nearly identical to that observed in controls (Terao and Shen, 1985). This work implicates the presence of rapidly acting substances in uremic blood that decrease the function of metabolizing enzymes in the liver.

Comparable findings have been observed in microsomal incubations. Metabolism of the angiotensin II receptor antagonist losartan, a substrate of CYP2C9 and CYP3A4, in hepatic microsomes prepared from normal rats was decreased by nearly 50% in the presence of uremic serum obtained from rats in two different experimental models of AKI (ureteral ligation or uranyl nitrate). Moreover, losartan metabolism was decreased by about 30% in the presence of the uremic toxin indoxyl sulfate alone (Yoshitani et al., 2002). Similarly, healthy human liver microsomes were incubated with the CYP2C9 probe tolbutamide and the CYP3A4 probe midazolam in the presence of uremic human plasma obtained from patients with

ESRD. The activities of CYPs 3A4 and 2C9 were decreased 80% and nearly 40%, respectively, compared with control (Taburet et al., 1996).

Data derived from humans provide additional evidence of posttranslational modifications of nonrenal clearance pathways in kidney disease. As described previously, studies using the EBT showed hemodialysis significantly improves $^{14}CO_2$ excretion in patients with ESRD, indicating that erythromycin clearance is increased postdialysis (Nolin et al., 2006). This phenomenon has also been reported with the CYP3A4 substrate telithromycin (Shi et al., 2004) and the CYP2D6 substrate propranolol (Bianchetti et al., 1976). The acuity of the response suggests that improvements in hepatic clearance, likely reflecting drug metabolism and/or transport, occur independent of transcriptional or translational modification, and therefore that a rapidly acting, dialyzable by-product of uremia acutely inhibits hepatic clearance pathways (Nolin et al., 2006).

SUMMARY

The nonrenal clearance of many drugs is altered in patients with CKD, which may be due to selective modulation of metabolizing enzyme activity and expression. Transcriptional, translational, and posttranslational modification, perhaps induced by uremic toxins, have been reported. Patients with CKD are prescribed numerous medications, and commonly receive treatment with drugs that are predominantly cleared by nonrenal metabolic pathways. For example, according to the 2015 United States Renal Data System Annual Data Report, statins and beta blockers were each prescribed to more than 50% of patients with CKD enrolled in Medicare Part D stand-alone prescription drug plans during 2013, and over one-third received a calcium channel blocker (United States Renal Data System, 2015). Thus, the likelihood of adverse consequences from medication use may be extraordinarily high. The US FDA has substantiated the significance of this issue in 2010. The FDA, in a guidance document providing recommendations regarding the conduction of PK studies in patients with impaired kidney function, now advise that studies be conducted for investigational compounds eliminated primarily via hepatic metabolism as well as those eliminated predominantly unchanged in the urine (U.S. Food and Drug Administration, 2010). Nevertheless, current data are limited regarding drug metabolism in humans with kidney disease. Knowledge of the impact and nature of the alterations in metabolism induced by kidney disease will hopefully enhance the safe and effective use of drugs in this patient population.

References

Akchurin, O.M., Kaskel, F., 2015. Update on inflammation in chronic kidney disease. Blood Purif. 39, 84–92.

Alshogran, O.Y., Naud, J., Ocque, A.J., Leblond, F.A., Pichette, V., Nolin, T.D., 2015a. Effect of experimental kidney disease on the functional expression of hepatic reductases. Drug Metab. Dispos. 43, 100–106.

Alshogran, O.Y., Urquhart, B.L., Nolin, T.D., 2015b. Downregulation of hepatic carbonyl reductase type 1 in end-stage renal disease. Drug Metab. Lett. 9, 111–118.

Atkinson Jr., A.J., Huang, S.M., 2009. Nephropharmacology: drugs and the kidney. Clin. Pharmacol. Ther. 86, 453–456.

Balant, L.P., Dayer, P., Fabre, J., 1983. Consequences of renal insufficiency on the hepatic clearance of some drugs. Int. J. Clin. Pharmacol. Res. 3, 459–474.

Barski, O.A., Tipparaju, S.M., Bhatnagar, A., 2008. The aldo-keto reductase superfamily and its role in drug metabolism and detoxification. Drug Metab. Rev. 40, 553–624.

Bates, D.W., Miller, E.B., Cullen, D.J., et al., 1999. Patient risk factors for adverse drug events in hospitalized patients. ADE Prevention Study Group. Arch. Intern. Med. 159, 2553–2560.

Beigneux, A.P., Moser, A.H., Shigenaga, J.K., Grunfeld, C., Feingold, K.R., 2002. Reduction in cytochrome P-450 enzyme expression is associated with repression of CAR (constitutive androstane receptor) and PXR (pregnane X receptor) in mouse liver during the acute phase response. Biochem. Biophys. Res. Commun. 293, 145–149.

Benet, L.Z., Cummins, C.L., Wu, C.Y., 2003. Transporter-enzyme interactions: implications for predicting drug-drug interactions from in vitro data. Curr. Drug Metab. 4, 393–398.

Benet, L.Z., Cummins, C.L., Wu, C.Y., 2004. Unmasking the dynamic interplay between efflux transporters and metabolic enzymes. Int. J. Pharm. 277, 3–9.

Benet, L.Z., 2009. The drug transporter-metabolism alliance: uncovering and defining the interplay. Mol. Pharm. 6, 1631–1643.

Bennett, W.M., Singer, I., Coggins, C.H., 1970. A practical guide to drug usage in adult patients with impaired renal function. JAMA 214, 1468–1475.

Bennett, W.M., 1988. Guide to drug dosage in renal failure. Clin. Pharmacokinet. 15, 326–354.

Bianchetti, G., Graziani, G., Brancaccio, D., et al., 1976. Pharmacokinetics and effects of propranolol in terminal uraemic patients and in patients undergoing regular dialysis treatment. Clin. Pharmacokinet. 1, 373–384.

Camaggi, C.M., Strocchi, E., Carisi, P., et al., 1992. Idarubicin metabolism and pharmacokinetics after intravenous and oral administration in cancer patients: a crossover study. Cancer Chemother. Pharmacol. 30, 307–316.

Chan, K.K., Lewis, R.J., Trager, W.F., 1972. Absolute configurations of the four warfarin alcohols. J. Med. Chem. 15, 1265–1270.

Chiu, Y.W., Teitelbaum, I., Misra, M., de Leon, E.M., Adzize, T., Mehrotra, R., 2009. Pill burden, adherence, hyperphosphatemia, and quality of life in maintenance dialysis patients. Clin. J. Am. Soc. Nephrol. 4, 1089–1096.

Choi, J.S., Lee, J.H., Burm, J.P., 2001. Pharmacokinetics of diltiazem and its major metabolite, deacetyldiltiazem after oral administration of diltiazem in mild and medium folate-induced renal failure rabbits. Arch. Pharm. Res. 24, 333–337.

Choi, Y.H., Lee, Y.S., Kim, T.K., Lee, B.Y., Lee, M.G., 2009. Faster clearance of mirodenafil in rats with acute renal failure induced by uranyl nitrate: contribution of increased protein expression of hepatic CYP3A1 and intestinal CYP1A1 and 3A1/2. J. Pharm. Pharmacol. 61, 1325–1332.

Chung, H.C., Kim, S.H., Lee, M.G., Kim, S.G., 2002. Increase in urea in conjunction with L-arginine metabolism in the liver leads to induction of cytochrome P450 2E1 (CYP2E1): the role of urea in CYP2E1 induction by acute renal failure. Drug Metab. Dispos. 30, 739–746.

Coulomb, F., Ducret, F., Laneury, J.P., et al., 2000. Pharmacokinetics of single-dose reboxetine in volunteers with renal insufficiency. J. Clin. Pharmacol. 40, 482–487.

Debord, P., Louchahi, K., Tod, M., Cournot, A., Perret, G., Petitjean, O., 1994. Influence of renal function on the pharmacokinetics of diacerein after a single oral dose. Eur. J. Drug Metab. Pharmacokinet. 19, 13–19.

Dettli, L., Spring, P., Habersang, R., 1970. Drug dosage in patients with impaired renal function. Postgrad. Med. J. 32–35. Suppl.

Dettli, L., 1973. Translation of pharmacokinetics to clinical medicine. J. Pharmacokinet. Biopharm. 1, 403–418.

Dettli, L., 1974. Individualization of drug dosage in patients with renal disease. Med. Clin. North Am. 58, 977–985.

Dettli, L., 1976. Drug dosage in renal disease. Clin. Pharmacokinet. 1, 126–134.

Dowling, T.C., Briglia, A.E., Fink, J.C., et al., 2003. Characterization of hepatic cytochrome P4503A activity in patients with end-stage renal disease. Clin. Pharmacol. Ther. 73, 427–434.

Dreisbach, A.W., Japa, S., Gebrekal, A.B., et al., 2003. Cytochrome P4502C9 activity in end-stage renal disease. Clin. Pharmacol. Ther. 73, 475–477.

Edwards, D.M., Pellizzoni, C., Breuel, H.P., et al., 1995. Pharmacokinetics of reboxetine in healthy volunteers. Single oral doses, linearity and plasma protein binding. Biopharm. Drug Dispos. 16, 443–460.

Elston, A.C., Bayliss, M.K., Park, G.R., 1993. Effect of renal failure on drug metabolism by the liver. Br. J. Anaesth. 71, 282–290.

Faucette, S.R., Hawke, R.L., Lecluyse, E.L., et al., 2000. Validation of bupropion hydroxylation as a selective marker of human cytochrome P450 2B6 catalytic activity. Drug Metab. Dispos. 28, 1222–1230.

Frassetto, L.A., Poon, S., Tsourounis, C., Valera, C., Benet, L.Z., 2007. Effects of uptake and efflux transporter inhibition on erythromycin breath test results. Clin. Pharmacol. Ther. 81, 828–832.

Gibson, T.P., Atkinson Jr., A.J., Matusik, E., Nelson, L.D., Briggs, W.A., 1977. Kinetics of procainamide and N-acetylprocainamide in renal failure. Kidney Int. 12, 422–429.

Gibson, T.P., 1986. Renal disease and drug metabolism: an overview. Am. J. Kidney Dis. 8, 7–17.

Goldstein, J.A., Faletto, M.B., Romkes-Sparks, M., et al., 1994. Evidence that CYP2C19 is the major (S)-mephenytoin 4'-hydroxylase in humans. Biochemistry 33, 1743–1752.

Guay, D.R., 1998. Repaglinide, a novel, short-acting hypoglycemic agent for type 2 diabetes mellitus. Pharmacotherapy 18, 1195–1204.

Guevin, C., Michaud, J., Naud, J., Leblond, F.A., Pichette, V., 2002. Down-regulation of hepatic cytochrome P450 in chronic renal failure: role of uremic mediators. Br. J. Pharmacol. 137, 1039–1046.

Gurley, B.J., Barone, G.W., Yamashita, K., Polston, S., Estes, M., Harden, A., 1997. Extrahepatic ischemia-reperfusion injury reduces hepatic oxidative drug metabolism as determined by serial antipyrine clearance. Pharm. Res. 14, 67–72.

Huang, S.M., Temple, R., Xiao, S., Zhang, L., Lesko, L.J., 2009. When to conduct a renal impairment study during drug development: US Food and Drug Administration perspective. Clin. Pharmacol. Ther. 86, 475–479.

Hug, B.L., Witkowski, D.J., Sox, C.M., et al., 2009. Occurrence of adverse, often preventable, events in community hospitals involving nephrotoxic drugs or those excreted by the kidney. Kidney Int. 76, 1192–1198.

Ikemoto, S., Imaoka, S., Hayahara, N., Maekawa, M., Funae, Y., 1992. Expression of hepatic microsomal cytochrome P450s as altered by uremia. Biochem. Pharmacol. 43, 2407–2412.

Izuwa, Y., Kusaba, J., Horiuchi, M., Aiba, T., Kawasaki, H., Kurosaki, Y., 2009. Comparative study of increased plasma quinidine concentration in rats with glycerol- and cisplatin-induced acute renal failure. Drug Metab. Pharmacokinet. 24, 451–457.

Joy, M.S., Frye, R.F., Stubbert, K., Brouwer, K.R., Falk, R.J., Kharasch, E.D., 2010. Use of enantiomeric bupropion and hydroxybupropion to assess CYP2B6 activity in glomerular kidney diseases. J. Clin. Pharmacol. 50, 714–720.

Kang, W., Weiss, M., 2003. Modeling the metabolism of idarubicin to idarubicinol in rat heart: effect of rutin and phenobarbital. Drug Metab. Dispos. 31, 462–468.

Karim, M.S., Wood, R.F., Dawnay, A.B., Fulton, P.A., 1990. The effect of renal ischemia on cyclosporine clearance in rabbits. Transplantation 49, 500–502.

Kassner, N., Huse, K., Martin, H.J., et al., 2008. Carbonyl reductase 1 is a predominant doxorubicin reductase in the human liver. Drug Metab. Dispos. 36, 2113–2120.

Kevorkian, J.P., Michel, C., Hofmann, U., et al., 1996. Assessment of individual CYP2D6 activity in extensive metabolizers with renal failure: comparison of sparteine and dextromethorphan. Clin. Pharmacol. Ther. 59, 583–592.

Kim, Y.G., Shin, J.G., Shin, S.G., et al., 1993. Decreased acetylation of isoniazid in chronic renal failure. Clin. Pharmacol. Ther. 54, 612–620.

Kim, R.B., Wandel, C., Leake, B., et al., 1999. Interrelationship between substrates and inhibitors of human CYP3A and P-glycoprotein. Pharm. Res. 16, 408–414.

Kirwan, C.J., MacPhee, I.A., Lee, T., Holt, D.W., Philips, B.J., 2012. Acute kidney injury reduces the hepatic metabolism of midazolam in critically ill patients. Intensive Care Med. 38, 76–84.

Kunin, C.M., 1967. A guide to use of antibiotics in patients with renal disease. A table of recommended doses and factors governing serum levels. Ann. Intern. Med. 67, 151–158.

Kurnik, D., Wood, A.J., Wilkinson, G.R., 2006. The erythromycin breath test reflects P-glycoprotein function independently of cytochrome P450 3A activity. Clin. Pharmacol. Ther. 80, 228–234.

Lai, A.A., Schroeder, D.H., 1983. Clinical pharmacokinetics of bupropion: a review. J. Clin. Psychiatry 44, 82–84.

Lam, J.L., Okochi, H., Huang, Y., Benet, L.Z., 2006. In vitro and in vivo correlation of hepatic transporter effects on erythromycin metabolism: characterizing the importance of transporter-enzyme interplay. Drug Metab. Dispos. 34, 1336–1344.

Lanchote, V.L., Ping, W.C., Santos, S.R., 1996. Influence of renal failure on cytochrome P450 activity in hypertensive patients using a "cocktail" of antipyrine and nifedipine. Eur. J. Clin. Pharmacol. 50, 83–89.

Lane, K., Dixon, J.J., MacPhee, I.A., Philips, B.J., 2013. Renohepatic crosstalk: does acute kidney injury cause liver dysfunction? Nephrol. Dial. Transplant. 28, 1634–1647.

Lau, Y.Y., Huang, Y., Frassetto, L., Benet, L.Z., 2007. Effect of OATP1B transporter inhibition on the pharmacokinetics of atorvastatin in healthy volunteers. Clin. Pharmacol. Ther. 81, 194–204.

Leber, H.W., Schutterle, G., 1972. Oxidative drug metabolism in liver microsomes from uremic rats. Kidney Int. 2, 152—158.

Leber, H.W., Gleumes, L., Schutterle, G., 1978. Enzyme induction in the uremic liver. Kidney Int. 13, S43—S48.

Leblond, F.A., Giroux, L., Villeneuve, J.P., Pichette, V., 2000. Decreased in vivo metabolism of drugs in chronic renal failure. Drug Metab. Dispos. 28, 1317—1320.

Leblond, F., Guevin, C., Demers, C., Pellerin, I., Gascon-Barre, M., Pichette, V., 2001. Downregulation of hepatic cytochrome P450 in chronic renal failure. J. Am. Soc. Nephrol. 12, 326—332.

Leblond, F.A., Petrucci, M., Dube, P., Bernier, G., Bonnardeaux, A., Pichette, V., 2002. Downregulation of intestinal cytochrome P450 in chronic renal failure. J. Am. Soc. Nephrol. 13, 1579—1585.

Lee, J.H., Lee, M.G., 2007. Effects of acute renal failure on the pharmacokinetics of telithromycin in rats: negligible effects of increase in CYP3A1 on the metabolism of telithromycin. Biopharm. Drug Dispos. 28, 157—166.

Lee, Y.H., Lee, M.H., Shim, C.K., 1992. Decreased systemic clearance of diltiazem with increased hepatic metabolism in rats with uranyl nitrate-induced acute renal failure. Pharm. Res. 9, 1599—1606.

Lee, A.K., Lee, J.H., Kwon, J.W., et al., 2004. Pharmacokinetics of clarithromycin in rats with acute renal failure induced by uranyl nitrate. Biopharm. Drug Dispos. 25, 273—282.

Levey, A.S., Inker, L.A., Coresh, J., 2015. Chronic kidney disease in older people. JAMA 314, 557—558.

Liddle, C., Goodwin, B., 2002. Regulation of hepatic drug metabolism: role of the nuclear receptors PXR and CAR. Semin. Liver Dis. 22, 115—122.

Lucas, D., Ferrara, R., Gonzalez, E., et al., 1999. Chlorzoxazone, a selective probe for phenotyping CYP2E1 in humans. Pharmacogenetics 9, 377—388.

Macias, W.L., Mueller, B.A., Scarim, S.K., 1991. Vancomycin pharmacokinetics in acute renal failure: preservation of nonrenal clearance. Clin. Pharmacol. Ther. 50, 688—694.

Malatkova, P., Wsol, V., 2014. Carbonyl reduction pathways in drug metabolism. Drug Metab. Rev. 46, 96—123.

Marbury, T.C., Ruckle, J.L., Hatorp, V., et al., 2000. Pharmacokinetics of repaglinide in subjects with renal impairment. Clin. Pharmacol. Ther. 67, 7—15.

Matzke, G.R., McGory, R.W., Halstenson, C.E., Keane, W.F., 1984. Pharmacokinetics of vancomycin in patients with various degrees of renal function. Antimicrob. Agents Chemother. 25, 433—437.

Michaud, J., Dube, P., Naud, J., et al., 2005. Effects of serum from patients with chronic renal failure on rat hepatic cytochrome P450. Br. J. Pharmacol. 144, 1067—1077.

Michaud, J., Naud, J., Chouinard, J., et al., 2006. Role of parathyroid hormone in the downregulation of liver cytochrome P450 in chronic renal failure. J. Am. Soc. Nephrol. 17, 3041—3048.

Michaud, J., Nolin, T.D., Naud, J., et al., 2008. Effect of hemodialysis on hepatic cytochrome P450 functional expression. J. Pharmacol. Sci. 108, 157—163.

Molnari, J.C., Myers, A.L., 2012. Carbonyl reduction of bupropion in human liver. Xenobiotica 42, 550—561.

Momper, J.D., Venkataramanan, R., Nolin, T.D., 2010. Nonrenal drug clearance in CKD: searching for the path less traveled. Adv. Chronic Kidney Dis. 17, 384—391.

Morgan, E.T., Goralski, K.B., Piquette-Miller, M., et al., 2008. Regulation of drug-metabolizing enzymes and transporters in infection, inflammation, and cancer. Drug Metab. Dispos. 36, 205—216.

Mueller, B.A., Scarim, S.K., Macias, W.L., 1993. Comparison of imipenem pharmacokinetics in patients with acute or chronic renal failure treated with continuous hemofiltration. Am. J. Kidney Dis. 21, 172—179.

Naud, J., Michaud, J., Boisvert, C., et al., 2007. Down-regulation of intestinal drug transporters in chronic renal failure in rats. J. Pharmacol. Exp. Ther. 320, 978—985.

Neirynck, N., Vanholder, R., Schepers, E., Eloot, S., Pletinck, A., Glorieux, G., 2013. An update on uremic toxins. Int. Urol. Nephrol. 45, 139—150.

Nicolas, P., Tod, M., Padoin, C., Petitjean, O., 1998. Clinical pharmacokinetics of diacerein. Clin. Pharmacokinet. 35, 347—359.

Niemi, M., Neuvonen, P.J., Kivisto, K.T., 2001. The cytochrome P4503A4 inhibitor clarithromycin increases the plasma concentrations and effects of repaglinide. Clin. Pharmacol. Ther. 70, 58—65.

Niemi, M., Backman, J.T., Neuvonen, M., Neuvonen, P.J., 2003. Effects of gemfibrozil, itraconazole, and their combination on the pharmacokinetics and pharmacodynamics of repaglinide: potentially hazardous interaction between gemfibrozil and repaglinide. Diabetologia 46, 347—351.

Nolin, T.D., Gastonguay, M.R., Bies, R.R., Matzke, G.R., Frye, R.F., 2003. Impaired 6-hydroxychlorzoxazone elimination in patients with kidney disease: implication for cytochrome P450 2E1 pharmacogenetic studies. Clin. Pharmacol. Ther. 74, 555—568.

Nolin, T.D., Appiah, K., Kendrick, S.A., Le, P., McMonagle, E., Himmelfarb, J., 2006. Hemodialysis acutely improves hepatic CYP3A4 metabolic activity. J. Am. Soc. Nephrol. 17, 2363–2367.

Nolin, T.D., Matzke, G.R., Barker, T.J., Frye, R.F., 2007. Effect of chronic kidney disease on cytochrome P450 2C19 activity and 4-hydroxymephenytoin urinary recovery. Clin. Pharmacol. Ther. 81 (Suppl. 1), S56.

Nolin, T.D., Naud, J., Leblond, F.A., Pichette, V., 2008. Emerging evidence of the impact of kidney disease on drug metabolism and transport. Clin. Pharmacol. Ther. 83, 898–903.

Nolin, T.D., Frye, R.F., Le, P., et al., 2009. ESRD impairs nonrenal clearance of fexofenadine but not midazolam. J. Am. Soc. Nephrol. 20, 2269–2276.

Nolin, T.D., 2008. Altered nonrenal drug clearance in ESRD. Curr. Opin. Nephrol. Hypertens. 17, 555–559.

Ohishi, N., Imaoka, S., Funae, Y., 1994. Changes in content of P450 isozymes in hepatic and renal microsomes of the male rat treated with cis-diamminedichloroplatinum. Xenobiotica 24, 873–880.

Okabe, H., Yano, I., Hashimoto, Y., Saito, H., Inui, K., 2002. Evaluation of increased bioavailability of tacrolimus in rats with experimental renal dysfunction. J. Pharm. Pharmacol. 54, 65–70.

Okabe, H., Hasunuma, M., Hashimoto, Y., 2003. The hepatic and intestinal metabolic activities of P450 in rats with surgery- and drug-induced renal dysfunction. Pharm. Res. 20, 1591–1594.

Okabe, H., Higashi, T., Ohta, T., Hashimoto, Y., 2004. Intestinal absorption and hepatic extraction of propranolol and metoprolol in rats with bilateral ureteral ligation. Biol. Pharm. Bull. 27, 1422–1427.

Osborne, R., Joel, S., Grebenik, K., Trew, D., Slevin, M., 1993. The pharmacokinetics of morphine and morphine glucuronides in kidney failure. Clin. Pharmacol. Ther. 54, 158–167.

Patterson, S.E., Cohn, V.H., 1984. Hepatic drug metabolism in rats with experimental chronic renal failure. Biochem. Pharmacol. 33, 711–716.

Portilla, D., Dai, G., McClure, T., et al., 2002. Alterations of PPARalpha and its coactivator PGC-1 in cisplatin-induced acute renal failure. Kidney Int. 62, 1208–1218.

Rege, B., Krieg, R., Gao, N., Sarkar, M.A., 2003. Down-regulation of hepatic CYP3A in chronic renal insufficiency. Pharm. Res. 20, 1600–1606.

Rivory, L.P., Watkins, P.B., 2001. Erythromycin breath test. Clin. Pharmacol. Ther. 70, 395–399.

Rivory, L.P., Slaviero, K.A., Hoskins, J.M., Clarke, S.J., 2001. The erythromycin breath test for the prediction of drug clearance. Clin. Pharmacokinet. 40, 151–158.

Robert, J., 1993. Clinical pharmacokinetics of idarubicin. Clin. Pharmacokinet. 24, 275–288.

Rostami-Hodjegan, A., Kroemer, H.K., Tucker, G.T., 1999. In-vivo indices of enzyme activity: the effect of renal impairment on the assessment of CYP2D6 activity. Pharmacogenetics 9, 277–286.

Schmiedlin-Ren, P., Thummel, K.E., Fisher, J.M., Paine, M.F., Watkins, P.B., 2001. Induction of CYP3A4 by 1 alpha,25-dihydroxyvitamin D3 is human cell line-specific and is unlikely to involve pregnane X receptor. Drug Metab. Dispos. 29, 1446–1453.

Schumacher, S., Abbasi, I., Weise, D., et al., 2001. Single- and multiple-dose pharmacokinetics of repaglinide in patients with type 2 diabetes and renal impairment. Eur. J. Clin. Pharmacol. 57, 147–152.

Shi, J., Montay, G., Chapel, S., et al., 2004. Pharmacokinetics and safety of the ketolide telithromycin in patients with renal impairment. J. Clin. Pharmacol. 44, 234–244.

Shibata, N., Inoue, Y., Fukumoto, K., et al., 2004. Evaluation of factors to decrease bioavailability of cyclosporin A in rats with gentamicin-induced acute renal failure. Biol. Pharm. Bull. 27, 384–391.

Simard, E., Naud, J., Michaud, J., et al., 2008. Downregulation of hepatic acetylation of drugs in chronic renal failure. J. Am. Soc. Nephrol. 19, 1352–1359.

Singlas, E., Pioger, J.C., Taburet, A.M., Colin, J.N., Fillastre, J.P., 1989. Zidovudine disposition in patients with severe renal impairment: influence of hemodialysis. Clin. Pharmacol. Ther. 46, 190–197.

Skarydova, L., Tomanova, R., Havlikova, L., Stambergova, H., Solich, P., Wsol, V., 2014. Deeper insight into the reducing biotransformation of bupropion in the human liver. Drug Metab. Pharmacokinet. 29, 177–184.

St Peter, W.L., 2015. Management of polypharmacy in dialysis patients. Semin. Dial. 28, 427–432.

Streetman, D.S., Bertino Jr., J.S., Nafziger, A.N., 2000. Phenotyping of drug-metabolizing enzymes in adults: a review of in-vivo cytochrome P450 phenotyping probes. Pharmacogenetics 10, 187–216.

Sun, H., Huang, Y., Frassetto, L., Benet, L.Z., 2004. Effects of uremic toxins on hepatic uptake and metabolism of erythromycin. Drug Metab. Dispos. 32, 1239–1246.

Sun, H., Frassetto, L.A., Huang, Y., Benet, L.Z., 2010. Hepatic clearance, but not gut availability, of erythromycin is altered in patients with end-stage renal disease. Clin. Pharmacol. Ther. 87, 465–472.

Taburet, A.M., Vincent, I., Perello, L., Coret, B., Baune, B., Furlan, V., 1996. Impairment of drug biotransformation in renal disease: an in vitro model. Clin. Pharmacol. Ther. 59, 136.

Talbert, R.L., 1994. Drug dosing in renal insufficiency. J. Clin. Pharmacol. 34, 99–110.

Tamassia, V., Pacciarini, M.A., Moro, E., Piazza, E., Vago, G., Libretti, A., 1987. Pharmacokinetic study of intravenous and oral idarubicin in cancer patients. Int. J. Clin. Pharmacol. Res. 7, 419–426.

Tanabe, H., Taira, S., Taguchi, M., Hashimoto, Y., 2007. Pharmacokinetics and hepatic extraction of metoprolol in rats with glycerol-induced acute renal failure. Biol. Pharm. Bull. 30, 552–555.

Terao, N., Shen, D.D., 1985. Reduced extraction of I-propranolol by perfused rat liver in the presence of uremic blood. J. Pharmacol. Exp. Ther. 233, 277–284.

Teunissen, M.W., Kampf, D., Roots, I., Vermeulen, N.P., Breimer, D.D., 1985. Antipyrine metabolite formation and excretion in patients with chronic renal failure. Eur. J. Clin. Pharmacol. 28, 589–595.

Thomson, B.K., Nolin, T.D., Velenosi, T.J., et al., 2015. Effect of CKD and dialysis modality on exposure to drugs cleared by nonrenal mechanisms. Am. J. Kidney Dis. 65, 574–582.

Toell, A., Degenhardt, S., Grabensee, B., Carlberg, C., 1999. Inhibitory effect of uremic solutions on protein-DNA-complex formation of the vitamin D receptor and other members of the nuclear receptor superfamily. J. Cell. Biochem. 74, 386–394.

Touchette, M.A., Slaughter, R.L., 1991. The effect of renal failure on hepatic drug clearance. DICP 25, 1214–1224.

Tucker, G.T., Houston, J.B., Huang, S.M., 2001. Optimizing drug development: strategies to assess drug metabolism/transporter interaction potential-toward a consensus. Clin. Pharmacol. Ther. 70, 103–114.

Turpeinen, M., Koivuviita, N., Tolonen, A., et al., 2007. Effect of renal impairment on the pharmacokinetics of bupropion and its metabolites. Br. J. Clin. Pharmacol. 64, 165–173.

U.S. Food and Drug Administration, March 2010. Guidance for Industry: Pharmacokinetics in Patients with Impaired Renal Function—study Design, Data Analysis, and Impact on Dosing and Labeling, Draft Guidance. Available from: http://www.fda.gov/downloads/Drugs/GuidanceComplianceRegulatoryInformation/Guidances/UCM204959.pdf.

Uchida, N., Kurata, N., Shimada, K., et al., 1995. Changes of hepatic microsomal oxidative drug metabolizing enzymes in chronic renal failure (CRF) rats by partial nephrectomy. Jpn. J. Pharmacol. 68, 431–439.

United States Renal Data System, 2015. 2015 USRDS Annual Data Report: Epidemiology of Kidney Disease in the United States. National Institutes of Health, National Institute of Diabetes and Digestive and Kidney Diseases, Bethesda, MD. Available at: http://www.usrds.org/adr.aspx.

van Heiningen, P.N., Hatorp, V., Kramer, N.K., et al., 1999. Absorption, metabolism and excretion of a single oral dose of (14)C-repaglinide during repaglinide multiple dosing. Eur. J. Clin. Pharmacol. 55, 521–525.

Van Peer, A.P., Belpaire, F.M., 1977. Hepatic oxidative drug metabolism in rats with experimental renal failure. Arch. Int. Pharmacodyn. Ther. 228, 180–183.

Velenosi, T.J., Urquhart, B.L., 2014. Pharmacokinetic considerations in chronic kidney disease and patients requiring dialysis. Expert Opin. Drug Metab. Toxicol. 10, 1131–1143.

Velenosi, T.J., Fu, A.Y., Luo, S., Wang, H., Urquhart, B.L., 2012. Down-regulation of hepatic CYP3A and CYP2C mediated metabolism in rats with moderate chronic kidney disease. Drug Metab. Dispos. 40, 1508–1514.

Velenosi, T.J., Feere, D.A., Sohi, G., Hardy, D.B., Urquhart, B.L., 2014. Decreased nuclear receptor activity and epigenetic modulation associates with down-regulation of hepatic drug-metabolizing enzymes in chronic kidney disease. FASEB J. 28, 5388–5397.

Venkatesh, P., Harisudhan, T., Choudhury, H., Mullangi, R., Srinivas, N.R., 2007. Pharmacokinetics of etoposide in rats with uranyl nitrate (UN)-induced acute renal failure (ARF): optimization of the duration of UN dosing. Eur. J. Drug Metab. Pharmacokinet. 32, 189–196.

Wienkers, L.C., Allievi, C., Hauer, M.J., Wynalda, M.A., 1999. Cytochrome P-450-mediated metabolism of the individual enantiomers of the antidepressant agent reboxetine in human liver microsomes. Drug Metab. Dispos. 27, 1334–1340.

Wilkinson, G.R., Guengerich, F.P., Branch, R.A., 1989. Genetic polymorphism of S-mephenytoin hydroxylation. Pharmacol. Ther. 43, 53–76.

Yeung, C.K., Shen, D.D., Thummel, K.E., Himmelfarb, J., 2014. Effects of chronic kidney disease and uremia on hepatic drug metabolism and transport. Kidney Int. 85, 522–528.

Yoshida, H., Goto, M., Honda, A., et al., 1994. Pharmacokinetics of doxorubicin and its active metabolite in patients with normal renal function and in patients on hemodialysis. Cancer Chemother. Pharmacol. 33, 450–454.

Yoshida, T., Kurella, M., Beato, F., et al., 2002. Monitoring changes in gene expression in renal ischemia-reperfusion in the rat. Kidney Int. 61, 1646–1654.

Yoshida, K., Sun, B., Zhang, L., et al., 2016. Systematic and quantitative assessment of the effect of chronic kidney disease on CYP2D6 and CYP3A4/5. Clin. Pharmacol. Ther.

Yoshitani, T., Yagi, H., Inotsume, N., Yasuhara, M., 2002. Effect of experimental renal failure on the pharmacokinetics of losartan in rats. Biol. Pharm. Bull. 25, 1077–1083.

Yu, C., Ritter, J.K., Krieg, R.J., Rege, B., Karnes, T.H., Sarkar, M.A., 2006. Effect of chronic renal insufficiency on hepatic and renal UDP-glucuronyltransferases in rats. Drug Metab. Dispos. 34, 621–627.

Yu, S.Y., 2002. Effects of acute renal failure induced by uranyl nitrate on the pharmacokinetics of intravenous theophylline in rats: the role of CYP2E1 induction in 1,3-dimethyluric acid formation. J. Pharm. Pharmacol. 54, 1687–1692.

Zaidenstein, R., Eyal, S., Efrati, S., et al., 2002. Adverse drug events in hospitalized patients treated with cardiovascular drugs and anticoagulants. Pharmacoepidemiol. Drug Saf. 11, 235–238.

Zhang, Y., Zhang, L., Abraham, S., et al., 2009. Assessment of the impact of renal impairment on systemic exposure of new molecular entities: evaluation of recent new drug applications. Clin. Pharmacol. Ther. 85, 305–311.

Drug and Fatty Acid Cytochrome P450 Metabolism in Critical Care

S.M. Poloyac

University of Pittsburgh, Pittsburgh, PA, United States

O U T L I N E

Introduction	115	Cardiac Arrest	127
Stroke	118	Summary	133
Traumatic Brain Injury	123	References	133

INTRODUCTION

Critical care medicine (also known as intensive care medicine) is focused on the diagnosis and management of life-threatening conditions. There are multiple intensive care units (ICUs) that cover a wide array of critical care conditions, which are organized by specialized medical units such as pediatric, neonatal, coronary, neurological, and surgical intensive care. Critical illness pathogenesis encompasses a wide array of insults that include tissue ischemia, reperfusion injury, immune system activation, and large organ failure that occur both within the primary acute insult and in the secondary postinjury phase of the disease. Patients under ICU care are facing the fragility of life and require precise, individualized care during both primary and secondary injuries by skilled intensivists to improve from their critically ill state and increase successful transition to the step down units. Interventions may include surgery, respiratory support, dialysis, and extensive use of drug therapeutic interventions. Although each critically ill disease state could encompass its own review, for the purposes of this chapter, the review will be focused on the neurological and neurovascular critical care illnesses of

Drug Metabolism in Diseases
http://dx.doi.org/10.1016/B978-0-12-802949-7.00005-5

stroke (both hemorrhagic and thromboembolic), traumatic brain injury (TBI), and cardiac arrest (CA). This review will also focus on the important role of the cytochrome P450 (CYP) enzyme system both in the metabolism of drug compounds to optimize patient care and also in small molecule fatty acid metabolites involved in critical insult pathogenesis.

In assessing the effects of stroke, TBI, and CA on drug-metabolizing enzymes, several factors should be considered. First of all, unlike chronic disease progression, critical illness has a rapid highly dynamic early phase, a later secondary injury phase, and a recovery phase after the initial insult. The primary pathogenic and recovery processes differ within each phase and therefore, have time and insult-dependent differential effects on enzyme regulation, including the P450 enzyme system, therefore, require the evaluation over time to account for the rapidly changing cellular milieu after insult. Second, the primary organ of insult (based on type of injury) will produce differential local and systemic effects after insult. For example, the brain is the primary organ of insult after TBI and stroke. There are known systemic alterations in the progression of the disease on other organ systems (liver, kidney, etc.) that accompany these insults; however, differential effects with respect to timing and magnitude of alterations require evaluation of tissue-specific changes in functional activity. In contrast, CA produces whole body anoxia during the period of asystole prior to resuscitation. The long-term ramifications for recovery postresuscitation are focused on brain recovery; however, it is important to differentiate that liver and other organ ischemia are involved in the overall insult for CA, but not for stroke and TBI. Finally, the importance of P450 alterations in each of these disease states includes alterations in drug concentrations (therefore optimal dosing of patients) and alterations in endogenous P450 substrate metabolism (which is involved with pathogenesis and recovery from insult).

In addition to their role in drug metabolism, CYP enzymes are also important in the bioactivation and inactivation of endogenous substrates. These endogenous substrates include cholesterol side-chain cleavage, estradiol formation, and vitamin D bioactivation. In addition to steroid structures, CYP enzymes bioactivate free fatty acids, particularly arachidonic acid (AA), to produce potent vasoactive metabolites. Growing evidence suggests that eicosanoids derived from the CYP pathway of AA metabolism are key regulators of cerebrovascular tone and vascular homeostasis with comparable potency as metabolites from the prostaglandin, leukotriene, and thromboxane pathways. Fig. 5.1 depicts the bioactivation pathways of AA by cyclooxygenase, lipoxygenase, and CYP enzyme pathways. In brain tissues, free arachidonic can be oxidized by CYP enzymes to form 20-hydroxyeicosatetraenoic acid (20-HETE) and epoxyeicosatrienoic acids (EETs). In humans, 20-HETE is formed primarily by CYP4F2 and CYP4A11 enzymes (Powell et al., 1998). 20-HETE constricts cerebral arteries and promotes angiogenesis, inflammation, apoptosis, and platelet aggregation (Imig et al., 2011). EETs consist of four regioselective isoforms (14,15-, 11,12-, 8,9-, and 5,6-EET) formed primarily by CYP2J2 and CYP2C8/9 enzymes. EETs dilate cerebral arteries, promote angiogenesis, and inhibit inflammation, apoptosis, and platelet aggregation (Imig et al., 2011). EETs can be further metabolized to inactive dihydroxyeicosatetraenoic acids (DHETs) by soluble epoxide hydrolase (sEH) which is present in neurons, astrocytes, oligodendrocytes, and cerebral vasculature (Sura et al., 2008). In addition, the CYP isoforms that form 20-HETE and EET metabolites are found in multiple other tissues, including liver and kidney, and have been implicated in blood pressure regulation and other physiologic and pathologic processes in these

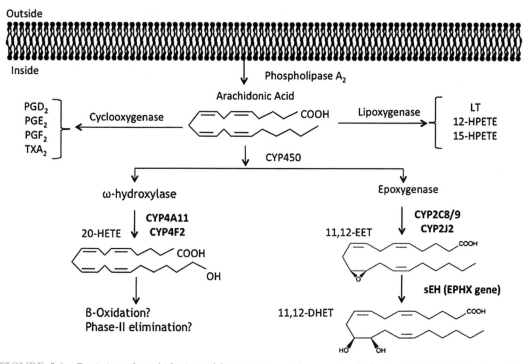

FIGURE 5.1 Depiction of arachidonic acid bioactivation pathways. Arachidonic acid is typically released by phospholipase A2 from the plasma membrane after which it is metabolized by cyclooxygenase, lipoxygenase, or cytochrome P450 (CYP) enzymes to produce a wide array of potent active metabolites. In particular, CYP4A11 and CYP4F2 produce the potent vasoconstrictive metabolite 20-hydroxyeicosatetraenoic acid (20-HETE), whereas CYP2C and CYP2J produce the vasodilatory epoxyeicosatrienoic acid (EET) metabolites. *sEH*, soluble epoxide hydrolase.

organs (Capdevila et al., 2015; Fan et al., 2015; Wu et al., 2014). Collectively, these studies demonstrate that CYP—eicosanoids may play an important role in the physiologic regulation of microvascular blood flow and inflammatory processes.

In this chapter, we will highlight how alterations in CYP metabolism alter the metabolism of drugs and endogenous substrates. This chapter will also illustrate the known role of these alterations in the pathogenesis of stroke, TBI, and CA. We will explore what is known about drug metabolic enzyme functionality and endogenous substrate P450 fatty acid metabolism for stroke, TBI, and CA. This chapter will not discuss the evolving literature concerning inherited genetic variant effects on CYP drug or endogenous fatty acid metabolism. We will discuss the specific role of these endogenous metabolites and highlight the potential expanded role of targeting specific CYP isoforms as a therapeutic intervention to improve disease outcomes within the field of critical care medicine. Fig. 5.2 illustrates the role of CYP enzymes in both the drug and endogenous substrate metabolisms and depicts the potential role that disease-mediated alterations in functional regulation may play both in effective therapeutic intervention and in the pathogenesis of the disease itself.

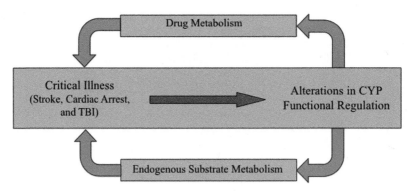

FIGURE 5.2   Cytochrome P450 (CYP) enzyme activity is altered by acute critical illness. Such changes in activity have implications in metabolism of several drugs commonly used in critically ill patients. In addition, endogenous P450 substrate (such as fatty acids) metabolism is similarly altered, thereby, affecting the overall disease pathogenesis. As a result, P450 metabolism serves as both a barrier to existing effective drug therapy and a potential new drug discovery target. *TBI*, traumatic brain injury.

STROKE

Stroke is typically classified into major subtypes based on its etiology. Strokes caused by occlusion of a blood vessel are referred to as "ischemic," whereas those caused by the rupture of a blood vessel are referred to as "hemorrhagic." Hemorrhagic strokes are further classified into intracerebral hemorrhage (ICH), which is characterized by bleeds in the brain parenchyma, and subarachnoid hemorrhage (SAH), which is characterized by bleeds into the subarachnoid cavity between the arachnoid membrane and pia matter. Ischemic strokes are the most common type accounting for 87% of all strokes with the remaining 10% and 3% of strokes accounted for by ICH and SAH, respectively (Go et al., 2013). Although hemorrhagic stroke is a less common type of stroke, it is associated with significantly higher cost and mortality rates (Bronnum-Hansen et al., 2001; Taylor, 1997). Evaluations of altered drug metabolizing enzymes after stroke have focused on the effects on endogenous CYP fatty acid metabolism and the potential role in disease pathogenesis. The effects of stroke on drug metabolism have been largely unstudied and remain an area of future evaluation for optimization of drug therapy. This section will focus on the known preclinical and clinical discoveries on the role of CYP fatty acid metabolism on both hemorrhagic and thromboembolic stroke pathogeneses.

Cerebral hypoperfusion is a mechanism of secondary brain injury in multiple neuronal insults including SAH, stroke, TBI, and CA. CYP enzymes produce mono-oxygenated metabolites of AA that are highly vasoactive and have been implicated as critical regulators of microvascular tone. Specifically, the terminal hydroxylation of AA to form 20-HETE is catalyzed by members of the CYP4 family (Nguyen et al., 1999; Sundseth and Waxman, 1992; Xu et al., 2004). In humans, the CYP4F2, CYP4A11, and CYP4F3B isoforms have been implicated in 20-HETE formation (Imaoka et al., 2005; Lasker et al., 2000; Powell et al., 1998). CYP4F2 and CYP4F3B have demonstrated the greatest catalytic activity in vitro at physiologically relevant AA substrate concentrations (Fer et al., 2008; Powell et al., 1998). The CYP4A and CYP4F subfamilies have also been shown to form 20-HETE in preclinical studies in rats and mice through transgenic and antisense inhibition studies (Cheng et al., 2014;

Kaide et al., 2003). The effects of 20-HETE on the microvasculature are opposed by mono-oxygenated AA metabolites known as EETs and the cyclooxygenase product prostaglandin E_2 (PGE_2) (Dhanasekaran et al., 2006; Liu et al., 2005). EETs are formed by the CYP2J and CYP2C isoforms and have been implicated as a counter-regulatory pathway to 20-HETE activity (Garcia et al., 2015). In vivo and in vitro studies have demonstrated that 20-HETE is one of the most potent vasoconstrictive eicosanoids. Direct application of 20-HETE onto pressurized 100–200 μm cat and rat pial arteries significantly reduced the internal diameter at concentrations of 10^{-9} and 10^{-10} M (Gebremedhin et al., 2000; Harder et al., 1994). 20-HETE-mediated vasoconstriction is of equal or greater potency as other known vasoconstrictive AA metabolites such as $PGF_{2\alpha}$, which produces constrictive effects at 10^{-8} M (Bednar et al., 2000). The role of 20-HETE formation on cerebrovascular tone was evaluated by Gebremedhin et al. (2000), who demonstrated that 20-HETE concentrations in middle cerebral arteries (150–200 μm) increased sixfold when vascular pressure is increased from 20 to 140 mmHg. Additional evidence in this study demonstrates that cerebral arteriolar autoregulation of cerebral blood flow (CBF) is impaired in the presence of the N-methylsulfonyl-12,12-dibromododec-11-enamide (DDMS) inhibitor of 20-HETE formation; thereby, suggesting that 20-HETE is important in cerebromicrovascular autoregulation. A recent study by Hall et al. (2014) published in *Nature* demonstrated that dilation by glutamate requires nitric oxide inhibition of 20-HETE formation to allow for PGE_2 to mediate dilation by binding to its EP4 receptors. This finding was particularly important given that the inhibition of nitric oxide synthase prevented glutamate vasodilation and the use of a 20-HETE formation inhibitor restored vasodilation even in the presence of the nitric oxide synthase inhibitor, thereby implicating 20-HETE in microvascular regulation. This work is consistent with prior work implicating 20-HETE as the mediator of nitric oxide dilation and autoregulatory control (Alonso-Galicia et al., 1998; Sun et al., 2000; Wink et al., 1993).

Several studies have demonstrated that inhibition of 20-HETE formation or EET degradation is neuroprotective in stroke animal models (Table 5.1). Studies have evaluated animal modes of SAH and temporary focal ischemia (TFI) with pre- and post-treatment with either 20-HETE formation (CYP4 inhibitors) or EET degradation (sEH inhibitors). With respect to 20-HETE in SAH models, Kehl et al. (2002) examined the effects of 20-HETE on CBF after SAH in the rat. This study found that the introduction of blood into the cisterna magna reduced regional CBF ~30% over 120 min, reduced the red blood cell supply rate, and increased 20-HETE 17-fold in the cerebral spinal fluid (CSF). Pretreatment of rats with the selective inhibitor of 20-HETE formation, N-hydroxy-N'(4-butyl-2methylphenyl)-formamidine (HET0016) 30 min prior to induction of SAH prevented the rise in CSF 20-HETE and attenuated the reduction in regional CBF with baseline values returning by 60 min. These data suggest that 20-HETE-induced myogenic cerebral vasoconstriction is important in autoregulation of CBF and maintenance of adequate cerebral perfusion in the rat SAH model. Another study by this group implicated 5-hydroxytryptamine-1B receptors in mediating the rise in 20-HETE observed after induction of SAH (Cambj-Sapunar et al., 2003). Similarly, it has been shown that the purported antagonist of 20-HETE improves CBF and agonists of the 20-HETE effects worsen CBF in this same SAH model (Yu et al., 2004). In addition, chronic administration the 20-HETE formation inhibitor TS-011 was shown to attenuate the development of delayed vasospasm and improve CBF in the rat (Takeuchi et al., 2005, 2006) and the dog SAH models (Hacein-Bey et al., 2006). These studies demonstrate that 20-HETE is a potent vasoconstrictor

TABLE 5.1   Stroke and CYP4 20-HETE Metabolism

Injury	Species	Items Assessed	Overall Effect and Likely Cause	References
SAH	Rat	20-HETE in CSF and effects of CYP4 inhibitors (HET0016 and 17-ODYA) on blood flow	20-HETE increased and inhibitors of 20-HETE formation improved CBF.	Kehl et al. (2002)
SAH	Rat	20-HETE in CSF and effects of CYP4 inhibitor (HET0016) and 5-hydroxy-tryptamine (5HT) on CBF	20-HETE increased by SAH and 5-HT. Inhibitors of CYP4 and 5-HT receptor blockade improve CBF.	Cambj-Sapunar et al. (2003)
SAH	Rat	Effects of 20-HETE agonists (WIT003 and ABSA) and 20-HETE antagonist (WIT002) on vessel diameter and CBF	20-HETE agonists decreased vessel diameter and reduced CBF after SAH, whereas 20-HETE antagonist increased diameter and CBF.	Yu et al. (2004)
SAH	Rat	Effects of CYP4 inhibitor (TS-011) on vessel diameter and CBF	CYP4 inhibitor, TS-011, significantly increased arterial diameter and CBF.	Takeuchi et al. (2005, 2006)
SAH	Dog	20-HETE in CSF and effects of CYP4 inhibitor (TS-011) on basilar artery diameter	20-HETE increased on day 7 and correlated with reduced artery diameter. TS-011 significantly increased artery diameter.	Hacein-Bey et al. (2006)
SAH	Human	20-HETE in CSF over 14 days in 108 SAH patients. Evaluated 20-HETE detection with vasospasm and delayed cerebral ischemia (DCI)	20-HETE was detectible in human CSF. Detectible 20-HETE was not associated with vasospasm but was associated with DCI.	Crago et al. (2011)
SAH	Human	20-HETE in CSF in 363 SAH patients. Evaluated quantified 20-HETE DCI, clinical neurologic deterioration (CND), modified Rankin Scores (MRS) and mortality at 3 and 12 months	20-HETE levels were higher in patients with CND and lower MRS. Patients with high to moderate 20-HETE levels more likely to have CND, lower MRS (2.1- to 2.5-fold), and were 3.3-fold more likely to have died at 12 months when controlling for age, sex, and bleed severity.	Donnelly et al. (2015b)
SAH	Human	20-HETE and EET CSF concentrations in 10 age and sex-matched control and 34 SAH patients. Evaluated levels relative to DCI, disposition, and mortality	Both 20-HETE and 14,15-EET CSF levels were higher in SAH over control and were higher on days 1—4 in patients with DCI. No level differences were observed with mortality. Whereas, 20-HETE levels were increased in patients with the disposition of a skilled nursing facility, rehab, or death when compared with home after SAH.	Siler et al. (2014)
TFI	Rat	Rats were treated with vehicle control or TS-011 at 60 min after artery occlusion. Infarct volume at 24 h after MCAO	Lesion volume was significantly decreased by 35% in TS-011 treated rats.	Miyata et al. (2005)

TABLE 5.1   Stroke and CYP4 20-HETE Metabolism—cont'd

Injury	Species	Items Assessed	Overall Effect and Likely Cause	References
TFI	Rat	Rats were pretreated with vehicle control or HET0016 for 3 days prior to and 3 days after MCAO. Infarct volume was assessed at 72 h and CBF was assessed by laser Doppler from baseline through 4 h after MCAO	Lesion volume was reduced by 84% in HET0016 treated rats. A significant improvement in postreperfusion CBF was observed at 3 and 4 h in HET0016 vs vehicle control treated rats.	Poloyac et al. (2006)
TFI	Rat and Monkey	Rats were treated TS-011 at 1, 2, and 4 h after MCAO with assessment of lesion volume and neurological deficits. Monkeys received TS-011 1 h after embolization with and without TPA	Infarct volume was significantly reduced in rats treated with TS-011 up to 4 h after MCAO. TS-011 also improved neurological deficits. Monkeys had no significant change in infarct size but a reduction in neurological deficits when TS-011 was administered with TPA.	Omura et al. (2006), Tanaka et al. (2007)
TFI	Rat	Effects of MCAO on lesion volume and CBF were evaluated in SHR, SHRSP, and WKY rats	20-HETE in the cerebral vasculature of SHRSP was about twice that seen in WKY rats. Infarct volume was greater in SHRSP than in SHR or WKY, which was associated with a greater reduction in CBF. SHR and SHRSP exhibited a sustained postischemic hyperperfusion. HET0016 reduced infarct size in SHR and SHRSP.	Dunn et al. (2008)
TFI	Rat	Rats were treated with TS-011 at 30 min after initiation of MCAO. Effects on infarct volume, volume at risk, and CBF were assessed	TS-011 reduced infarct volume by 70% (cortical) and 55% (total). TS-011 had no effect on the volume at risk or CBF up to 30 min after ischemia. TS-011 reduced the delayed fall in CBF 2 h after reperfusion.	Renic et al. (2009)
TFI	Mouse	Mice were treated with TS-011 IV for 1 h every 6 h. CBF and the vascular perfusion area were assessed	TS-011 significantly improved blood flow and perfusion in peri-infarct region. TS-011 also significantly reduced the infarct volume.	Marumo et al. (2010)

CBF, cerebral blood flow; CYP, cytochrome P450; EET, epoxyeicosatrienoic acids; HETE, hydroxyeicosatetraenoic acid; MCAO, middle cerebral artery occlusion; SAH, subarachnoid hemorrhage; SHR, spontaneously hypertensive; SHRSP, spontaneously hypertensive stroke prone; TFI, temporary focal ischemia; TPA, tissue plasminogen activator; WKY, Wistar–Kyoto.

in the microvasculature and that inhibition of 20-HETE formation attenuates the pathogenic mechanisms of vasoconstriction in the cerebral vasculature during SAH in the rat and dog SAH model, thereby, implicating CYP-mediated formation of 20-HETE as a target for interventional drug development.

Studies in ischemic stroke have evaluated both 20-HETE formation inhibitors and inhibitors of EET degradation (sEH inhibitors). 20-HETE formation inhibitors have demonstrated significant reductions in lesion volume in the TFI model. Miyata et al. (2005) reported that the 20-HETE formation inhibitor TS-011 decreased lesion volume by 35% in the ischemic stroke model. Our laboratory demonstrated that pretreatment with HET0016 significantly reduced lesion volume to $9.1 \pm 4.9\%$ when compared with $57.4 \pm 9.8\%$ in vehicle control animals after TFI (Poloyac et al., 2006). We also demonstrated an improvement in CBF with HET0016 administration as determined by laser Doppler blood flow. Subsequent studies in rats demonstrated similar reductions in overall lesion volume after ischemia and reperfusion brain injury (Omura et al., 2006; Tanaka et al., 2007) and Omura et al. demonstrated no significant change in lesion volume but improved neurological deficits in monkeys during coadministration of TS-011 with tissue plasminogen activator (TPA). Renic and colleagues further evaluated TS-011 neuroprotection in which they demonstrated reduced infarct size after cerebral ischemia, but did not observe differences in area at risk for injury or the overall CBF, thereby, suggesting that 20-HETE inhibition decreases overall injury by reducing neuronal damage (Dunn et al., 2008; Renic et al., 2009). In contrast, Marumo et al. (2010) demonstrated that the TS-011 inhibitor also improved peri-infarct vascular perfusion area and also decreased overall lesion volume after TFI. Studies have also demonstrated that 20-HETE synthesis is increased after ischemia (Fordsmann et al., 2013; Kawasaki et al., 2012) and that inhibitors prevent secondary impairment of CBF, brain edema, and blood brain barrier dysfunction that occur after injury (Liu et al., 2014; Miyata and Roman, 2005; Takeuchi et al., 2005). Overall, it has been universally demonstrated by multiple laboratories that administration of 20-HETE formation inhibitors decrease lesion volume in the rat TFI model. The mechanism of this protection remains in question with evidence in support and against either cerebrovascular and/or direct neuroprotective mechanisms.

Clinical studies by our laboratory have demonstrated that 20-HETE is found in human CSF (Miller et al., 2009; Poloyac et al., 2005) and that high 20-HETE CSF concentrations are associated with higher mortality and poor outcomes in patients with SAH (Table 5.1). Our early study in a small cohort of patients with SAH demonstrated that CSF 20-HETE levels were elevated early (days 3–5) in some patients and that the patients with detectible 20-HETE levels had a higher rate of complications (Crago et al., 2011). Most recently we evaluated the relationship between 20-HETE CSF levels and acute/long-term outcomes after aneurysmal SAH (aSAH) in 363 adult patients over 14-days (Donnelly et al., 2015b). Patients with clinical neurological deterioration and unfavorable 3-month Modified Rankin Scores had 2.6-fold higher maximum 20-HETE CSF levels for both outcome measures. Patients with high-to-moderate 20-HETE levels (35.7%) were 2.1- to 2.5-fold more likely to have acute clinical neurological deterioration (95% confidence interval [CI] 1.16–3.96) and lower Modified Rankin Scores at 3 months (95% CI 1.16–4.93) and 12 months (95% CI 1.05–4.06). Patients with high/moderate 20-HETE in CSF were 3.3-fold (95% CI 1.51–7.26) more likely to have died at 12 months after controlling for age, sex, and Fisher grade. Importantly, the results of our study were consistent with the findings by Siler et al. (2014), who demonstrated that 20-HETE levels were higher in aSAH versus controls. Since 20-HETE effects are opposed by the effects of EET metabolites, both inhibition of 20-HETE formation and inhibition of EET degradation have been proposed as therapeutic approaches (Siler et al., 2014). Although both approaches are theoretically viable, our clinical data suggest stronger associations with 20-HETE (Donnelly et al., 2015b) over EETs (Donnelly et al., 2015a) in SAH, however, these results will require a second validation cohort in a future study. Overall, these results by independent laboratories demonstrate that 20-HETE is found in human CSF and that the levels of 20-HETE are associated with acute complications and poor outcomes after aSAH. These results provide additional evidence of the translational potential for development of 20-HETE formation inhibitors given the association with poor patient outcomes.

CYP enzymes also form epoxide metabolites of AA that produce the opposite physiologic and pathophysiologic effects of 20-HETE. There are four metabolites that arise from epoxidation at each of the double bond sites of AA primarily by the CYP2J2 and CYP2C8/9 isoforms to produce 5,6-EET, 8,9-EET, 11,12-EET, and 14,15-EET (Fleming, 2001). The most potent of these epoxide metabolites are the 11,12-EET and 14,15-EET that have been shown to dilate cerebral arteries, inhibit inflammation, decrease apoptosis, and inhibit platelet aggregation (Imig et al., 2011). EETs can be further metabolized to the predominantly less active DHETs by sEH (Sura et al., 2008). Preclinical evidence has demonstrated that EETs are protective against neuronal injury after ischemic or hemorrhagic stroke. Increasing EET concentrations by sEH inhibition or sEH gene deletion reduce infarct size and increase CBF in animal models of TFI (Zhang et al., 2007, 2008). In vitro studies demonstrate that EETs protect astrocytes against ischemic cell death (Liu and Alkayed, 2005). Also, variants in the EPHX2 gene, which codes for sEH, have been shown to affect sEH activity and neuronal survival after ischemic injury (Koerner et al., 2007). Furthermore, clinical evaluations have demonstrated that patients with certain allelic variants in CYP2C8 are associated with EET levels and that EET CSF levels are elevated in patients with SAH (Donnelly et al., 2015a; Siler et al., 2014). Since the EETs are protective, the primary interventional strategy has been to decrease sEH activity to decrease damage after stroke (Huang et al., 2016; Imig et al., 2011). The development and utility of sEH inhibitors is being extensively evaluated and sEH inhibitors are currently in clinical trials for safety and efficacy for a variety of disease states (Morisseau and Hammock, 2013).

Collectively, the research findings have demonstrated that CYP metabolites of AA are important mediators of stroke pathogenesis. The preponderance of evidence to date has particularly implicated 20-HETE as a pathogenic mediator and EETs as a protective mediator of stroke pathogenesis. Preclinical studies have demonstrated in SAH and ischemic stroke models in rats, dogs, and piglets that 20-HETE formation inhibition is an effective intervention to decrease overall lesion volume and improve neurological outcomes. In addition, the clinical studies have also associated 20-HETE concentrations with poor outcomes in patients with SAH. These combined results implicate this pathway as a pathogenic mediator in preclinical studies and as a biomarker of poor outcomes in patients with SAH. Future research will likely elucidate the viability of CYP4 inhibition and/or 20-HETE receptor blockade as well as sEH inhibition as novel therapeutic interventions to improve outcomes in these patients.

TRAUMATIC BRAIN INJURY

Studies evaluating the effects of TBI on CYP activity have predominantly focused on the evaluation of hepatic drug metabolism. In contrast to the reports in the stroke literature, relatively few studies have evaluated the effects of TBI on CYP-mediated fatty acid metabolism. This section will review the known alterations in CYP drug metabolism after TBI in both preclinical and clinical studies and will also discuss the limited known alterations in CYP fatty acid metabolism after TBI.

TBI produces a systemic inflammatory response that includes increased cytokine concentrations after injury. It has been well known through the seminal work of Morgan and others, that proinflammatory cytokines produce transcriptional downregulation of the expression of several CYP isoforms. To date, alterations in functional CYP regulation have been evaluated in two different rat models of TBI: cortical concussive and blast-induced brain injury (Table 5.2). An original evaluation of the temporal effects of TBI on CYP3A and CYP2C11 expression and functional activity in the rat cortical concussive model was conducted by Toler et al. (1993). This study demonstrated significant reductions in CYP3A and CYP2C11 mRNA at 24 h after injury and also similar reductions due to craniotomy without cortical impact. Neither CYP3A or CYP2C11 activity nor protein levels were significantly altered by cortical injury. Subsequent to this analysis, evaluation of CYP2E1 functional regulation after cortical concussive injury was assessed in the liver, kidney, and brain (Poloyac et al., 2000). This study demonstrated a significant reduction in CYP2E1 activity, assessed by 6OH-CZN formation, in the liver at 48 h after injury and a similar nonsignificant trend in CYP2E1 protein as assessed by Western blot. A significant increase in CYP2E1 activity was observed in the kidney at 24 h after insult with a similar nonsignificant trend in CYP2E1 protein. TBI effects on CYP functional regulation was also conducted by Kalsotra et al. (2003). This study demonstrated a reduction in total P450 at 24 h followed by an increase at 2 weeks. Hepatic CYP1A protein and activity were reduced at 24 h and 2 weeks after injury. Conversely, CYP3A activity (assessed by erythromycin N-demethylation) was increased at both 24 h

TABLE 5.2   Effects of Traumatic Brain Injury on Cytochrome P450 (CYP) Isoform Expression and Function

CYP Enzyme Evaluated	Animal	Injury/Model	Items Assessed	Overall Effect on Drug Metabolism and Likely Cause	References
CYP3A and 2C11	Rat	Cortical concussion	mRNA, protein, and microsome activity by testosterone hydroxylation	50% reduced CYP3A and CYP2C11 mRNA at 24 h with craniotomy or brain injury. No significant alteration in protein expression or activity (testosterone hydroxylation) were observed.	Toler et al. (1993)
Total P450 and CYP2E1	Rat	Cortical concussion	Total P450, microsome activity by chlorzoxazone hydroxylation, and protein content	Total P450 reduced to 86% at 24 h and CYP2E1 activity reduced to 74% at 48 h. No significant change in CYP2E1 protein observed.	Poloyac et al. (2000)
Total P450, CYP1A, 2B, 2D, 3A, and 4F	Rat	Cortical concussion	Total P450, protein, and activity by individual isoform probe substrates	Total P450 reduced at 24 h and increased at 2 weeks. CYP1A activity reduced at 2 weeks. CYP3A activity increased at 24 h and 2 weeks.	Kalsotra et al. (2003)

TABLE 5.2   Effects of Traumatic Brain Injury on Cytochrome P450 (CYP) Isoform Expression and Function—cont'd

CYP Enzyme Evaluated	Animal	Injury/Model	Items Assessed	Overall Effect on Drug Metabolism and Likely Cause	References
Microarray mRNA expression and CYP2D4 and CYP3A1	Rat	Cortical concussion	Microarray mRNA expression and liver protein analysis	CYP4A1, 4A2, and CYP4A8 mRNA upregulated (1.60- to 1.65-fold) at 24 h. No alteration in CYP2D6 or CYP3A1 protein.	Anderson et al. (2015)
CYP1A2, 2B1, 2D6, and 3A2	Rat	Blast injury	mRNA and protein	CYP1A2, 3A2, and 2D1 mRNA reduced at 24 h, 48 h, and 1 week (no mRNA change in CYP2B1). CYP1A2 protein significantly reduced at 24 h. CYP2B1, 2D1, and 3A2 protein most significantly reduced at 24 and 48 h.	Ma et al. (2016)
CYP3A4	Human	Adult patients with TBI randomized to receive cyclosporine	Patients randomized to receive placebo or one of three doses of cyclosporine every 12 h for 72 h. Cyclosporine whole blood concentrations were evaluated	Pharmacokinetic analysis revealed that patients with TBI had higher clearance and a larger volume of distribution when compared with reports from other patient populations.	Empey et al. (2006)
CYP2C9, CYP3A4, CYP2C19, CYP2E1	Human	Adult critical injury (brain and other with 3 of 23 patients with TBI)	CYP metabolizing activity was assessed via mephenytoin (2C19), chlorzoxazone (2E1), dapsone (3A4 and 2C9), and flurbiprofen (2C9)	Mephenytoin metabolism was suppressed after injury and increased during postinjury, chlorzoxazone metabolism was also suppressed. Measures of dapsone and flurbiprofen metabolism were elevated throughout the study.	Harbrecht et al. (2005)
CYP2C9, CYP2C19	Human	Pediatric TBI patients receiving normo-thermia vs therapeutic hypothermia	Phenytoin free and total concentrations evaluated over time in 10 hypothermic and 9 normothermic children	Therapeutic hypothermia decreased the time-variant component of the V_{max} metabolism (V_{max}) 4.6-fold and reduced the overall V_{max} by $\sim$50%. Simulations showed that the risk for drug toxicity extends for days beyond the end of cooling.	Empey et al. (2013)

and 2 weeks with a comparable increase in CYP3A protein at 2 weeks. These results suggest isoform-specific alterations in CYP regulation that differ from the more universal downregulation of CYP functional expression observed after inflammatory insults such as lipopolysaccharide (LPS) injection. Anderson et al. (2015) used microarray and enzyme-linked immunosorbent assay (ELISA) analysis to evaluate cortical concussive injury changes in inflammatory mediators and CYP mRNA and protein changes in the rat. The mRNA microarray analyses showed an ~1.6-fold increase in CYP4A1, 4A2, and 4A8 expression. No differences in CYP2D4 or CYP3A1 protein content were observed after TBI. Finally, a recent study by Ma et al. (2016) evaluated the effects of blast injury on liver CYP mRNA and protein expression. Significant reductions in CYP1A2, 3A2, and 2D1 mRNA were observed at 24 h, 48 h, and 1 week with no significant mRNA changes in CYP2B1. Western blot analysis showed significant reductions in CYP1A2 protein at 24 h only, whereas CYP2B1, CYP2D1, and CYP3A2 proteins were most significantly reduced at 24 and 48 h after injury. These studies suggest that CYP regulation is modestly altered in an isoform-specific manner by cortical concussive brain injury with relatively minor reductions in activity. One recent study has suggested more significant alterations in CYP expression in the blast injury model; however, the magnitude of the blast injury mediated alterations on functional CYP activity remains to be elucidated. Overall it can be concluded that preclinical models of brain injury do demonstrate altered CYP expression; however, the magnitude of altered CYP metabolism after brain injury is not as great as the alterations observed after LPS and other inflammatory preclinical models.

Clinically, few studies have been conducted to evaluate alterations in CYP metabolism after TBI. Patients who suffer a TBI have been shown to enter a hypermetabolic state with ranges from 32% to 200% above noninjured levels. This hypermetabolic state includes energy expenditure during the first 30 days after TBI and has been reviewed previously by Foley et al. (2008). If this hypermetabolic energy expenditure is also seen with hepatic drug metabolism is largely unknown and is not necessarily reflected in the preclinical studies, suggesting downregulation after TBI. One clinical study demonstrating increased drug clearance after TBI was reported by Empey et al. (2006). This study evaluated cyclosporine concentrations as part of a randomized dose escalation study in adult patients with TBI. Results from the pharmacokinetic analyses suggested higher systemic cyclosporine clearance and a larger volume of distribution in patients with TBI when compared with other patient populations. These results suggest that drug metabolism may be increased in patients with TBI. Another clinical study by Harbrecht et al. (2005) showed isoform-specific alteration in drug metabolism after severe critical injury. The effects of critical illness on the metabolism of the probe substrates mephenytoin (CYP2C19), chlorzoxazone (CZN) (CYP2E1), dapsone (CYP3A4 and CYP2C9), and flurbiprofen (CYP2C9) were evaluated. Mephenytoin metabolism was suppressed after injury and increased during postinjury, CZN metabolism was suppressed to a smaller degree. The metabolism of dapsone and flurbiprofen was elevated throughout, also suggesting some elevations in metabolism. It is important to note that only 3 of the 23 patients studied suffered a TBI; however, these results do suggest isoform-specific alterations after severe critical injury. Empey et al. (2013) also later evaluated the effects of therapeutic hypothermia on phenytoin elimination in children suffering TBI. A total of 29 children with severe TBI were randomized to receive either normothermia or 48 h of induced hypothermia (32–33°C) followed by slow rewarming. Phenytoin was administered to these patients for seizure prophylaxis, and both total and free phenytoin levels were assessed as part of routine care. This study demonstrated that use of therapeutic hypothermia decreased the maximum velocity of phenytoin metabolism (V_{max}) by ~50% and demonstrated that the elevations in concentration extended several days after the end of cooling, thereby suggesting that the later time window has the highest risk for drug toxicity. Hypothermia and TBI in pediatric patients increased phenytoin concentrations above the acceptable therapeutic window, thereby warranting careful therapeutic drug monitoring in these highly vulnerable patients. Overall, the effects of TBI in patients do not entirely support prior observations of decreased drug metabolism in preclinical studies. Instead, these results suggest isoform-specific regulation with some evidence of increased metabolism in patients with TBI. Future studies are needed to clarify both the time course of such alterations and the magnitude of these changes to clearly delineate suggested alterations in drug dosing in patients with TBI. Furthermore, consideration of interventions, such as therapeutic hypothermia, that have direct actions on enzyme activity are needed for a full understanding of drug dose optimization in critically ill patients.

The effects of TBI on endogenous CYP fatty acid metabolism have not been extensively evaluated. In an early study, Kalsotra et al. (2007) evaluated the regulation of CYP4F in the lung in the rat concussive TBI model at 24 h and 2 weeks after injury. Specifically, this study demonstrated that the CYP4F-mediated hydroxylation of leukotriene B4 was increased at 2 weeks, thereby, suggesting mechanistic CYP4F upregulation to mediate resolution of inflammation in the lung after TBI. Similarly, this same group evaluated CYP4F regulation of leukotriene B4 levels in the rat brain after TBI (Wang et al., 2008). In the brain, CYP4F mRNA expression was reduced at 24 h postinjury and was increased at 2 weeks. Also, leukotriene B4 levels in the brain inversely correlated with the CYP4F expression, thereby, suggesting that CYP4F-mediated leukotriene B4 metabolism alterations are temporally regulated after TBI. Another study by Birnie et al. (2013) evaluated the transcriptional regulation of multiple AA CYP isoforms after TBI in the cortical contusion model with differential regulation of several CYP isoforms in a time- and brain region—dependent manner. Overall, few studies have been conducted to evaluate the effects of TBI on CYP fatty acid metabolism and the definitive role of these metabolites in secondary damage after TBI remains an important area of future evaluation.

CARDIAC ARREST

Over 300,000 patients suffer a CA each year in the United States with approximately a 10% overall survival rate. Of the patients who are resuscitated and survive, brain injury is the primary factor determining overall recovery. Unlike TBI and stroke, CA involves whole-body ischemia, thereby directly injuring all organ systems during the periods of asystole and reperfusion. With respect to hepatic drug metabolism, the net effects of CA include both the direct ischemic and reperfusion injury coupled with the overall systemic mediators of inflammation, all of which can alter CYP functional regulation. One common therapeutic intervention after CA is the purposeful reduction in body temperature, known as either targeted temperature management or therapeutic hypothermia. Therapeutic hypothermia has been shown to improve neurological recovery in patients after out-of-hospital CA (Bernard et al., 2002;

Shankaran and Laptook, 2007). Typically body temperature is reduced from 37°C to 33–34°C for 24–48 h after resuscitation from CA. More recent studies also suggest that targeting 36°C does not differ from 33°C in terms of neurological outcomes in CA patients (Moler et al., 2015); however, future studies are needed to delineate the ideal temperature and duration of temperature regulation after CA. The use of therapeutic hypothermia has been extensively evaluated and reviewed in both preclinical and clinical studies and is known to reduce CYP metabolism in an isoform-specific manner (Sunjic et al., 2015; Tortorici et al., 2007; van den Broek et al., 2010; Zhou and Poloyac, 2011). For the purposes of this chapter, we will discuss the effects of therapeutic hypothermia with a focus on the disease-mediated effects of CA on specific CYP probe drug metabolism in both preclinical and patient studies (Table 5.3). This section of the chapter will also discuss the role of CYP fatty acid metabolites in the pathogenesis of secondary brain injury after CA.

Hepatic ischemia that accompanies CA is known to decrease liver metabolism. Preclinical studies have evaluated alterations in the metabolism of known CYP probe drugs. Our laboratory also evaluated the mRNA and microsomal formation rates of 6-hydroxychlorzoxazone (6OH-CZN) and 6β-hydroxytestosterone to assess CYP2E1 and CYP3A2 activity, respectively (Tortorici et al., 2009). At 24 h after CA, 6β-hydroxytestosterone and 6OH-CZN microsomal formation rates were decreased, $55.7 \pm 12.8\%$ and $46.8 \pm 29.7\%$ of control, respectively. CA also significantly decreased CYP3A2 mRNA, but not CYP2E1 mRNA. CA also produced an ~10-fold increase in plasma IL-6. Therapeutic hypothermia prevented the CA-mediated inhibition of CYP3A2 and CYP2E1 and also attenuated the observed rise in IL-6 after resuscitation. Similarly, the effects of CA on the in vivo pharmacokinetics of P450 probe drugs have been evaluated by our group. In a series of two studies, we first evaluated the probe drug CZN (Tortorici et al., 2006), and in the second study, we evaluated the effects on multiple P450 microdosed probe drugs after CA (Zhou et al., 2011). CZN clearance was reduced in rats receiving CA and therapeutic hypothermia to either 30°C or 33°C in these studies. The study by Zhou et al. evaluated the pharmacokinetics of four simultaneously microdosed probe drugs in rats receiving either sham surgery or asphyxia CA under either normothermic (37.5–38°C) or mild hypothermic (32.5–33°C) conditions. Probe drugs, midazolam (CYP3A), CZN (CYP2E1), diclofenac (CYP2C), and dextromethorphan (CYP2D) were administered intravenously after temperature stabilization. We observed isoform-specific alterations in CYP activity. No significant changes were observed with either diclofenac or dextromethorphan clearance, whereas significant reductions in clearance were observed with midazolam and CZN in the CA hypothermia rats when compared with sham normothermia rats. Two important findings from this study are that (1) the CA and hypothermia-mediated changes are specific to a given CYP450 isoform and (2) ischemic injury is a significant contributor to reduced metabolism in this injury model producing decreased clearance of CZN and midazolam.

A study by Empey et al. evaluated the prolonged use of mild hypothermia (33°C) up to 10 h on fentanyl and midazolam steady-state pharmacokinetics in the rat model of asphyxial CA (Empey et al., 2011). Fentanyl and midazolam were administered via a continuous intravenous infusion and both drugs are metabolized by the CYP3A2 isoform in rats. The clearance of fentanyl and midazolam was significantly decreased by mild hypothermia by 27.5% and 17% of CA normothermic rats, respectively. The independent effects of CA were not assessed in this study. Additionally, no differences were observed in the blood to brain ratio for either drug or CYP3A expression between experimental groups.

TABLE 5.3 Effects of Cardiac Arrest on CYP Isoform Expression and Function

CYP Enzyme/Pathway Evaluated	Animal	Injury/Model	Items Assessed	Overall Effect on Drug Metabolism and Likely Cause	References
CYP2E1 and CYP3A2	Rat	Asphyxial cardiac arrest with moderate hypothermia (30°C)	Rat received asphyxial arrest with cooling maintained for 3 h. Animals were sacrificed at 5 or 24 h. Microsomal activity and mRNA expression of CYP3A2 and CYP2E1. Plasma interleukin-6 levels were determined	At 24 h, cardiac arrest decreased CYP3A2 and CYP2E1 activity by 55.7% and 46.8% of control, respectively. CA decreased CYP3A2 mRNA but not CYP2E1 mRNA. CA also produced a ~10-fold increase in plasma IL-6. CA mediated inhibition of CYP3A2 and CYP2E1 was attenuated by hypothermia, as was the increase in IL-6.	Tortorici et al. (2009)
CYP2E1	Rat	Asphyxial cardiac arrest with moderate hypothermia (30°C)	All rats received asphyxial arrest and moderate hypothermia (30°C) vs normothermia (37°C) was evaluated. Chlorozoxazone IV pharmacokinetics and protein binding were assessed	Hypothermia after cardiac arrest in rats decreased the systemic clearance of chlorzoxazone. No changes in chlorzoxazone protein binding were observed. This suggests that cardiac arrest and moderate hypothermia to 30°C decrease CYP2E1 activity.	Tortorici et al. (2006)
CYP3A, CYP2C, CYP2D, CYP2E1	Rat	Asphyxial cardiac arrest with mild hypothermia (33°C)	Rats received sham normothermia, CA normothermia, sham hypothermia, and CA hypothermia. Probe drugs (midazolam, diclofenac, dextromethorphan, and chlorzoxazone) were given IV simultaneously after temperature stabilization	The clearance of midazolam (CYP3A) in CA hypothermia was reduced from sham normothermia rats. Chlorzoxazone (CYP2E) clearance was similarly reduced. Population PK analysis further demonstrated the decreased clearance of midazolam (CYP3A) and chlorxozaxone was associated with CA injury. CYP2C and CYP2D were not significantly altered, thereby, suggesting drug/isoform-specific effects.	Zhou et al. (2011)
CYP3A	Rat	Asphyxial cardiac arrest with mild hypothermia (33°C)	Rats received cardiac arrest and mild hypothermia (33°C) for 10 h. Fentanyl and midazolam were administered by IV infusion for plasma and brain analysis. CYP3A2 microsomal protein and activity were analyzed at 37°C and 33°C	Mild hypothermia decreased the systemic clearance of both fentanyl and midazolam after cardiac arrest. The elevated systemic concentrations did not lead to parallel increased brain exposures of either drug. Mechanistically, no differences in CYP3A2 expression was observed, but the in vitro metabolism of both drugs was decreased at 33°C vs 37°C.	Empey et al. (2011)

(Continued)

TABLE 5.3 Effects of Cardiac Arrest on CYP Isoform Expression and Function—cont'd

CYP Enzyme/ Pathway Evaluated	Animal	Injury/Model	Items Assessed	Overall Effect on Drug Metabolism and Likely Cause	References
20-HETE	Piglet	Cardiac arrest	Effects of CYP4 inhibitor (HET0016) on neuronal recovery after cardiac arrest	HET0016 inhibited ischemia-induced phosphorylation and improved Na^+, K^+-ATPase activity. HET0016 also suppressed Erk1/2 activation and nitrosative/oxidative stress.	Yang et al. (2012)
20-HETE	Piglet	Cardiac arrest with hypothermia	Effects of CYP4 inhibitor (HET0016) administered 5 min after resuscitation on neuronal recovery in hypothermic (34°C for 24 h) and normothermic piglets after cardiac arrest.	Therapeutic hypothermia increased viable neuronal density when compared with normothermic animals. HET0016 further increased neuronal viability in hypothermic animals greater than that observed in hypothermia alone. This suggests that HET0016 augments the neuroprotective effects of hypothermia in the piglet cardiac arrest model.	Zhu et al. (2015)
20-HETE and EETs	Rat	Pediatric cardiac arrest	20-HETE, EET, and DHET levels in the brain and the effects of HET0016 were evaluated in after 9 and 12 min of cardiac arrest. Cortical perfusion, neurodegeneration, and short-term neurological outcomes were assessed.	After 9 min of CA, EETs increased vs sham. Conversely, after 12 min of CA, 20-HETE increased, without compensatory increases in EETs. Inhibition of 20-HETE synthesis after 12 min of CA decreased cortical 20-HETE levels, increased CBF, reduced neurologic deficits, and reduced neurodegeneration and edema.	Shaik et al. (2015)
EETs	Mouse	Cardiac arrest	Evaluated the role of EETs by assessing the effects of sEH gene deletion on survival, renal function, and ischemic renal damage following cardiac arrest.	Unexpectedly, the sEH knockout mice required significantly higher doses of epinephrine, longer CPR, delayed blood pressure recovery, and had significantly higher mortality compared with wild-type controls. These data suggest that increased EETs due to sEH deletion decrease mortality after cardiac arrest.	Hutchens et al. (2008)

CA, cardiac arrest; DHET, dihydroxyeicosatrienoic acid; EET, expoxyeicosatrienoic acid; HETE, hydroxyeicosatetraenoic acid; sEH, soluble epoxide hydrolase.

As detailed in our and others published reviews on the effects of therapeutic hypothermia on drug metabolism (Sunjic et al., 2015; Tortorici et al., 2007; van den Broek et al., 2010; Zhou and Poloyac, 2011), several small clinical and preclinical studies have consistently demonstrated increased plasma concentrations during hypothermia of various drugs that rely on CYP enzymes as their pathway of elimination. Most notably, therapeutic hypothermia increased morphine concentrations in neonates with hypoxic ischemic encephalopathy above toxic concentrations (Roka et al., 2008). Similarly, up to five-fold elevations in concentrations have been reported with phenytoin (Iida et al., 2001) and midazolam (Fukuoka et al., 2004) in brain injured hypothermia-treated patients. Alterations in drug elimination due to therapeutic hypothermia have been shown to be dependent on the route of elimination. In addition, some studies have shown that drugs that require active renal secretion are also significantly altered by therapeutic hypothermia in preclinical animal models (Koren et al., 1985; Nishida et al., 2007). Collectively, these results suggest that hypothermia alters active routes of renal and hepatic elimination, whereas passive renal filtration is likely unchanged.

Although alterations in drug disposition after therapeutic hypothermia have been reported, the translation of this research into meaningful recommendations for patients with CA remains to be elucidated. A few clinical studies have proposed dosage recommendations during cooling, and fewer studies have evaluated the effects of CA and hypothermia in patients. Currently, dosage recommendations have been proposed for remifentanil (Michelsen et al., 2001) in coronary artery bypass patients (30% clearance decrease/5°C change), for vecuronium (Caldwell et al., 2000) in normal healthy volunteers ($\sim$55% clearance decrease/5°C change), and for midazolam (Hostler et al., 2010) in normal healthy volunteers ($\sim$11% clearance change/1°C change). Whether or not the effects of short duration hypothermia translate to patients with CA receiving longer durations of cooling are currently unknown. In addition, these recommendations are across a wide array of disease states for the use of therapeutic hypothermia. The specific CA disease-mediated effects coupled with therapeutic hypothermia effects are currently unknown. Since CA represents the primary application of therapeutic hypothermia in adults, future studies to elucidate the specific changes in hepatic metabolism due to the CA event with and without clinical use of therapeutic hypothermia would greatly aid in determining dosing guidelines for drugs requiring CYP metabolism as a major route of elimination.

Studies have also been conducted to evaluate the role of CYP AA metabolites in the pathogenesis of CA. Studies have demonstrated that after resuscitation from CA, the brain undergoes an early hyperemia followed by secondary hypoperfusion period, which is brain region, injury type, and injury duration dependent (Drabek et al., 2014; He et al., 2015; Manole et al., 2014). Furthermore, it has been suggested that these secondary alterations in brain blood flow lead to secondary neuronal damage and poor neurofunctional outcome after arrest. The remaining research question is if the derangements in brain blood flow are mediated by CYP fatty acid metabolites involved in microvascular autoregulation. Some studies have been conducted to evaluate the role of CYP metabolites in both rat and mouse models, as well as studies in neonatal piglets. In a study by Shaik et al. (2015), our group evaluated the effect of 9 and 12 min of asphyxial CA and resuscitation on brain CYP AA metabolite concentrations in the postnatal day 17 pediatric rat model. This study demonstrated that CA increased EET levels in the brain when compared with sham animals after

9 min of arrest. However, after 12 min of CA prior to resuscitation, 20-HETE was highly elevated without a compensatory increase in EET levels in the brain. This increase in the vasoconstrictive 20-HETE metabolite is consistent with the significant reduction in cortical blood flow that has been observed with 12 min of asystole. Furthermore, this study evaluated the effects of the CYP4F inhibitor, HET0016 on brain CYP AA metabolite concentrations and the resultant effects on neurodegeneration and short-term neurological function. The CA-induced increased cortical 20-HETE was inhibited by the administration of HET0016 (0.9 mg/kg IV) at the time of resuscitation, and the inhibition of 20-HETE formation did not produce shunting of AA down either EET or prostaglandin metabolic pathways. This study also demonstrated that HET0016 reduced cortical neurodegeneration and decreased the percentage of brain tissue water ($84 \pm 0.13\%$ vs $83.43 \pm 0.24\%$, vehicle vs HET0016, $p < .05$), thereby suggesting neuroprotection and reduced brain edema. Additionally, neurologic deficits were greater in rats receiving the vehicle when compared with the observed reduction in neurologic deficits in rats treated with HET0016. Overall, these data demonstrate that inhibition of CYP4 by HET0016 is neuroprotective after CA and reduces edema and improves CBF early after insult in the rat. In the piglet hypoxia-ischemia model, it has been shown that 20-HETE formation inhibition by HET0016 protected neurons in the putamen 4 days after recovery and reduced markers of oxidative stress without alterations in CBF (Yang et al., 2012). More recently, Zhu et al. (2015) demonstrated that HET0016 was protective with the use of therapeutic hypothermia (34°C for 20 h) in the neonatal piglet hypoxia—ischemia model. HET0016 (1 mg/kg) administered at resuscitation significantly increased viable neurons in the putamen, somatosensory cortex, and thalamus over the protective benefits of therapeutic hypothermia in the piglet. Collectively, these data indicate that inhibition of 20-HETE formation is protective after neuronal ischemia in rats and piglets and also suggest that the protective benefits complement the protection afforded by therapeutic hypothermia.

Few studies have been conducted to evaluate the role of EETs in the pathogenesis of CA. As previously stated, increases in brain EET levels were observed after 9 min of asphyxial CA (Shaik et al., 2015); however, such elevations in EETs were not observed in more severe insults as 12 min of asystole. Thereby, these data suggest that severe injury-mediated reductions in blood flow may be mediated by 20-HETE elevations in the absence of counter-regulatory EET metabolites. Another study by Hutchens et al. (2008) evaluated the role of EETs in CA pathogenesis by evaluating CA-mediated brain and kidney damage in the soluble epoxide gene knockout mice. sEH converts EETs to the presumably less active DHET metabolites; therefore the knockout animals have been shown to have elevations in EETs. This study hypothesized that the elevation in EETs would be protective from CA-mediated tissue damage. Unexpectedly, this study demonstrated that the knockout mice had higher mortality, required higher doses of epinephrine during resuscitation, had longer periods of CPR prior to resuscitation and had a delayed blood pressure recovery when compared with wild-type control animals. These results suggest that either EETs worsened the CA recovery, that DHETs have other currently unrecognized effects important to recovery, or that developmental compensatory pathways in the knockout animals yield worse recovery. Additional studies in conditional knockout animals and with sEH inhibitor compounds are needed to truly delineate the reasons for the observed increase in mortality in sEH animals after CA.

SUMMARY

CYP enzymes are important in both drug metabolism and bioactivation of AA in several critically ill disease states. Within the field of stroke research, P450-mediated formation of 20-HETE and EET metabolites has been shown to play an important role in the resultant brain damage and secondary injury after either hemorrhagic or thromboembolic stroke. Inhibitors of CYP4 enzymatic formation of 20-HETE decrease neurodegeneration and neurological injury after stroke in preclinical animal studies. Conversely, EET metabolites that are formed by CYP2C and CYP2J isoforms are protective; therefore prevention of EET degradation by sEH also affords protection. Within TBI, the role of 20-HETE and EETs has not been extensively studied. However, the effects of TBI on P450-mediated drug metabolism have been the focus of both preclinical and clinical evaluations. Overall, preclinical studies in TBI suggest relatively minor reductions in P450 enzyme activity that is likely due to cytokine-mediated decreases in expression. Conversely, the few clinical studies that have been conducted to date suggest that patients have increased P450 metabolism due to a hypermetabolic state after brain injury. Finally, the effect of whole body insult during CA is also known to affect both drug metabolism and AA bioactivation by P450 enzymes. Differences in regulation after CA have been shown to be both isoform and drug specific after resuscitation. P450 formation of 20-HETE has also been shown to be a mechanism of secondary neuronal injury. Collectively, these studies highlight the importance of understanding alterations in P450 metabolism after critical illness. Future studies will likely elucidate both the drug dosing optimization in these patients, as well as the potential to target P450 isoforms that bioactivate AA as a novel therapeutic approach to improve disease outcomes.

References

Alonso-Galicia, M., Sun, C.W., Falck, J.R., Harder, D.R., Roman, R.J., 1998. Contribution of 20-HETE to the vasodilator actions of nitric oxide in renal arteries. Am. J. Physiol. 275 (3 Pt 2), F370–F378.

Anderson, G.D., Peterson, T.C., Vonder Haar, C., Farin, F.M., Bammler, T.K., MacDonald, J.W., et al., 2015. Effect of traumatic brain injury, erythropoietin, and anakinra on hepatic metabolizing enzymes and transporters in an experimental rat model. AAPS J. 17 (5), 1255–1267. http://dx.doi.org/10.1208/s12248-015-9792-y.

Bednar, M.M., Gross, C.E., Russell, S.R., Fuller, S.P., Ahern, T.P., Howard, D.B., et al., 2000. 16(R)-hydroxyeicosatetraenoic acid, a novel cytochrome P450 product of arachidonic acid, suppresses activation of human polymorphonuclear leukocyte and reduces intracranial pressure in a rabbit model of thromboembolic stroke. Neurosurgery 47 (6), 1410–1418.

Bernard, S.A., Gray, T.W., Buist, M.D., Jones, B.M., Silvester, W., Gutteridge, G., Smith, K., 2002. Treatment of comatose survivors of out-of-hospital cardiac arrest with induced hypothermia. New Engl. J. Med. 346 (8), 557–563. http://dx.doi.org/10.1056/NEJMoa003289.

Birnie, M., Morrison, R., Camara, R., Strauss, K.I., 2013. Temporal changes of cytochrome P450 (Cyp) and eicosanoid-related gene expression in the rat brain after traumatic brain injury. BMC Genomics 14, 303. http://dx.doi.org/10.1186/1471-2164-14-303.

Bronnum-Hansen, H., Davidsen, M., Thorvaldsen, P., Danish, Monica Study Group, 2001. Long-term survival and causes of death after stroke. Stroke 32 (9), 2131–2136.

Caldwell, J.E., Heier, T., Wright, P.M., Lin, S., McCarthy, G., Szenohradszky, J., et al., 2000. Temperature-dependent pharmacokinetics and pharmacodynamics of vecuronium. Anesthesiology 92 (1), 84–93.

Cambj-Sapunar, L., Yu, M., Harder, D.R., Roman, R.J., 2003. Contribution of 5-hydroxytryptamine1B receptors and 20-hydroxyeicosatetraenoic acid to fall in cerebral blood flow after subarachnoid hemorrhage. Stroke 34 (5), 1269–1275.

Capdevila, J.H., Wang, W., Falck, J.R., 2015. Arachidonic acid monooxygenase: genetic and biochemical approaches to physiological/pathophysiological relevance. Prostaglandins Other Lipid Mediat. 120, 40–49. http://dx.doi.org/10.1016/j.prostaglandins.2015.05.004.

Cheng, J., Edin, M.L., Hoopes, S.L., Li, H., Bradbury, J.A., Graves, J.P., et al., 2014. Vascular characterization of mice with endothelial expression of cytochrome P450 4F2. FASEB J. 7, 2915–2931. http://dx.doi.org/10.1096/fj.13-241927.

Crago, E.A., Thampatty, B.P., Sherwood, P.R., Kuo, C.W., Bender, C., Balzer, J., et al., 2011. Cerebrospinal fluid 20-HETE is associated with delayed cerebral ischemia and poor outcomes after aneurysmal subarachnoid hemorrhage. Stroke 42 (7), 1872–1877. http://dx.doi.org/10.1161/STROKEAHA.110.605816. STROKEAHA.110.605816 [pii].

Dhanasekaran, A., Al-Saghir, R., Lopez, B., Zhu, D., Gutterman, D.D., Jacobs, E.R., Medhora, M., 2006. Protective effects of epoxyeicosatrienoic acids on human endothelial cells from the pulmonary and coronary vasculature. Am. J. Physiol. Heart Circ. Physiol. 291 (2), H517–H531.

Donnelly, M.K., Conley, Y.P., Crago, E.A., Ren, D., Sherwood, P.R., Balzer, J.R., Poloyac, S.M., 2015a. Genetic markers in the EET metabolic pathway are associated with outcomes in patients with aneurysmal subarachnoid hemorrhage. J. Cereb. Blood Flow Metab. 35 (2), 267–276. http://dx.doi.org/10.1038/jcbfm.2014.195.

Donnelly, M.K., Crago, E.A., Conley, Y.P., Balzer, J.R., Ren, D., Ducruet, A.F., et al., 2015b. 20-HETE is associated with unfavorable outcomes in subarachnoid hemorrhage patients. J. Cereb. Blood Flow Metab. http://dx.doi.org/10.1038/jcbfm.2015.75.

Drabek, T., Foley, L.M., Janata, A., Stezoski, J., Kevin Hitchens, T., Manole, M.D., Kochanek, P.M., 2014. Global and regional differences in cerebral blood flow after asphyxial versus ventricular fibrillation cardiac arrest in rats using ASL-MRI. Resuscitation 85 (7), 964–971. http://dx.doi.org/10.1016/j.resuscitation.2014.03.314.

Dunn, K.M., Renic, M., Flasch, A.K., Harder, D.R., Falck, J., Roman, R.J., 2008. Elevated production of 20-HETE in the cerebral vasculature contributes to severity of ischemic stroke and oxidative stress in spontaneously hypertensive rats. Am. J. Physiol. Heart Circ. Physiol. 295 (6), H2455–H2465. http://dx.doi.org/10.1152/ajpheart.00512.2008.

Empey, P.E., McNamara, P.J., Young, B., Rosbolt, M.B., Hatton, J., 2006. Cyclosporin A disposition following acute traumatic brain injury. J. Neurotrauma 23 (1), 109–116. http://dx.doi.org/10.1089/neu.2006.23.109.

Empey, P.E., Miller, T.M., Philbrick, A.H., Melick, J., Kochanek, P.M., Poloyac, S.M., 2011. Mild hypothermia decreases fentanyl and midazolam steady-state clearance in a rat model of cardiac arrest. Crit. Care Med. http://dx.doi.org/10.1097/CCM.0b013e31823779f9.

Empey, P.E., Velez de Mendizabal, N., Bell, M.J., Bies, R.R., Anderson, K., Kochanek, P.M., et al., 2013. Therapeutic hypothermia decreases phenytoin elimination in children with traumatic brain injury. Crit. Care Med. 41 (10), 2379–2387.

Fan, F., Muroya, Y., Roman, R.J., 2015. Cytochrome P450 eicosanoids in hypertension and renal disease. Curr. Opin. Nephrol. Hypertens. 24 (1), 37–46. http://dx.doi.org/10.1097/MNH.0000000000000088.

Fer, M., Corcos, L., Dreano, Y., Plee-Gautier, E., Salaun, J.P., Berthou, F., Amet, Y., 2008. Cytochromes P450 from family 4 are the main omega hydroxylating enzymes in humans: CYP4F3B is the prominent player in PUFA metabolism. J. Lipid Res. 49 (11), 2379–2389. http://dx.doi.org/10.1194/jlr.M800199-JLR200.

Fleming, I., 2001. Cytochrome p450 and vascular homeostasis. Circ. Res. 89 (9), 753–762.

Foley, N., Marshall, S., Pikul, J., Salter, K., Teasell, R., 2008. Hypermetabolism following moderate to severe traumatic acute brain injury: a systematic review. J. Neurotrauma 25 (12), 1415–1431. http://dx.doi.org/10.1089/neu.2008.0628.

Fordsmann, J.C., Ko, R.W., Choi, H.B., Thomsen, K., Witgen, B.M., Mathiesen, C., et al., 2013. Increased 20-HETE synthesis explains reduced cerebral blood flow but not impaired neurovascular coupling after cortical spreading depression in rat cerebral cortex. J. Neurosci. 33 (6), 2562–2570. http://dx.doi.org/10.1523/JNEUROSCI.2308-12.2013.

Fukuoka, N., Aibiki, M., Tsukamoto, T., Seki, K., Morita, S., 2004. Biphasic concentration change during continuous midazolam administration in brain-injured patients undergoing therapeutic moderate hypothermia. Resuscitation 60 (2), 225–230.

Garcia, V., Cheng, J., Weidenhammer, A., Ding, Y., Wu, C.C., Zhang, F., et al., 2015. Androgen-induced hypertension in angiotensinogen deficient mice: role of 20-HETE and EETS. Prostaglandins Other Lipid Mediat. 116–117, 124–130. http://dx.doi.org/10.1016/j.prostaglandins.2014.12.001.

Gebremedhin, D., Lange, A.R., Lowry, T.F., Taheri, M.R., Birks, E.K., Hudetz, A.G., et al., 2000. Production of 20-HETE and its role in autoregulation of cerebral blood flow. Circ. Res. 87 (1), 60—65.

Go, A.S., Mozaffarian, D., Roger, V.L., Benjamin, E.J., Berry, J.D., Borden, W.B., et al., 2013. Heart disease and stroke statistics—2013 update: a report from the American Heart Association. Circulation 127 (1), e6—e245. http://dx.doi.org/10.1161/CIR.0b013e31828124ad.

Hacein-Bey, L., Harder, D.R., Meier, H.T., Varelas, P.N., Miyata, N., Lauer, K.K., et al., 2006. Reversal of delayed vasospasm by TS-011 in the dual hemorrhage dog model of subarachnoid hemorrhage. AJNR Am. J. Neuroradiol. 27 (6), 1350—1354.

Hall, C.N., Reynell, C., Gesslein, B., Hamilton, N.B., Mishra, A., Sutherland, B.A., et al., 2014. Capillary pericytes regulate cerebral blood flow in health and disease. Nature 508 (7494), 55—60. http://dx.doi.org/10.1038/nature13165.

Harbrecht, B.G., Frye, R.F., Zenati, M.S., Branch, R.A., Peitzman, A.B., 2005. Cytochrome P-450 activity is differentially altered in severely injured patients. Crit. Care Med. 33 (3), 541—546.

Harder, D.R., Gebremedhin, D., Narayanan, J., Jefcoat, C., Falck, J.R., Campbell, W.B., Roman, R.J., 1994. Formation and action of a P-450 4A metabolite of arachidonic acid in cat cerebral microvessels. Am. J. Physiol. 266, H2098—H2107.

He, J., Lu, H., Deng, R., Young, L., Tong, S., Jia, X., 2015. Real-time monitoring of cerebral blood flow by laser speckle contrast imaging after cardiac arrest in rat. Conf. Proc. IEEE Eng. Med. Biol. Soc. 2015, 6971—6974. http://dx.doi.org/10.1109/EMBC.2015.7319996.

Hostler, D., Zhou, J., Tortorici, M.A., Bies, R.R., Rittenberger, J.C., Empey, P.E., et al., 2010. Mild hypothermia alters midazolam pharmacokinetics in normal healthy volunteers. Drug Metab. Dispos. 38 (5), 781—788. http://dx.doi.org/10.1124/dmd.109.031377 dmd.109.031377 [pii].

Huang, H., Al-Shabrawey, M., Wang, M.H., 2016. Cyclooxygenase- and cytochrome P450-derived eicosanoids in stroke. Prostaglandins Other Lipid Mediat. 122, 45—53. http://dx.doi.org/10.1016/j.prostaglandins.2015.12.007.

Hutchens, M.P., Nakano, T., Dunlap, J., Traystman, R.J., Hurn, P.D., Alkayed, N.J., 2008. Soluble epoxide hydrolase gene deletion reduces survival after cardiac arrest and cardiopulmonary resuscitation. Resuscitation 76 (1), 89—94. http://dx.doi.org/10.1016/j.resuscitation.2007.06.031.

Iida, Y., Nishi, S., Asada, A., 2001. Effect of mild therapeutic hypothermia on phenytoin pharmacokinetics. Ther. Drug Monit. 23 (3), 192—197.

Imaoka, S., Hashizume, T., Funae, Y., 2005. Localization of rat cytochrome P450 in various tissues and comparison of arachidonic acid metabolism by rat P450 with that by human P450 orthologs. Drug Metab. Pharmacokinet. 20 (6), 478—484.

Imig, J.D., Simpkins, A.N., Renic, M., Harder, D.R., 2011. Cytochrome P450 eicosanoids and cerebral vascular function. Expert Rev. Mol. Med. 13, e7. http://dx.doi.org/10.1017/S1462399411001773.

Kaide, J., Wang, M.H., Wang, J.S., Zhang, F., Gopal, V.R., Falck, J.R., et al., 2003. Transfection of CYP4A1 cDNA increases vascular reactivity in renal interlobar arteries. Am. J. Physiol. Ren. Physiol. 284 (1), F51—F56.

Kalsotra, A., Turman, C.M., Dash, P.K., Strobel, H.W., 2003. Differential effects of traumatic brain injury on the cytochrome p450 system: a perspective into hepatic and renal drug metabolism. J. Neurotrauma 20 (12), 1339—1350.

Kalsotra, A., Zhao, J., Anakk, S., Dash, P.K., Strobel, H.W., 2007. Brain trauma leads to enhanced lung inflammation and injury: evidence for role of P4504Fs in resolution. J. Cereb. Blood Flow Metab. 27 (5), 963—974. http://dx.doi.org/10.1038/sj.jcbfm.9600396.

Kawasaki, T., Marumo, T., Shirakami, K., Mori, T., Doi, H., Suzuki, M., et al., 2012. Increase of 20-HETE synthase after brain ischemia in rats revealed by PET study with 11C-labeled 20-HETE synthase-specific inhibitor. J. Cereb. Blood Flow Metab. 32 (9), 1737—1746. http://dx.doi.org/10.1038/jcbfm.2012.68.

Kehl, F., Cambj-Sapunar, L., Maier, K.G., Miyata, N., Kametani, S., Okamoto, H., et al., 2002. 20-HETE contributes to the acute fall in cerebral blood flow after subarachnoid hemorrhage in the rat. Am. J. Physiol. Heart Circ. Physiol. 282 (4), H1556—H1565.

Koerner, I.P., Jacks, R., DeBarber, A.E., Koop, D., Mao, P., Grant, D.F., Alkayed, N.J., 2007. Polymorphisms in the human soluble epoxide hydrolase gene EPHX2 linked to neuronal survival after ischemic injury. J. Neurosci. 27 (17), 4642—4649. http://dx.doi.org/10.1523/JNEUROSCI.0056-07.2007.

Koren, G., Barker, C., Bohn, D., Kent, G., Biggar, W.D., 1985. Influence of hypothermia on the pharmacokinetics of gentamicin and theophylline in piglets. Crit. Care Med. 13 (10), 844—847.

Lasker, J.M., Chen, W.B., Wolf, I., Bloswick, B.P., Wilson, P.D., Powell, P.K., 2000. Formation of 20-hydroxyeicosatetraenoic acid, a vasoactive and natriuretic eicosanoid, in human kidney. Role of Cyp4F2 and Cyp4A11. J. Biol. Chem. 275 (6), 4118–4126.

Liu, M., Alkayed, N.J., 2005. Hypoxic preconditioning and tolerance via hypoxia inducible factor (HIF) 1alpha-linked induction of P450 2C11 epoxygenase in astrocytes. J. Cereb. Blood Flow Metab. 25 (8), 939–948.

Liu, Y., Wang, D., Wang, H., Qu, Y., Xiao, X., Zhu, Y., 2014. The protective effect of HET0016 on brain edema and blood—brain barrier dysfunction after cerebral ischemia/reperfusion. Brain Res. 1544, 45–53. http://dx.doi.org/10.1016/j.brainres.2013.11.031.

Liu, Y., Zhang, Y., Schmelzer, K., Lee, T.S., Fang, X., Zhu, Y., et al., 2005. The antiinflammatory effect of laminar flow: the role of PPARgamma, epoxyeicosatrienoic acids, and soluble epoxide hydrolase. Proc. Natl. Acad. Sci. USA 102 (46), 16747–16752.

Ma, J., Wang, J., Cheng, J., Xiao, W., Fan, K., Gu, J., et al., 2016. Impacts of blast-induced traumatic brain injury on expressions of hepatic cytochrome P450 1A2, 2B1, 2D1, and 3A2 in rats. Cell Mol. Neurobiol. http://dx.doi.org/10.1007/s10571-016-0351-6.

Manole, M.D., Kochanek, P.M., Bayir, H., Alexander, H., Dezfulian, C., Fink, E.L., et al., 2014. Brain tissue oxygen monitoring identifies cortical hypoxia and thalamic hyperoxia after experimental cardiac arrest in rats. Pediatr. Res. 75 (2), 295–301. http://dx.doi.org/10.1038/pr.2013.220.

Marumo, T., Eto, K., Wake, H., Omura, T., Nabekura, J., 2010. The inhibitor of 20-HETE synthesis, TS-011, improves cerebral microcirculatory autoregulation impaired by middle cerebral artery occlusion in mice. Br. J. Pharmacol. 161 (6), 1391–1402. http://dx.doi.org/10.1111/j.1476-5381.2010.00973.x.

Michelsen, L.G., Holford, N.H., Lu, W., Hoke, J.F., Hug, C.C., Bailey, J.M., 2001. The pharmacokinetics of remifentanil in patients undergoing coronary artery bypass grafting with cardiopulmonary bypass. Anesth. Analg. 93 (5), 1100–1105.

Miller, T.M., Donnelly, M.K., Crago, E.A., Roman, D.M., Sherwood, P.R., Horowitz, M.B., Poloyac, S.M., 2009. Rapid, simultaneous quantitation of mono and dioxygenated metabolites of arachidonic acid in human CSF and rat brain. J. Chromatogr. B Analyt. Technol. Biomed. Life Sci. 877 (31), 3991–4000. http://dx.doi.org/10.1016/j.jchromb.2009.10.012. S1570-0232(09)00715-6 [pii].

Miyata, N., Roman, R.J., 2005. Role of 20-hydroxyeicosatetraenoic acid (20-HETE) in vascular system. J. Smooth Muscle Res. 41 (4), 175–193.

Miyata, N., Seki, T., Tanaka, Y., Omura, T., Taniguchi, K., Doi, M., et al., 2005. Beneficial effects of a new 20-hydroxyeicosatetraenoic acid synthesis inhibitor, TS-011 [N-(3-chloro-4-morpholin-4-yl) phenyl-N′-hydroxyimido formamide], on hemorrhagic and ischemic stroke. J. Pharmacol. Exp. Ther. 314 (1), 77–85.

Moler, F.W., Silverstein, F.S., Holubkov, R., Slomine, B.S., Christensen, J.R., Nadkarni, V.M., et al., 2015. Therapeutic hypothermia after out-of-hospital cardiac arrest in children. N. Engl. J. Med. 372 (20), 1898–1908. http://dx.doi.org/10.1056/NEJMoa1411480.

Morisseau, C., Hammock, B.D., 2013. Impact of soluble epoxide hydrolase and epoxyeicosanoids on human health. Annu. Rev. Pharmacol. Toxicol. 53, 37–58. http://dx.doi.org/10.1146/annurev-pharmtox-011112-140244.

Nguyen, X., Wang, M.H., Reddy, K.M., Falck, J.R., Schwartzman, M.L., 1999. Kinetic profile of the rat CYP4A isoforms: arachidonic acid metabolism and isoform-specific inhibitors. Am. J. Physiol. 276 (6 Pt 2), R1691–R1700.

Nishida, K., Okazaki, M., Sakamoto, R., Inaoka, N., Miyake, H., Fumoto, S., et al., 2007. Change in pharmacokinetics of model compounds with different elimination processes in rats during hypothermia. Biol. Pharm. Bull. 30 (9), 1763–1767.

Omura, T., Tanaka, Y., Miyata, N., Koizumi, C., Sakurai, T., Fukasawa, M., et al., 2006. Effect of a new inhibitor of the synthesis of 20-HETE on cerebral ischemia reperfusion injury. Stroke 37 (5), 1307–1313.

Poloyac, S.M., Reynolds, R.B., Yonas, H., Kerr, M.E., 2005. Identification and quantification of the hydroxyeicosatetraenoic acids, 20-HETE and 12-HETE, in the cerebrospinal fluid after subarachnoid hemorrhage. J. Neurosci. Methods 144 (2), 257–263. http://dx.doi.org/10.1016/j.jneumeth.2004.11.015. S0165-0270(04)00425-X [pii].

Poloyac, S.M., Zhang, Y., Bies, R.R., Kochanek, P.M., Graham, S.H., 2006. Protective effect of the 20-HETE inhibitor HET0016 on brain damage after temporary focal ischemia. J. Cereb. Blood Flow Metab. 26 (12), 1551–1561. http://dx.doi.org/10.1038/sj.jcbfm.9600309, 9600309 [pii].

Poloyac, S.M., Perez, A., Blouin, R.A., 2000. Tissue specific alterations in the 6-hydroxylation of chlorzoxazone following traumatic brain injury in the rat. Drug Metab. Dispos. 29 (3), 296–298.

Powell, P.K., Wolf, I., Jin, R., Lasker, J.M., 1998. Metabolism of arachidonic acid to 20-hydroxy-5,8,11, 14-eicosatetraenoic acid by P450 enzymes in human liver: involvement of CYP4F2 and CYP4A11. J. Pharmacol. Exp. Ther. 285 (3), 1327−1336.

Renic, M., Klaus, J.A., Omura, T., Kawashima, N., Onishi, M., Miyata, N., et al., 2009. Effect of 20-HETE inhibition on infarct volume and cerebral blood flow after transient middle cerebral artery occlusion. J. Cereb. Blood Flow Metab. 29 (3), 629−639. http://dx.doi.org/10.1038/jcbfm.2008.156.

Roka, A., Melinda, K.T., Vasarhelyi, B., Machay, T., Azzopardi, D., Szabo, M., 2008. Elevated morphine concentrations in neonates treated with morphine and prolonged hypothermia for hypoxic ischemic encephalopathy. Pediatrics 121 (4), e844−849. http://dx.doi.org/10.1542/peds.2007-1987, 121/4/e844 [pii].

Shaik, J.S., Poloyac, S.M., Kochanek, P.M., Alexander, H., Tudorascu, D.L., Clark, R.S., Manole, M.D., 2015. 20-Hydroxyeicosatetraenoic acid inhibition by HET0016 offers neuroprotection, decreases edema, and increases cortical cerebral blood flow in a pediatric asphyxial cardiac arrest model in rats. J. Cereb. Blood Flow Metab. http://dx.doi.org/10.1038/jcbfm.2015.117.

Shankaran, S., Laptook, A.R., 2007. Hypothermia as a treatment for birth asphyxia. Clin. Obstet. Gynecol. 50 (3), 624−635. http://dx.doi.org/10.1097/GRF.0b013e31811eba5e.

Siler, D.A., Martini, R.P., Ward, J.P., Nelson, J.W., Borkar, R.N., Zuloaga, K.L., et al., 2014. Protective role of P450 epoxyeicosanoids in subarachnoid hemorrhage. Neurocrit. Care. http://dx.doi.org/10.1007/s12028-014-0011-y.

Sun, C.W., Falck, J.R., Okamoto, H., Harder, D.R., Roman, R.J., 2000. Role of cGMP versus 20-HETE in the vasodilator response to nitric oxide in rat cerebral arteries. Am. J. Physiol. Heart Circ. Physiol. 279 (1), H339−H350.

Sundseth, S.S., Waxman, D.J., 1992. Sex-dependent expression and clofibrate inducibility of cytochrome P450 4A fatty acid omega-hydroxylases. Male specificity of liver and kidney CYP4A2 mRNA and tissue-specific regulation by growth hormone and testosterone. J. Biol. Chem. 267 (6), 3915−3921.

Sunjic, K.M., Webb, A.C., Sunjic, I., Pala Creus, M., Folse, S.L., 2015. Pharmacokinetic and other considerations for drug therapy during targeted temperature management. Crit. Care Med. 43 (10), 2228−2238. http://dx.doi.org/10.1097/CCM.0000000000001223.

Sura, P., Sura, R., Enayetallah, A.E., Grant, D.F., 2008. Distribution and expression of soluble epoxide hydrolase in human brain. J. Histochem. Cytochem. 56 (6), 551−559. http://dx.doi.org/10.1369/jhc.2008.950659.

Takeuchi, K., Miyata, N., Renic, M., Harder, D.R., Roman, R.J., 2006. Hemoglobin, NO, and 20-HETE interactions in mediating cerebral vasoconstriction following SAH. Am. J. Physiol. Regul. Integr. Comp. Physiol. 290 (1), R84−R89.

Takeuchi, K., Renic, M., Bohman, Q.C., Harder, D.R., Miyata, N., Roman, R.J., 2005. Reversal of delayed vasospasm by an inhibitor of the synthesis of 20-HETE. Am. J. Physiol. Heart Circ. Physiol. 289 (5), H2203−H2211.

Tanaka, Y., Omura, T., Fukasawa, M., Horiuchi, N., Miyata, N., Minagawa, T., et al., 2007. Continuous inhibition of 20-HETE synthesis by TS-011 improves neurological and functional outcomes after transient focal cerebral ischemia in rats. Neurosci. Res. 59 (4), 475−480.

Taylor, T.N., 1997. The medical economics of stroke. Drugs 54 (Suppl. 3), 51−57 discussion 57−58.

Toler, S.M., Young, A.B., McClain, C.J., Shedlofsky, S.I., Bandyopadhyay, A.M., Blouin, R.A., 1993. Head injury and cytochrome P-450 enzymes. Differential effect on mRNA and protein expression in the Fischer-344 rat. Drug Metab. Dispos. 21 (6), 1064−1069.

Tortorici, M.A., Kochanek, P.M., Bies, R.R., Poloyac, S.M., 2006. Therapeutic hypothermia-induced pharmacokinetic alterations on CYP2E1 chlorzoxazone-mediated metabolism in a cardiac arrest rat model. Crit. Care Med. 34 (3), 785−791.

Tortorici, M.A., Kochanek, P.M., Poloyac, S.M., 2007. Effects of hypothermia on drug disposition, metabolism, and response: a focus of hypothermia-mediated alterations on the cytochrome P450 enzyme system. Crit. Care Med. 35 (9), 2196−2204.

Tortorici, M.A., Mu, Y., Kochanek, P.M., Xie, W., Poloyac, S.M., 2009. Moderate hypothermia prevents cardiac arrest-mediated suppression of drug metabolism and induction of interleukin-6 in rats. Crit. Care Med. 37 (1), 263−269. http://dx.doi.org/10.1097/CCM.0b013e3181931ed3.

van den Broek, M.P., Groenendaal, F., Egberts, A.C., Rademaker, C.M., 2010. Effects of hypothermia on pharmacokinetics and pharmacodynamics: a systematic review of preclinical and clinical studies. Clin. Pharmacokinet. 49 (5), 277−294. http://dx.doi.org/10.2165/11319360-000000000-00000.

Wang, Y., Zhao, J., Kalsotra, A., Turman, C.M., Grill, R.J., Dash, P.K., Strobel, H.W., 2008. CYP4Fs expression in rat brain correlates with changes in LTB4 levels after traumatic brain injury. J. Neurotrauma 25 (10), 1187–1194. http://dx.doi.org/10.1089/neu.2008.0542.

Wink, D.A., Osawa, Y., Darbyshire, J.F., Jones, C.R., Eshnaur, S.C., Nims, R.W., 1993. Inhibition of cytochromes P450 by nitric oxide and nitric oxide-releasing agent. Arch. Biochem. Biophys. 300, 115–123.

Wu, C.C., Gupta, T., Garcia, V., Ding, Y., Schwartzman, M.L., 2014. 20-HETE and blood pressure regulation: clinical implications. Cardiol. Rev. 22 (1), 1–12. http://dx.doi.org/10.1097/CRD.0b013e3182961659.

Xu, F., Falck, J.R., Ortiz De Montellano, P.R., Kroetz, D.L., 2004. Catalytic activity and isoform specific inhibition of rat CYP4F isoforms. J. Pharmacol. Exp. Ther. 308 (3), 887–895.

Yang, Z.J., Carter, E.L., Kibler, K.K., Kwansa, H., Crafa, D.A., Martin, L.J., et al., 2012. Attenuation of neonatal ischemic brain damage using a 20-HETE synthesis inhibitor. J. Neurochem. 121 (1), 168–179. http://dx.doi.org/10.1111/j.1471-4159.2012.07666.x.

Yu, M., Cambj-Sapunar, L., Kehl, F., Maier, K.G., Takeuchi, K., Miyata, N., et al., 2004. Effects of a 20-HETE antagonist and agonists on cerebral vascular tone. Eur. J. Pharmacol. 486 (3), 297–306. http://dx.doi.org/10.1016/j.ejphar.2004.01.009.

Zhang, W., Koerner, I.P., Noppens, R., Grafe, M., Tsai, H.J., Morisseau, C., et al., 2007. Soluble epoxide hydrolase: a novel therapeutic target in stroke. J. Cereb. Blood Flow Metab. 27 (12), 1931–1940.

Zhang, W., Otsuka, T., Sugo, N., Ardeshiri, A., Alhadid, Y.K., Iliff, J.J., et al., 2008. Soluble epoxide hydrolase gene deletion is protective against experimental cerebral ischemia. Stroke 39 (7), 2073–2078.

Zhou, J., Empey, P.E., Bies, R.R., Kochanek, P.M., Poloyac, S.M., 2011. Cardiac arrest and therapeutic hypothermia decrease isoform-specific cytochrome P450 drug metabolism. Drug Metab. Dispos. 39 (12), 2209–2218. http://dx.doi.org/10.1124/dmd.111.040642 dmd.111.040642 [pii].

Zhou, J., Poloyac, S.M., 2011. The effect of therapeutic hypothermia on drug metabolism and response: cellular mechanisms to organ function. Expert Opin. Drug Metab. Toxicol. 7 (7), 803–816.

Zhu, J., Wang, B., Lee, J.H., Armstrong, J.S., Kulikowicz, E., Bhalala, U.S., et al., 2015. Additive neuroprotection of a 20-HETE inhibitor with delayed therapeutic hypothermia after hypoxia-ischemia in neonatal piglets. Dev. Neurosci. 37 (4–5), 376–389. http://dx.doi.org/10.1159/000369007.

CHAPTER

6

Drug Metabolism in Cardiovascular Disease

J.C. Coons, P. Empey

University of Pittsburgh, Pittsburgh, PA, United States

OUTLINE

Introduction   139

Cardiovascular Diseases   140
  Heart Failure   140
  Cardiorenal Syndrome   141
  Cardiohepatic Syndrome   143
  Cardiac Arrest   146
    Therapeutic Hypothermia   146

Cytochrome P-450 Expression in
Cardiovascular Disease   147

Pharmacogenomics Related to
Cardiovascular Drugs and
Disease   148
  Variation in Drug Metabolism   148
  Heart Failure and Hypertension   148
    β-Blockers and CYP2D6   148

Angiotensin Receptor Blockers and
  CYP2C9   149
Digoxin and ATP-Binding Cassette
  B1   150
Acute Coronary Syndrome and
  Percutaneous Coronary Intervention 150
  Clopidogrel and CYP2C19   150
Thromboembolism   151
  Warfarin and CYP2C9, VKORC1   151
  Dabigatran and Carboxylesterase-1   152
Dyslipidemia   152
  HMG-CoA Reductase Inhibitors
    and SLCO1B1   152

Conclusion   153

References   153

INTRODUCTION

Cardiovascular (CV) diseases are the leading cause of death globally, representing ∼30% of all mortality (Mozaffarian et al., 2015). Over 85 million adults in the United States (US) have at least one form of CV disease, and more than half of these cases occur in those $\geq$60 years of age (Mozaffarian et al., 2015). CV drugs represent the most prevalent pharmacologic category in polypharmacy cohorts and rank among the top 20 most prescribed drugs in the US (antiplatelets, statins, β-blockers [BBs], and renin–angiotensin system inhibitors) (Qato et al., 2008). Not surprisingly, several common CV conditions were associated with the highest levels of prescribing (heart failure [HF], ischemic heart disease, and atrial fibrillation) (Payne et al., 2014). Polypharmacy with these drugs increases the risks of drug–drug interactions and adverse events (AEs). In fact, CV drugs are the most frequent cause of AEs in older ambulatory patients (Payne et al., 2014). Several examples of CV drugs (i.e., antiarrhythmics, anticoagulants) have narrow therapeutic indices, and their dosing is sufficiently complex that knowledge of relevant pharmacokinetic (PK) changes is essential.

The PK and pharmacodynamics (PD) of CV drugs may be altered in the context of the CV disease itself or its associated comorbidities (Mukhtar and Jackson, 2015). Physiologic changes also play an important role, most notably the effects of aging. Examples of PK changes seen in elderly patients include: reduction in kidney function, hepatic metabolism, less protein binding, increased body fat, and fewer target cell receptor sites (Rossello et al., 2015; Kowey et al., 2000). Interindividual variability in drug response seen as a result of pharmacogenetic differences in drug metabolism and transport are also important factors to consider. In summary, each of these factors changes the distribution, metabolism, and elimination of CV drugs (Mukhtar and Jackson, 2015; Rossello et al., 2015). Consequently, an understanding of the implications of CV disease and its associated conditions on drug metabolism and disposition is paramount. In many instances, therapeutic regimens are adjusted to account for these changes in an effort to optimize efficacy and minimize the risk for toxicity.

CARDIOVASCULAR DISEASES

Heart Failure

HF is a complex clinical syndrome which affects an estimated 5.1 million patients annually in the US (Yancy et al., 2013). The incidence of HF increases with each decade of life, such that by 2050 one in five persons over the age of 65 will develop this condition. The central pathophysiologic tenet of HF is an inability to meet the metabolic demands of the body on the basis of impaired cardiac structure and/or function. Consequently, reductions in end-organ function due to HF have a direct impact on drug disposition and elimination. The most compelling examples are progressive declines in hepatic and renal blood flow which impair drug elimination (Kowey et al., 2000). Other PK changes seen with HF include a reduction in the volume of distribution (V_d) due to inadequate organ perfusion. Reduced absorption can also be expected with HF but may limit or prevent drug accumulation as a result of the lower V_d (Kowey et al., 2000). Ultimately, most CV drugs are dependent upon hepatic or renal function (or both) and thus generally require lower doses to maintain a steady-state plasma concentration. The specific effects of HF on the liver and kidneys are further described in the subsequent sections with notable examples of known or anticipated changes in PK for commonly used drugs in this setting.

Cardiorenal Syndrome

Cardiorenal syndrome (CRS) is a poignant example of organ cross talk whereby interdependency exists between the function of the heart and kidneys, and vice versa (Ronco et al., 2008). These interactions are a result of complex communications involving humoral, cellular, and other mechanical mechanisms. Five types of CRSs have been recognized: (1) acute CRS, seen when rapid worsening of cardiac function leads to acute kidney injury (AKI); (2) chronic CRS, due to chronic worsening in cardiac function which causes progressive chronic kidney disease (CKD); (3) acute renocardiac syndrome, characterized by abrupt and primary worsening of kidney function leading to acute cardiac dysfunction; (4) chronic renocardiac syndrome, where primary CKD leads to decreased cardiac function; and (5) secondary CRS, or combined cardiac and renal dysfunction, due to acute or chronic systemic disorders (Ronco et al., 2008).

The most relevant example of a CV condition that causes or is directly affected by CRS is HF. Manifestations of HF may include: chronic HF with either reduced or preserved left ventricular function, acutely decompensated HF, cardiogenic shock, and predominant right ventricular failure (Ronco et al., 2008). Type 1 CRS is frequently seen in the inpatient setting, where more than 1 million patients in the US are hospitalized each year with either new onset acute HF or acutely decompensated chronic HF (Ronco et al., 2008; Yancy et al., 2013). The onset of AKI in this setting is likely a result of inadequate kidney perfusion due to poor cardiac output and/or significant elevation in venous pressure which leads to congestion of the kidney (Ronco et al., 2008). Type II CRS is another frequently encountered clinical problem in which chronic HF is accompanied by a 25% prevalence of chronic kidney dysfunction. In these patients, reduced kidney perfusion is likely superimposed on microvascular and macrovascular diseases (Ronco et al., 2008). Changes in kidney function seen in types I and II CRS would be expected to cause alternations in drug metabolism and/or disposition. However, little data are available on the PK of medications used in the context of CRS.

A notable example of variability in drug response in the setting of HF includes the loop diuretics. Table 6.1 describes the known PK changes with this class of drugs in HF. The presence of HF itself slows the rate of absorption of loop diuretics, resulting in a delayed peak response of at least 4 h after the last dose was administered (Brater, 1998; Vasko et al., 1985). Additionally, renal responsiveness to diuretics may also be decreased in HF (Brater et al., 1980; Vargo et al., 1995; Brater, 1998). For example, patients with New York Heart Association class II or III HF have 1/4 to 1/3 the natriuretic response compared with normal subjects. This difference is even greater for patients with more severe HF symptoms (Brater et al., 1980, 1998; Vargo et al., 1995). The delivery of loop diuretic to the site of action is generally not affected directly by HF; however, it is impaired in the presence of kidney dysfunction such as in CRS. In fact, patients with a creatinine clearance <15 mL/min have only 1/5 to 1/10 the secretion of loop diuretic into tubular fluid as normal subjects (Brater, 1998; Beermann, 1984). Since patients with CRS have coexisting cardiac and kidney impairment, changes in these PK parameters with loop diuretics could be anticipated. Because of the inadequacy of diuretic delivery to the nephron in patients with kidney impairment, larger doses are frequently required. In contrast, the delayed and decreased responsiveness to diuretics in HF typically requires more frequent

TABLE 6.1 Pharmacokinetics of Commonly Used Diuretics in Heart Failure

		Elimination Half-Life (h)			
Drug	Bioavailability (%)	Normal Subjects	Patients With Congestive Heart Failure	Patients With Renal Insufficiency	Patients With Cirrhosis
LOOP DIURETICS					
Furosemide	10–100	1.5–2	2.7	2.8	2.5
Bumetanide	80–100	1	1.3	1.6	2.3
Torsemide	80–100	3–4	6	4–5	8
THIAZIDE DIURETICS					
Chlorthalidone	64	24–55	ND	ND	ND
Chlorothiazide	30–50	1.5	ND	ND	ND
Hydrochlorothiazide	65–75	2.5	ND	Increased	ND
Indapamide	93	15–25	ND	ND	ND
POTASSIUM SPARING					
Amiloride	Conflicting data	17–26	ND	100	Negligible change
Triamterene[a]	>80	2–5	ND	Prolonged	No change
Spironolactone	Conflicting data	1.5	ND	No change	No change

[a]Values for active metabolite.
ND, not determined.
Adapted from Brater, D.C., 1998. Diuretic therapy. N. Engl. J. Med. 339 (6), 387–395.

administration of moderate doses to attain the therapeutic response. In summary, patients with CRS may require both an increase in dose as well as frequency of loop diuretics to account for the known changes in PK.

Other medications susceptible to changes in PK in the context of CRS include certain hydrophilic β-adrenoreceptor antagonists (BBs), such as atenolol and sotalol. Atenolol is a cardioselective BB with limited hepatic metabolism. The elimination half-life of atenolol is significantly prolonged in kidney impairment, particularly in patients with end-stage kidney disease (half-life 15–35 h when compared with 6–7 h in normal kidney function) (Product Information, 2012). Sotalol is a nonselective BB that also exhibits potassium channel–blocking properties. Sotalol is not metabolized and is eliminated almost entirely by the kidneys (90%). The half-life in normal kidney function is 12 h but progressively increases with worsening kidney function (Kowey et al., 2000). The risks with unadjusted dose or dosing intervals of these BB in patients with kidney impairment or CRS include: bradycardia, heart block, hypotension, and shock. In the case of sotalol, inappropriate adjustment of dose could also lead to QT interval prolongation and risk for Torsade de pointes (TdP). Dofetilide is another example of an antiarrhythmic, similar to sotalol, which must be dose adjusted in the presence of renal insufficiency to avoid QT prolongation and TdP. Elderly patients are at excess risk for these effects not only based on the decline in kidney function, but also due to a reduced number of β-adrenergic receptors (Vestal et al., 1979; Kowey et al., 2000). This latter effect may be especially important because the usual physiologic response to β-blockade is to upregulate β-adrenergic receptors and compensate for the initial reduction in cardiac output. In summary, patients with CRS would be safest to use alternative BBs that are more lipophilic with greater dependency on hepatic metabolism, such as carvedilol, metoprolol, or propranolol.

Digoxin is a classic example of a CV drug which is primarily eliminated by the kidneys as unchanged drug. Its elimination closely aligns with glomerular filtration rate (GFR). The elimination half-life in healthy volunteers is approximately 26–45 h, but progressively increases with decrements in GFR (Iisalo, 1977). Digoxin also possesses a large V_d with high concentrations found in cardiac and kidney tissues as well as in skeletal muscle. The PD and clinical responses to digoxin are correlated with uptake into cardiac tissue acutely and with steady-state serum concentrations in the maintenance phase (Iisalo, 1977). Therefore, changes in digoxin PK in the context of CRS would necessitate adjustments in dosing and/or frequency to avoid toxicity. A secondary analysis of the landmark Digoxin Investigation Group (DIG) study found that kidney dysfunction was strongly linked to mortality in stable outpatients with HF, particularly when the estimated GFR was <50 mL/min per 1.73 m^2 (Shlipak et al., 2004). Consequently, digoxin may be best avoided altogether in advanced stages of kidney impairment. Table 6.2 outlines the PK of various antiarrhythmics, including agents discussed in this section as well as others seen in clinical practice.

Cardiohepatic Syndrome

The liver is well perfused under normal physiology circumstances owing to the rich dual supply of blood from the portal vein and hepatic artery. Because of these features, the liver is generally protected against ischemia during periods of brief hypotension (Weisberg and Jacobson, 2011). However, there are a number of CV conditions which make the liver susceptible to injury and predispose to alterations in drug metabolism. Ischemic hepatitis, also referred to as shock liver or hypoxic hepatitis, is one type of diffuse injury that can occur as a result of impaired oxygen delivery (Weisberg and Jacobson, 2011). Common underlying causes of shock liver are acute myocardial infarction (MI) and acute HF complicated by systemic hypotension and/or shock. Cardiogenic shock occurs in approximately 5–10% of patients with extensive acute MI but can also be seen in smaller infarctions among patients with poor left ventricular systolic function (Hollenberg et al., 1999). Other causes of shock may include: myocarditis, end-stage cardiomyopathy, valvular heart disease, pulmonary embolism, and myocardial dysfunction after prolonged cardiopulmonary bypass (Hollenberg et al., 1999). Another mechanism by which shock liver can occur is through chronic passive congestion of the liver (congestive hepatopathy) or preexisting portal hypertension (Weisberg and Jacobson, 2011). Congestive hepatopathy refers to chronic liver changes seen in the context of right-sided HF and any disease which results in an increase in right-sided filling pressures (i.e., central venous pressure): right ventricular infarction, biventricular failure due to cardiomyopathy, severe pulmonary hypertension, cor pulmonale, and valvulopathies

TABLE 6.2   Pharmacokinetics of Antiarrhythmics

Drug	Major Route of Elimination (%)	Elimination Half-Life	Active Metabolites
Quinidine	Hepatic (50–90)	7–18 h	3-Hydroxy quinidine
	Renal (10–30)		
Procainamide	Hepatic (40–70)	2.5–4.7 h	N-acetyl procainamide
	Renal (30–60)		
Disopyramide	Renal (36–77)	7–9 h	Mono-N-dealkyl disopyramide
	Hepatic (11–37)		
Lidocaine	Hepatic (90)	1.5–4 h	MEGX, GX
Mexiletine	Hepatic (90)	8–12 h	None
Flecainide	Hepatic (70)	8–14 h	Meta-O-dealkylated flecainide
	Renal (25)		
Propafenone	Hepatic (99)	2–32 h	5-Hydroxy-propafenone; N-depropylpropafenone
Sotalol	Renal (90)	10–20 h	None
Dofetilide	Renal (70)	8–10 h	None
	Hepatic (30)		
Amiodarone	Hepatic (99)	3–15 weeks	Desethyl amiodarone
Ibutilide	Hepatic (75)	6 h	Alpha-hydroxy
Diltiazem	Hepatic (90)	3–5 h	Desacetyl and demethyldiltiazem
Verapamil	Hepatic (70)	4 h	Norverapamil
Digoxin	Renal (60)	30–50 h	None
Adenosine	Vascular endothelium, erythrocytes	<10 s	None

GX, glycylxylidide; MEGX, monoethylglycylxylidide.
Adapted from Kowey, P.R., Marinchak, R.A., Rials, S.J., Bharucha, D.B., 2000. Classification and pharmacology of antiarrhythmic drugs. Am. Heart J. 140 (1), 12–20.

(Weisberg and Jacobson, 2011). The common pathophysiologic disturbances found in both ischemic hepatitis and congestive hepatopathy are a reduction in cardiac output and hepatic blood flow (Giallourakis et al., 2002; Weisberg and Jacobson, 2011).

Chronic HF is key example of a condition in which both features of liver dysfunction are seen: ischemic hepatitis and congestive hepatopathy. Ischemic hepatitis generally presents as asymptomatic transaminitis after episodes of hypotension, and the clinical sequela is generally self-limiting (Giallourakis et al., 2002; Weisberg and Jacobson, 2011). The classic finding of ischemic hepatitis is a substantial, yet transient, increase in aminotransferase concentrations (concentrations more than 20 times the upper limit of normal) (Weisberg and Jacobson, 2011). These findings may be more commonly observed in patients with acute HF (Poelzl et al., 2012). In fact, ischemic hepatitis has been identified among 22% of all cardiac intensive care unit admissions with decreased cardiac output but may be even more common in elderly patients (Henrion et al., 1994; Weisberg and Jacobson, 2011). Chronic congestive hepatopathy that remains long standing and uncontrolled may lead to fibrotic changes of the liver and ultimately cardiac cirrhosis. These liver changes result from prolonged and/or recurrent episodes of HF (Weisberg and Jacobson, 2011). Patients with these congestive features are also usually asymptomatic but have laboratory evidence of liver dysfunction and physical evidence of right-sided HF (Weisberg and Jacobson, 2011). Unlike ischemic hepatitis, the aminotransferase concentrations are rarely two to three times greater than the upper limit of normal (Weisberg and Jacobson, 2011). Patients with chronic HF and congestive hepatopathy seem more likely to have cholestatic changes (increases in total bilirubin, alkaline phosphatase, and γ-glutamyltransferase) than aminotransferase changes which may predict disease severity. The term "cardiohepatic syndrome" has been proposed to describe these patients. The overall prevalence of congestive hepatopathy among patients with significant HF is quite varied based on the definition used but has been estimated to be 15–65% (van Deursen et al., 2010; Weisberg and Jacobson, 2011). In addition to congestive hepatopathy changes, acute liver injury may occur in any patient with preexisting severe chronic HF, cirrhosis, or sustained hepatic ischemia (Giallourakis et al., 2002).

Aberrations in liver function seen in the setting of CV disease would be expected to alter drug metabolism. The changes in liver function due to HF (i.e., reduction in hepatic blood flow) would be expected to significantly affect the PK of CV medications which undergo extensive first-pass metabolism. Some of these medications have substantial differences in intravenous and oral doses (i.e., propranolol, atenolol, metoprolol, propafenone, and verapamil) (Kowey et al., 2000). Conversely, other medications can only be given by the intravenous route since the high first-pass effect precludes oral administration (i.e., lidocaine, ibutilide) (Thomson et al., 1973; Kowey et al., 2000). Similar changes would be seen after a large acute MI, where cardiac output is compromised, and hepatic blood flow is reduced. However, another change described after an acute MI is an increased concentration of α-1 acid glycoprotein (Kessler et al., 1984; Kowey et al., 2000). The clinical consequence of this is an increased affinity of binding to certain drugs (i.e., propranolol and quinidine). Although there may be an increase in total plasma concentration, the concentration of unbound free drug may not change (Kowey et al., 2000). The increased protein binding of the drugs, however, could potentially lead to drug interactions that involve competition for binding sites for highly protein-bound drugs (i.e., amiodarone and warfarin) (Marcus, 1983; Kessler et al., 1984; Kowey et al., 2000). This interaction is highly clinically significant and requires the need to dose adjust warfarin to less the bleeding risk. Ultimately, though data which report on comprehensive and specific changes in PK among patients with acute CV conditions and reductions in hepatic function (i.e., cardiohepatic syndrome) are lacking and thus are urgently needed.

Currently, the mainstay of therapy for patients with acute ischemic hepatitis and/or congestive hepatopathy is to manage the underlying CV cause. Typically, this occurs in the form of treatment that augments cardiac output (inotropy via use of dobutamine or milrinone). Diuretics are frequently useful but must be used cautiously to avoid episodes of dehydration, hypotension, and hepatic ischemia (Kisloff and Schaffer, 1976; Weisberg and Jacobson, 2011). Anticoagulants may be indicated in this setting to manage coexisting conditions such as severe left ventricular dysfunction and atrial fibrillation but must also be used cautiously due to baseline increases in the international normalized ratio (INR) (Jafri, 1997). Therefore, patients would exhibit sensitivity to agents such as warfarin and unfractionated heparin with the potential for increased bleeding complications.

Cardiac Arrest

Therapeutic Hypothermia

Patients who suffer out-of-hospital or in-hospital cardiac arrest who are comatose, but have achieved return of spontaneous circulation, are recommended to have targeted temperature management (TTM) between 32°C and 36°C (Callaway et al., 2015). For both "shockable" (ventricular fibrillation/pulseless ventricular tachycardia) and "nonshockable" rhythms (asystole/pulseless electrical activity), TTM helps to improve neurologic recovery. The duration of TTM after cardiac arrest should be at least 24 h, once the goal temperature has been reached (Callaway et al., 2015). There are limited data that have described the impact of hypothermia on drug metabolism of CV drugs. Empiric adjustments in drug therapy may be warranted but are largely based on preclinical data, case reports, and human data which used moderate (28–32°C) to deep (<28°C) hypothermia (Arpino and Greer, 2008). An understanding of the physiologic effects of hypothermia on the CV system is also important to anticipate the overall response to CV drugs.

As most enzymatic-dependent processes in the body are determined by temperature, hypothermia causes a reduction in the clearance of any CV drug that relies upon metabolism (Arpino and Greer, 2008). Examples include propranolol and verapamil, in which reduced in vitro hepatic metabolism has been documented (Arpino and Greer, 2008). Nitroglycerin is another example where metabolism was shown to decrease by 66% with hypothermia (<32°C) (Arpino and Greer, 2008). The PK effects of P2Y12 platelet inhibitors have not been as well characterized, but reductions in their PD effects have been observed. Clopidogrel is a prodrug that must be metabolized to its active form via cytochrome P450 (CYP) enzymes, and PD data indicate high residual platelet reactivity (Bjelland et al., 2010). In fact, even higher potency P2Y12 inhibitors such as ticagrelor and prasugrel have demonstrated reduced platelet inhibition in the setting of therapeutic hypothermia postcardiac arrest (Ibrahim et al., 2014). Some CV drugs are metabolized through nontemperature-dependent chemical reactions and are thus not as vulnerable to the effects of hypothermia. One example is sodium nitroprusside, which is transformed to nitric oxide and cyanide (CN) through interactions with sulfhydryl groups. The formation of CN was not affected by temperature, but the subsequent reaction to metabolize CN to thiocyanate via the enzyme rhodanase resulted in a delayed clearance of CN which could still lead to toxicity (Arpino and Greer, 2008).

There are physiologic implications of hypothermia on the CV system which need to be considered in addition to the direct effects on drug metabolism. Some of these factors work in concert to change the drug effect and need to be considered when making dosage recommendations. A prime example is that hypothermia will redistribute blood flow away from muscle, skin, and fat. Therefore, drugs that have large V_d (i.e., propranolol) will distribute to a reduced volume and produce higher plasma concentrations which could result in toxicity (Arpino and Greer, 2008). Additionally, drugs with high V_d that are administered prior to hypothermia may become sequestered due to reduced blood flow. Upon rewarming, these drugs will redistribute from the tissues into the plasma compartment leading to potential toxicity. Other physiologic changes in the CV system that occur in response to hypothermia, and which should be considered in drug therapy, include: heart rate slowing; prolongation of the PR, QT, and QRS intervals; and provocation of a variety of arrhythmias (Arpino and Greer, 2008). These would necessitate empiric reductions in doses of BB, calcium channel blockers, digoxin, and a number of other antiarrhythmics such as amiodarone. Other physiologic changes with hypothermia include abnormal bleeding due to platelet dysfunction and slowing of the coagulation cascade that relies upon a series of enzymatic reactions (Arpino and Greer, 2008). Therefore, anticoagulation (i.e., heparin) and platelet aggregation inhibitors (i.e., glycoprotein IIb/IIIa inhibitors) must be used more cautiously to minimize the potential for bleeding. In the case of glycoprotein IIb/IIIa inhibitors, augmentation of antiplatelet effect has been demonstrated (Arpino and Greer, 2008). However, with all anticoagulants and antiplatelets, the extent to which a change in dose would mitigate bleeding risk is unknown. A better characterization of specific PK changes with different dose regimens with these medication classes, as well as others discussed in this section, are urgently needed.

CYTOCHROME P-450 EXPRESSION IN CARDIOVASCULAR DISEASE

The CYP superfamily of enzymes is the primary mediator of oxidative transformation of both exogenous and endogenous molecules and compounds. The expression of CYP is seen in both hepatic and extra-hepatic organs, including the CV system. In fact, CYP reaction products, or metabolites, have been identified in myocardium, endocardium, endothelium, vascular smooth muscle, and coronary arteries. CYP function and dysregulation are likely to serve an important role in the onset, progression, and outcome of CV disease in susceptible individuals. However, relatively little is known about the expression and regulation of CYP enzymes in both heart and blood vessels. The expression of CYP enzymes and production of their metabolites are altered in CV disease. Alterations in CYP expression have also been found in other pathologic conditions, such as hepatic and kidney diseases, which may be important in the context of CV disease as reviewed previously (Elbekai et al., 2004; Korashy et al., 2004; Elbekai and El-Kadi, 2006). By extension, it is hypothesized that interindividual differences in CYP enzyme activity seen in a population may be accounted for by genetic differences. Therefore, relevant changes in the metabolism and transport of drugs used to treat patients with CV medications are also likely to be a result of pharmacogenetic differences. There are numerous PK and therapeutic implications seen as a result of variable CYP expression and activity in patients with CV disease. The most pertinent examples will be reviewed in the following section.

PHARMACOGENOMICS RELATED TO CARDIOVASCULAR DRUGS AND DISEASE

Variation in Drug Metabolism

The therapeutic response to most CV drugs is determined by polygenic factors, or the interplay between several genes that determine PK and PD effects. Genetic differences in PK include drug-metabolizing enzymes and transporters, whereas PD factors include inherited differences in drug targets (receptors) (Evans and McLeod, 2003). The CYP pathway is responsible for metabolism of a large number of CV drugs. The CYP isoforms found to be most important for CV drug biotransformation include: CYP3A, CYP2D6, CYP2C19, CYP2C9, and CYP1A2 (Abernethy and Flockhart, 2000). However, the CYP2C19, CYP2C9, and CYP2D6 isoforms are most susceptible to genetic polymorphisms (Abernethy and Flockhart, 2000). The variable expressions of these enzymes have been attributed to the significant variability in plasma concentrations and therapeutic effects of a number of CV drugs (Cascorbi et al., 2004). Notable examples of these CV drugs where polymorphic enzymes affect drug disposition and response include: BBs (i.e., metoprolol and carvedilol), angiotensin receptor blockers (ARBs; i.e., losartan and irbesartan), propafenone, clopidogrel, and warfarin. These medications are used to treat a number of common CV conditions, including HF, arrhythmias, ischemic heart disease, and thromboembolism. Pharmacogenomics relevant to CV drug metabolism in the context of these conditions will be further highlighted.

Heart Failure and Hypertension

β-Blockers and CYP2D6

BB is the mainstay of therapy for management of patients with HF with a reduced ejection fraction (HFrEF) and also is used as adjuncts for treatment of hypertension. Among the most commonly used BB are carvedilol and metoprolol (Yancy et al., 2013). Each of these BB is a substrate of CYP2D6 (Cascorbi et al., 2004), but metoprolol is more extensively metabolized by this pathway than any other BB. As an example of the polymorphic nature of this isoenzyme, ~7–10% of Caucasians exhibit no CYP2D6 activity (Cascorbi et al., 2004; Pepper et al., 1991; Oldham and Clarke, 1997). In contrast to poor metabolizer (PM) status, CYP2D6 activity may also be enhanced through increased gene duplications. The incidence of this phenomenon has been observed at 1–3% for Middle Europeans but as high as 29% in Ethiopians (Aklillu et al., 1996; Cascorbi et al., 2004).

The polymorphic nature of CYP2D6 led to the observation that among PMs, there was a sixfold elevation in the metabolic ratio of metoprolol and an association between these patients and the presence of significant AEs (Rau et al., 2002; Wuttke et al., 2002; Cascorbi et al., 2004). Another study of metoprolol in hypertensive patients found that PMs of CYP2D6 had a significantly longer elimination half-life, higher S-metoprolol area under the plasma concentration–time curve (AUC), and lower oral clearance ($p \leq 0.07$) for each parameter compared with extensive and intermediate metabolizers (IMs) (Zineh et al., 2004). In terms of clinical response for this study, however, AEs did not differ between extensive, intermediate, or PMs. The antihypertensive response rate and change in blood pressure (BP) were also not different, despite the changes in PK (Zineh et al., 2004). Similar to the aforementioned metoprolol data, a study of carvedilol demonstrated an increased steady-state plasma concentration among CYP2D6 PMs (bioavailability 38% vs 25%; $p < .01$) (Giessmann et al., 2004; Cascorbi et al., 2004), although clinical response was not determined. A more recent and well-designed study of metoprolol tartrate in patients with hypertension ($n = 281$) evaluated clinical response and AEs in relation to CYP2D6 genotype status. After 8 weeks of treatment, the heart-rate response was more pronounced in the PM and IM groups, although BP response (systolic and diastolic) and AEs were not significantly different based on CYP2D6 genotype (Hamadeh et al., 2014). In summary, although the PK of BB are influenced by CYP2D6 genotype, this does not appear to translate to clinically important differences in overall efficacy or safety (Hamadeh et al., 2014; Johnson et al., 2011a).

Propafenone is another example of a CV drug whose metabolism is dependent primarily on the CYP2D6 isoenzyme (Abernethy and Flockhart, 2000). Propafenone exhibits its antiarrhythmic properties through inhibition of voltage-gated sodium channels and thus is useful for the cardioversion and maintenance of normal sinus rhythm in patients with atrial fibrillation. However, it should not be used in patients with structural heart disease, including HF due to worse clinical outcomes (Kowey et al., 2000). Nonetheless, the parent drug propafenone is structurally similar to propranolol and therefore exhibits β-blocking properties similar to metoprolol and carvedilol (Kowey et al., 2000). In fact, the degree of β-blockade is dependent upon CYP2D6 activity, as its active metabolite, 5-hydroxypropafenone, is relatively devoid of these effects (Kowey et al., 2000). Therefore, patients with genetically low levels of CYP2D6 activity would be expected to have significantly greater β-blockade and central nervous system adverse effects relative to patients with high CYP2D6 activity (Abernethy and Flockhart, 2000). The PK of propafenone is further complicated by its nonlinear dose response due to saturable metabolism, leading to exponential increases in plasma concentrations as the dose increases (Kowey et al., 2000).

Angiotensin Receptor Blockers and CYP2C9

In addition to BB, inhibitors of the renin—angiotensin—aldosterone (RAAS) pathway serve as the foundational pharmacotherapy for management of HFrEF (Yancy et al., 2013). These therapies include angiotensin-converting enzyme inhibitors and ARBs. Certain ARBs, such as losartan and irbesartan, have been associated with polymorphic metabolism in the CYP2C9 isoenzyme (Yasar et al., 2001; Hallberg et al., 2002; Lee et al., 2003; Cascorbi et al., 2004). Losartan is a prodrug that requires biotransformation by CYP2C9 to its active carboxylic acid form, EXP3174, whereas irbesartan is inactivated by CYP2C9 (Cascorbi et al., 2004). The two major polymorphisms in CYP2C9 lead to decreased enzyme activity by way of amino acid replacements (Cascorbi et al., 2004). In the case of losartan, a study of healthy Japanese subjects demonstrated that carriers of the wild-type allele have lower systolic BPs relative to their counterparts with PM activity (Sekino et al., 2003). Conversely, hypertensive patients with a reduced function allele for CYP2C9 treated with irbesartan showed significantly lower diastolic and systolic BP (Hallberg et al., 2002). Similar to BB and CYP2D6 polymorphisms, however, clinical outcomes associated with ARBs and CYP2C9 polymorphisms have not been sufficiently evaluated.

Digoxin and ATP-Binding Cassette B1

Digoxin is a substrate for the membrane efflux transporter, P-glycoprotein (P-gp), which is widely expressed in the duodenum, kidneys, liver, and the blood—brain barrier (Marzolini et al., 2004). The P-gp transporter is important in the uptake, distribution, and excretion of many drugs, including digoxin (Marzolini et al., 2004). The ATP-binding cassette B1 (ABCB1) or multidrug resistance 1 (MDR1) gene encodes for P-gp, and there have been several single-nucleotide polymorphism (SNPs) linked to altered expression of this gene. One of the main SNPs associated with decreased ABCB1 function and higher digoxin concentrations is the C3435T polymorphism (Aarnoudse et al., 2008; Chowbay et al., 2005). Most of the evidence for this association, however, was derived from small, single dose, studies of digoxin in healthy volunteers. A meta-analysis that evaluated the C3435T SNP showed no significant effect on digoxin AUC_{0-4} or AUC_{0-24}, but C_{max} values were lower in wild-type (CC) subjects among both Caucasian and Japanese subjects (Chowbay et al., 2005). However, other SNPs beyond C3435T have also been identified (C1236T, G2677T) (Aarnoudse et al., 2008).

A population-based cohort of elderly European patients in the general population who were taking digoxin demonstrated the strongest association between digoxin concentrations and the 1236-2677-3435 TTT haplotype allele (0.18—0.21 mcg/L per T allele), suggesting an interaction between the relevant individual SNPs (Aarnoudse et al., 2008). In contrast, other data have not demonstrated an association between digoxin PK and genotype in digoxin users (Kurzawski et al., 2007; DiDomenico et al., 2014). In summary, although variants in ABCB1 appear to explain some variability in digoxin concentrations, the evidence is mixed and incorporation of ABCB1 genotype does not seem to add significantly to dose prediction in the clinical setting.

Acute Coronary Syndrome and Percutaneous Coronary Intervention

Clopidogrel and CYP2C19

Clopidogrel is a thienopyridine prodrug that must be biotransformed by the liver to its active thiol metabolite (SR 26334) through CYP to irreversibly inhibit the platelet P2Y12 adenosine diphosphate receptor (Brandt et al., 2007; Johnson et al., 2011a). The majority of a clopidogrel dose (85%) is hydrolyzed by esterases to inactive metabolites. The remainder of the parent drug (15%) is metabolized through CYP in two successive steps. The first step converts clopidogrel to an intermediate, 2-oxo-clopidogrel, whereas the second step is responsible for conversion to the active metabolite. These latter CYP-dependent pathways are mediated by a number of isoenzymes (CYP1A2, CYP2B6, CYP2C9, CYP2C19, and CYP3A4/5) (Brandt et al., 2007). Wide interindividual variability in response to clopidogrel has been documented, largely based on genetic polymorphisms in CYP metabolism. Compelling evidence has shown that variants in CYP2C19 affect the metabolism of clopidogrel to its active form, and thus its platelet inhibitory effects and therapeutic response (Johnson et al., 2011a). The most common variant is the loss-of-function (LoF) CYP2C19*2 allele. The frequency of this variant has been reported to be 15% for both European and African ancestry, but as high as 29% for East Asian ancestry (Johnson et al., 2011a). Another common variant is the *17 gain-of-function allele. Other LoF alleles have been identified, including *3, but are far less common than *2 (Johnson et al., 2011a). From a PK perspective, presence of the *2 allele was significantly associated with lower AUC_{0-24} ($p = 0.043$) and C_{max} ($p = 0.006$) of the active metabolite of clopidogrel compared with those that were *1/*1 homozygotes (Brandt et al., 2007). Furthermore, carriers of LoF alleles have an increased risk of major adverse CV events and stent thrombosis compared with noncarriers among high-risk patients with acute coronary syndrome that were managed with percutaneous coronary intervention (PCI) (Mega et al., 2010).

In response to the evidence that genetic variation of CYP2C19 is strongly associated with PK, PDs, and clinical response, the clopidogrel label was updated to state that genetic testing is available to determine PM status in an effort to consider alternative therapy (Johnson et al., 2011a). The Clinical Pharmacogenetics Implementation Consortium (CPIC) provides guidance on genotype-directed antiplatelet therapy (Scott et al., 2013). For intermediate or PMs of CYP2C19, alternate therapy recommendations include higher potency antiplatelets such as prasugrel or ticagrelor. The benefits of these latter therapies have been shown to be most pronounced in patients with CYP2C19 LoF alleles among high-risk patients who undergo PCI (Scott et al., 2013).

Thromboembolism

Warfarin and CYP2C9, VKORC1

Warfarin is a vitamin K antagonist that exerts its effect by interfering with the hepatic carboxylation of vitamin K—dependent coagulation factors (e.g., factors II, VII, IX, X). Ultimately, reduction in these four factors is needed before the anticoagulant effect is observed. The antithrombotic effect, in particular, occurs after prothrombin (half-life of 60—72 h) has been sufficiently depleted (Johnson et al., 2011a). Warfarin is a racemic mixture of active isomers, both of which require biotransformation by the liver through the CYP isoenzyme system. The intra- and interindividual variability in response to warfarin is extensive. In fact, the initial dose required to achieve a therapeutic INR varies by 10- to 20-fold (Johnson et al., 2011a). It has been estimated that up to 35% of the variability in dose requirements can be attributed to genetic polymorphisms in the major metabolizing hepatic enzyme for S-warfarin (CYP2C9), and its protein target (vitamin K epoxide reductase [VKORC1]) (Johnson, 2012). The CYP2C9*2 and *3 alleles lead to 40—70% reductions in S-warfarin clearance and ~20—40% lower dosage requirements, respectively. The presence of these alleles also influences bleeding risk (Johnson et al., 2011b). The VKORC1-1639 G > A SNP augments sensitivity to warfarin at its binding site thus decreasing dosage requirements of warfarin (Johnson et al., 2011a,b).

When pharmacogenomic data (CYP2C9 *2 and *3 alleles coupled with VKORC1-1639 G > A) are coupled with common clinical variables, such as age, body weight, and drug—drug interactions (i.e., amiodarone), 50—60% of the maintenance dose variability in Caucasians can be explained. However, in African—Americans, only about 25% of the variability in maintenance dose can be accounted for (Johnson et al., 2011a). Although other genetic variants, such as CYP4F2, have been found to affect a small additional percentage of variability, VKORC1 is the major genetic determinant of dose across ethnicities (Johnson et al., 2011a). Of course, other nongenetic variables play a significant role in warfarin response, including environmental factors (e.g., vitamin K and herbal products) and other disease states (e.g., liver dysfunction, HF, and end-stage renal disease). Currently, the warfarin dosing label includes specific dosing recommendations based on validated algorithms that integrate genotype information to better predict dosing requirements. The CPIC guidelines endorse use of the Gage or International Warfarin Pharmacogenetics Consortium algorithm as being preferred for the integration of genetic data into dose prediction (Johnson et al., 2011b).

Dabigatran and Carboxylesterase-1

The direct-acting oral anticoagulants (DOACs) have been viewed as potential replacements for warfarin for several reasons, not the least of which is their more predictable dose–response relationship. However, the influence of pharmacogenomics on variability of DOACs, such as dabigatran, has recently been investigated. Dabigatran etexilate is a prodrug which is biotransformed by esterases, including liver carboxylesterase-1 (CES-1), to the active metabolite dabigatran. The prodrug is also a substrate of a P-GP (ABCB1). Each of these targets could be implicated in the significant interindividual variability in blood concentrations of the active metabolite (Liesenfeld et al., 2011). Consequently, investigators have conducted a genome-wide analysis of data from the RE-LY trial to determine possible associations with dabigatran (Pare et al., 2013). The study included 1694 patients and discovered the presence of a SNP, rs2244613, for CES-1 which resulted in lower trough concentrations of the active metabolite and less bleeding (relative risk 0.73, 95% confidence interval 0.63–0.86). Approximately 30% of the population studied was a carrier of this minor allele (Pare et al., 2013). Two other SNPs were identified, one each for CES-1 and ABCB1, which were associated with peak concentrations but not bleeding (Pare et al., 2013). These initial findings will likely promote future investigations into the feasibility of genotyping to identify the optimal patient-specific dabigatran dose.

Dyslipidemia

HMG-CoA Reductase Inhibitors and SLCO1B1

Simvastatin is among the most commonly prescribed CV drugs to treat dyslipidemia and to manage patients at risk for CV disease. A drug transporter, organic anion-transporting polypeptide 1B1 (encoded by SLCO1B1), facilitates the hepatic uptake of some statins and other compounds (Johnson et al., 2011a). The genetic association between the function of this transporter and statin-related skeletal muscle toxicity has been well documented. The minor C allele contained within SLCO1B1*5, *15, and *17 haplotypes has been associated with decreased transporter function and clearance of simvastatin (Ramsey et al., 2014). The presence of this allele is seen in ~5–20% of most populations (Ramsey et al., 2014). The overall PK profile of simvastatin is affected more by this transporter than for any other hydroxymethyl-glutaryl-coenzyme A (HMG-CoA) reductase inhibitor or statin (Johnson et al., 2011a). In fact, homozygotes for the C allele had greater exposure to the active simvastatin acid (AUC_{0-12}) than those homozygous for the T allele (Ramsey et al., 2014; Pasanen et al., 2006).

The Study of the Effectiveness of Additional Reductions in Cholesterol and Homocysteine (SEARCH) consortium evaluated more than 12,000 subjects that received low (20 mg) or high (80 mg) simvastatin. Among the subjects that were homozygous for the CC risk allele, the rate of muscle toxicity over 5 years was 18.6% versus 0.63% in the low-risk (TT) group. Overall, the odds ratio for myopathy was 4.5 per copy of the minor C allele (Group et al., 2008). Consequently, the FDA has advised against initiating simvastatin 80 mg and to only continue therapy in patients that have previously tolerated treatment for more than 1 year. The CPIC guidelines recommend a lower dose or an alternative statin (pravastatin or rosuvastatin) for patients who have one or two copies of the minor C allele, and thus are at intermediate to high risk of myopathy, respectively (Ramsey et al., 2014).

CONCLUSION

The preponderance of CV disease and the compelling indications for multiple drugs to treat these conditions often result in the need to adjust therapeutic regimens to attain efficacy while minimizing toxicity. Alterations in drug metabolism and transport occur due to the interplay of many factors, such as organ cross talk in the context of CV disease, the physiology of aging, and relevant pharmacogenomic considerations. Although much progress has been made in our understanding of these issues, this chapter also makes apparent the overall paucity of data which characterizes changes in PK in CV disease. Current practices frequently rely upon empiric dose adjustments based on an incomplete understanding of variability in drug response as a function of changes in metabolism. This is particularly germane knowing that approximately 20% of the US population will be 65 years or older by 2030 and commensurate increases in CV disease burden will also be seen (Fleg et al., 2011). In conclusion, recognition of factors that alter the metabolism of drugs used in CV disease is critical to making appropriate adjustments in therapy to optimize outcome. Future research is urgently needed to address these gaps in our understanding of drug metabolism in CV disease.

References

Aarnoudse, A.J., Dieleman, J.P., Visser, L.E., Arp, P.P., van der Heiden, I.P., van Schaik, R.H., Molokhia, M., Hofman, A., Uitterlinden, A.G., Stricker, B.H., 2008. Common ATP-binding cassette B1 variants are associated with increased digoxin serum concentration. Pharmacogenet. Genomics 18 (4), 299–305.

Abernethy, D.R., Flockhart, D.A., 2000. Molecular basis of cardiovascular drug metabolism: implications for predicting clinically important drug interactions. Circulation 101 (14), 1749–1753.

Aklillu, E., Persson, I., Bertilsson, L., Johansson, I., Rodrigues, F., Ingelman-Sundberg, M., 1996. Frequent distribution of ultrarapid metabolizers of debrisoquine in an Ethiopian population carrying duplicated and multiduplicated functional CYP2D6 alleles. J. Pharmacol. Exp. Ther. 278 (1), 441–446.

Arpino, P.A., Greer, D.M., 2008. Practical pharmacologic aspects of therapeutic hypothermia after cardiac arrest. Pharmacotherapy 28 (1), 102–111.

Beermann, B., 1984. Aspects on pharmacokinetics of some diuretics. Acta Pharmacol. Toxicol. (Copenh) 54 (Suppl. 1), 17–29.

Bjelland, T.W., Hjertner, O., Klepstad, P., Kaisen, K., Dale, O., Haugen, B.O., 2010. Antiplatelet effect of clopidogrel is reduced in patients treated with therapeutic hypothermia after cardiac arrest. Resuscitation 81 (12), 1627–1631.

Brandt, J.T., Close, S.L., Iturria, S.J., Payne, C.D., Farid, N.A., Ernest 2nd, C.S., Lachno, D.R., Salazar, D., Winters, K.J., 2007. Common polymorphisms of CYP2C19 and CYP2C9 affect the pharmacokinetic and pharmacodynamic response to clopidogrel but not prasugrel. J. Thromb. Haemost. 5 (12), 2429–2436.

Brater, D.C., 1998. Diuretic therapy. N. Engl. J. Med. 339 (6), 387–395.

Brater, D.C., Chennavasin, P., Seiwell, R., 1980. Furosemide in patients with heart failure: shift in dose-response curves. Clin. Pharmacol. Ther. 28 (2), 182–186.

Callaway, C.W., Donnino, M.W., Fink, E.L., Geocadin, R.G., Golan, E., Kern, K.B., Leary, M., Meurer, W.J., Peberdy, M.A., Thompson, T.M., Zimmerman, J.L., 2015. Part 8: post-cardiac arrest care: 2015 American Heart Association guidelines update for cardiopulmonary resuscitation and emergency cardiovascular care. Circulation 132 (18 Suppl. 2), S465–S482.

Cascorbi, I., Paul, M., Kroemer, H.K., 2004. Pharmacogenomics of heart failure – focus on drug disposition and action. Cardiovasc. Res. 64 (1), 32–39.

Chowbay, B., Li, H., David, M., Cheung, Y.B., Lee, E.J., 2005. Meta-analysis of the influence of MDR1 C3435T polymorphism on digoxin pharmacokinetics and MDR1 gene expression. Br. J. Clin. Pharmacol. 60 (2), 159–171.

DiDomenico, R.J., Bress, A.P., Na-Thalang, K., Tsao, Y.Y., Groo, V.L., Deyo, K.L., Patel, S.R., Bishop, J.R., Bauman, J.L., 2014. Use of a simplified nomogram to individualize digoxin dosing versus standard dosing practices in patients with heart failure. Pharmacotherapy 34 (11), 1121–1131.

van Deursen, V.M., Damman, K., Hillege, H.L., van Beek, A.P., van Veldhuisen, D.J., Voors, A.A., 2010. Abnormal liver function in relation to hemodynamic profile in heart failure patients. J. Card. Fail. 16 (1), 84–90.

Elbekai, R.H., El-Kadi, A.O., 2006. Cytochrome P450 enzymes: central players in cardiovascular health and disease. Pharmacol. Ther. 112 (2), 564–587.

Elbekai, R.H., Korashy, H.M., El-Kadi, A.O., 2004. The effect of liver cirrhosis on the regulation and expression of drug metabolizing enzymes. Curr. Drug Metab. 5 (2), 157–167.

Evans, W.E., McLeod, H.L., 2003. Pharmacogenomics–drug disposition, drug targets, and side effects. N. Engl. J. Med. 348 (6), 538–549.

Fleg, J.L., Aronow, W.S., Frishman, W.H., 2011. Cardiovascular drug therapy in the elderly: benefits and challenges. Nat. Rev. Cardiol. 8 (1), 13–28.

Giallourakis, C.C., Rosenberg, P.M., Friedman, L.S., 2002. The liver in heart failure. Clin. Liver Dis. 6 (4), 947–967 viii–ix.

Giessmann, T., Modess, C., Hecker, U., Zschiesche, M., Dazert, P., Kunert-Keil, C., Warzok, R., Engel, G., Weitschies, W., Cascorbi, I., Kroemer, H.K., Siegmund, W., 2004. CYP2D6 genotype and induction of intestinal drug transporters by rifampin predict presystemic clearance of carvedilol in healthy subjects. Clin. Pharmacol. Ther. 75 (3), 213–222.

Group, S.C., Link, E., Parish, S., Armitage, J., Bowman, L., Heath, S., Matsuda, F., Gut, I., Lathrop, M., Collins, R., 2008. SLCO1B1 variants and statin-induced myopathy—a genomewide study. N. Engl. J. Med. 359 (8), 789–799.

Hallberg, P., Karlsson, J., Kurland, L., Lind, L., Kahan, T., Malmqvist, K., Ohman, K.P., Nystrom, F., Melhus, H., 2002. The CYP2C9 genotype predicts the blood pressure response to irbesartan: results from the Swedish Irbesartan Left Ventricular Hypertrophy Investigation vs Atenolol (SILVHIA) trial. J. Hypertens. 20 (10), 2089–2093.

Hamadeh, I.S., Langaee, T.Y., Dwivedi, R., Garcia, S., Burkley, B.M., Skaar, T.C., Chapman, A.B., Gums, J.G., Turner, S.T., Gong, Y., Cooper-DeHoff, R.M., Johnson, J.A., 2014. Impact of CYP2D6 polymorphisms on clinical efficacy and tolerability of metoprolol tartrate. Clin. Pharmacol. Ther. 96 (2), 175–181.

Henrion, J., Descamps, O., Luwaert, R., Schapira, M., Parfonry, A., Heller, F., 1994. Hypoxic hepatitis in patients with cardiac failure: incidence in a coronary care unit and measurement of hepatic blood flow. J. Hepatol. 21 (5), 696–703.

Hollenberg, S.M., Kavinsky, C.J., Parrillo, J.E., 1999. Cardiogenic shock. Ann. Intern. Med. 131 (1), 47–59.

Ibrahim, K., Christoph, M., Schmeinck, S., Schmieder, K., Steiding, K., Schoener, L., Pfluecke, C., Quick, S., Mues, C., Jellinghaus, S., Wunderlich, C., Strasser, R.H., Kolschmann, S., 2014. High rates of prasugrel and ticagrelor non-responder in patients treated with therapeutic hypothermia after cardiac arrest. Resuscitation 85 (5), 649–656.

Iisalo, E., 1977. Clinical pharmacokinetics of digoxin. Clin. Pharmacokinet. 2 (1), 1–16.

Jafri, S.M., 1997. Hypercoagulability in heart failure. Semin. Thromb. Hemost. 23 (6), 543–545.

Johnson, J.A., 2012. Warfarin pharmacogenetics: a rising tide for its clinical value. Circulation 125 (16), 1964–1966.

Johnson, J.A., Cavallari, L.H., Beitelshees, A.L., Lewis, J.P., Shuldiner, A.R., Roden, D.M., 2011a. Pharmacogenomics: application to the management of cardiovascular disease. Clin. Pharmacol. Ther. 90 (4), 519–531.

Johnson, J.A., Gong, L., Whirl-Carrillo, M., Gage, B.F., Scott, S.A., Stein, C.M., Anderson, J.L., Kimmel, S.E., Lee, M.T., Pirmohamed, M., Wadelius, M., Klein, T.E., Altman, R.B., Clinical Pharmacogenetics Implementation Consortium, 2011b. Clinical pharmacogenetics implementation consortium guidelines for CYP2C9 and VKORC1 genotypes and warfarin dosing. Clin. Pharmacol. Ther. 90 (4), 625–629.

Kessler, K.M., Kissane, B., Cassidy, J., Pefkaros, K.C., Kozlovskis, P., Hamburg, C., Myerburg, R.J., 1984. Dynamic variability of binding of antiarrhythmic drugs during the evolution of acute myocardial infarction. Circulation 70 (3), 472–478.

Kisloff, B., Schaffer, G., 1976. Fulminant hepatic failure secondary to congestive heart failure. Am. J. Dig. Dis. 21 (10), 895–900.

Korashy, H.M., Elbekai, R.H., El-Kadi, A.O., 2004. Effects of renal diseases on the regulation and expression of renal and hepatic drug-metabolizing enzymes: a review. Xenobiotica 34 (1), 1–29.

Kowey, P.R., Marinchak, R.A., Rials, S.J., Bharucha, D.B., 2000. Classification and pharmacology of antiarrhythmic drugs. Am. Heart J. 140 (1), 12–20.

Kurzawski, M., Bartnicka, L., Florczak, M., Gornik, W., Drozdzik, M., 2007. Impact of ABCB1 (MDR1) gene polymorphism and P-glycoprotein inhibitors on digoxin serum concentration in congestive heart failure patients. Pharmacol. Rep. 59 (1), 107–111.

Lee, C.R., Pieper, J.A., Hinderliter, A.L., Blaisdell, J.A., Goldstein, J.A., 2003. Losartan and E3174 pharmacokinetics in cytochrome P450 2C9*1/*1, *1/*2, and *1/*3 individuals. Pharmacotherapy 23 (6), 720–725.

Liesenfeld, K.H., Lehr, T., Dansirikul, C., Reilly, P.A., Connolly, S.J., Ezekowitz, M.D., Yusuf, S., Wallentin, L., Haertter, S., Staab, A., 2011. Population pharmacokinetic analysis of the oral thrombin inhibitor dabigatran etexilate in patients with non-valvular atrial fibrillation from the RE-LY trial. J. Thromb. Haemost. 9 (11), 2168–2175.

Marcus, F.I., 1983. Drug interactions with amiodarone. Am. Heart J. 106 (4 Pt 2), 924–930.

Marzolini, C., Paus, E., Buclin, T., Kim, R.B., 2004. Polymorphisms in human MDR1 (P-glycoprotein): recent advances and clinical relevance. Clin. Pharmacol. Ther. 75 (1), 13–33.

Mega, J.L., Simon, T., Collet, J.P., Anderson, J.L., Antman, E.M., Bliden, K., Cannon, C.P., Danchin, N., Giusti, B., Gurbel, P., Horne, B.D., Hulot, J.S., Kastrati, A., Montalescot, G., Neumann, F.J., Shen, L., Sibbing, D., Steg, P.G., Trenk, D., Wiviott, S.D., Sabatine, M.S., 2010. Reduced-function CYP2C19 genotype and risk of adverse clinical outcomes among patients treated with clopidogrel predominantly for PCI: a meta-analysis. JAMA 304 (16), 1821–1830.

Mozaffarian, D., Benjamin, E.J., Go, A.S., Arnett, D.K., Blaha, M.J., Cushman, M., de Ferranti, S., Despres, J.P., Fullerton, H.J., Howard, V.J., Huffman, M.D., Judd, S.E., Kissela, B.M., Lackland, D.T., Lichtman, J.H., Lisabeth, L.D., Liu, S., Mackey, R.H., Matchar, D.B., McGuire, D.K., Mohler 3rd, E.R., Moy, C.S., Muntner, P., Mussolino, M.E., Nasir, K., Neumar, R.W., Nichol, G., Palaniappan, L., Pandey, D.K., Reeves, M.J., Rodriguez, C.J., Sorlie, P.D., Stein, J., Towfighi, A., Turan, T.N., Virani, S.S., Willey, J.Z., Woo, D., Yeh, R.W., Turner, M.B., American Heart Association Statistics Committee, Stroke Statistics Subcommittee, 2015. Heart disease and stroke statistics–2015 update: a report from the American Heart Association. Circulation 131 (4), e29–322.

Mukhtar, O., Jackson, S.H., 2015. Drug therapies in older adults (part 1). Clin. Med. 15 (1), 47–53.

Oldham, H.G., Clarke, S.E., 1997. In vitro identification of the human cytochrome P450 enzymes involved in the metabolism of R(+)- and S(-)-carvedilol. Drug Metab. Dispos. 25 (8), 970–977.

Pare, G., Eriksson, N., Lehr, T., Connolly, S., Eikelboom, J., Ezekowitz, M.D., Axelsson, T., Haertter, S., Oldgren, J., Reilly, P., Siegbahn, A., Syvanen, A.C., Wadelius, C., Wadelius, M., Zimdahl-Gelling, H., Yusuf, S., Wallentin, L., 2013. Genetic determinants of dabigatran plasma levels and their relation to bleeding. Circulation 127 (13), 1404–1412.

Pasanen, M.K., Neuvonen, M., Neuvonen, P.J., Niemi, M., 2006. SLCO1B1 polymorphism markedly affects the pharmacokinetics of simvastatin acid. Pharmacogenet. Genomics 16 (12), 873–879.

Payne, R.A., Avery, A.J., Duerden, M., Saunders, C.L., Simpson, C.R., Abel, G.A., 2014. Prevalence of polypharmacy in a Scottish primary care population. Eur. J. Clin. Pharmacol. 70 (5), 575–581.

Pepper, J.M., Lennard, M.S., Tucker, G.T., Woods, H.F., 1991. Effect of steroids on the cytochrome P4502D6-catalysed metabolism of metoprolol. Pharmacogenetics 1 (2), 119–122.

Poelzl, G., Ess, M., Mussner-Seeber, C., Pachinger, O., Frick, M., Ulmer, H., 2012. Liver dysfunction in chronic heart failure: prevalence, characteristics and prognostic significance. Eur. J. Clin. Invest. 42 (2), 153–163.

Product Information, 2012. Tenormin (Atenolol), AstraZeneca Pharmaceuticals. Wilmington, DE.

Qato, D.M., Alexander, G.C., Conti, R.M., Johnson, M., Schumm, P., Lindau, S.T., 2008. Use of prescription and over-the-counter medications and dietary supplements among older adults in the United States. JAMA 300 (24), 2867–2878.

Ramsey, L.B., Johnson, S.G., Caudle, K.E., Haidar, C.E., Voora, D., Wilke, R.A., Maxwell, W.D., McLeod, H.L., Krauss, R.M., Roden, D.M., Feng, Q., Cooper-DeHoff, R.M., Gong, L., Klein, T.E., Wadelius, M., Niemi, M., 2014. The clinical pharmacogenetics implementation consortium guideline for SLCO1B1 and simvastatin-induced myopathy: 2014 update. Clin. Pharmacol. Ther. 96 (4), 423–428.

Rau, T., Heide, R., Bergmann, K., Wuttke, H., Werner, U., Feifel, N., Eschenhagen, T., 2002. Effect of the CYP2D6 genotype on metoprolol metabolism persists during long-term treatment. Pharmacogenetics 12 (6), 465–472.

Ronco, C., Haapio, M., House, A.A., Anavekar, N., Bellomo, R., 2008. Cardiorenal syndrome. J. Am. Coll. Cardiol. 52 (19), 1527–1539.

Rossello, X., Pocock, S.J., Julian, D.G., 2015. Long-term use of cardiovascular drugs: challenges for research and for patient care. J. Am. Coll. Cardiol. 66 (11), 1273–1285.

Scott, S.A., Sangkuhl, K., Stein, C.M., Hulot, J.S., Mega, J.L., Roden, D.M., Klein, T.E., Sabatine, M.S., Johnson, J.A., Shuldiner, A.R., Clinical Pharmacogenetics Implementation Consortium, 2013. Clinical Pharmacogenetics Implementation Consortium guidelines for CYP2C19 genotype and clopidogrel therapy: 2013 update. Clin. Pharmacol. Ther. 94 (3), 317–323.

Sekino, K., Kubota, T., Okada, Y., Yamada, Y., Yamamoto, K., Horiuchi, R., Kimura, K., Iga, T., 2003. Effect of the single CYP2C9*3 allele on pharmacokinetics and pharmacodynamics of losartan in healthy Japanese subjects. Eur. J. Clin. Pharmacol. 59 (8–9), 589–592.

Shlipak, M.G., Smith, G.L., Rathore, S.S., Massie, B.M., Krumholz, H.M., 2004. Renal function, digoxin therapy, and heart failure outcomes: evidence from the digoxin intervention group trial. J. Am. Soc. Nephrol. 15 (8), 2195–2203.

Thomson, P.D., Melmon, K.L., Richardson, J.A., Cohn, K., Steinbrunn, W., Cudihee, R., Rowland, M., 1973. Lidocaine pharmacokinetics in advanced heart failure, liver disease, and renal failure in humans. Ann. Intern. Med. 78 (4), 499–508.

Vargo, D.L., Kramer, W.G., Black, P.K., Smith, W.B., Serpas, T., Brater, D.C., 1995. Bioavailability, pharmacokinetics, and pharmacodynamics of torsemide and furosemide in patients with congestive heart failure. Clin. Pharmacol. Ther. 57 (6), 601–609.

Vasko, M.R., Cartwright, D.B., Knochel, J.P., Nixon, J.V., Brater, D.C., 1985. Furosemide absorption altered in decompensated congestive heart failure. Ann. Intern. Med. 102 (3), 314–318.

Vestal, R.E., Wood, A.J., Shand, D.G., 1979. Reduced beta-adrenoceptor sensitivity in the elderly. Clin. Pharmacol. Ther. 26 (2), 181–186.

Weisberg, I.S., Jacobson, I.M., 2011. Cardiovascular diseases and the liver. Clin. Liver Dis. 15 (1), 1–20.

Wuttke, H., Rau, T., Heide, R., Bergmann, K., Bohm, M., Weil, J., Werner, D., Eschenhagen, T., 2002. Increased frequency of cytochrome P450 2D6 poor metabolizers among patients with metoprolol-associated adverse effects. Clin. Pharmacol. Ther. 72 (4), 429–437.

Yancy, C.W., Jessup, M., Bozkurt, B., Butler, J., Casey Jr., D.E., Drazner, M.H., Fonarow, G.C., Geraci, S.A., Horwich, T., Januzzi, J.L., Johnson, M.R., Kasper, E.K., Levy, W.C., Masoudi, F.A., McBride, P.E., McMurray, J.J., Mitchell, J.E., Peterson, P.N., Riegel, B., Sam, F., Stevenson, L.W., Tang, W.H., Tsai, E.J., Wilkoff, B.L., 2013. 2013 ACCF/AHA guideline for the management of heart failure: executive summary: a report of the American College of Cardiology Foundation/American Heart Association Task Force on practice guidelines. Circulation 128 (16), 1810–1852.

Yasar, U., Tybring, G., Hidestrand, M., Oscarson, M., Ingelman-Sundberg, M., Dahl, M.L., Eliasson, E., 2001. Role of CYP2C9 polymorphism in losartan oxidation. Drug Metab. Dispos. 29 (7), 1051–1056.

Zineh, I., Beitelshees, A.L., Gaedigk, A., Walker, J.R., Pauly, D.F., Eberst, K., Leeder, J.S., Phillips, M.S., Gelfand, C.A., Johnson, J.A., 2004. Pharmacokinetics and CYP2D6 genotypes do not predict metoprolol adverse events or efficacy in hypertension. Clin. Pharmacol. Ther. 76 (6), 536–544.

Pharmacogenetic Factors That Affect Drug Metabolism and Efficacy in Type 2 Diabetes Mellitus

X. Li, Z.Q. Liu

Xiangya Hospital Central South University, Changsha, China

O U T L I N E

Introduction   158

Sulfonylureas   158
Mechanism   158
Mutations in Drug-Metabolizing Enzyme
    Coding Genes   161
Mutations in Other Genes   162

Meglitinides   163
Mechanism   163
Mutations in Drug-Metabolizing Enzyme
    Coding Genes   164
Mutations in Drug Transporter Coding
    Genes   164
Mutations in the Other Genes   165

Metformin   166
Mechanism   166

Mutations in Drug Transporter Coding
    Genes   166
Mutations in the Other Genes   168

Thiazolidinediones   169
Mechanism   169
Mutations in Drug-Metabolizing
    Enzyme Coding Genes   169
Mutations in Drug Transporter Coding
    Genes   170
Mutations in the Other Genes   170

α-Glucosidase Inhibitors   172

DPP-4 Inhibitors   173

Conclusion   173

References   173

INTRODUCTION

Diabetes, characterized by high blood sugar levels over a prolonged period, is a group of metabolic diseases. Patients with high blood sugar levels may lead to symptoms like frequent urination, increased thirst, and increased hunger. Poorly controlled high blood sugar will lead to many acute and long-term complications for the patients with diabetes, including diabetic ketoacidosis, nonketotic hyperosmolar coma, possible blindness, foot ulcers, cardiovascular disease, stroke, and kidney failure (Kitabchi et al., 2009). According to the statistics, diabetes affects 347 million individuals worldwide in 2008 (Danaei et al., 2011) and is projected to be the seventh leading cause of death in 2030 (Mathers and Loncar, 2006). There are three types of diabetes: type 1 diabetes mellitus (T1DM), type 2 diabetes mellitus (T2DM), and gestational diabetes. The major type of diabetes is T2DM, also known as "noninsulin-dependent diabetes", which makes up to 90% of the cases (Shi and Hu, 2014).

Pharmacological approach is indispensable when lifestyle changes are not sufficient to alleviate the clinical symptoms for the patients with diabetes. Oral antidiabetic drugs (OADs) are the most important and first-line agents for patients with T2DM. The major OADs include hypoglycemic agents (sulfonylureas and meglitinides) that stimulate insulin secretion, antihyperglycemic agents that do not increase plasma insulin levels but act as the insulin sensitizers (metformin and thiazolidinediones, TZDs), drugs that reduce postprandial absorption of glucose (α-glucosidase inhibitors), and other agents (dipeptidyl peptidase-4 [DPP-4] inhibitors).

It has been reported that individually variable responses were observed in patients administrated with similar OADs. Generally, interindividual variability is mainly determined by genetic mutation. A significant number of studies found that the genetic mutations were associated with different response among patients with T2DM who received similar OADs. In this chapter, we will summarize the mutations of genes, especially the genes whose expression and activity are implicated in the pharmacokinetics (PK) and pharmacodynamics (PD) of OADs (Table 7.1).

SULFONYLUREAS

Mechanism

Sulfonylureas are the first OADs to be used but irrespective of novel pharmacological concepts. Sulfonylureas act at the pancreatic β-cell membrane by closing ATP-sensitive potassium channels, which leads to an enhanced insulin secretion independent of glucose. Sulfonylureas can dramatically improve glycemic control and should be considered as the initial treatment for patients with poor glycemic control on an appropriate diet (Pearson et al., 2000). Oral sulfonylurea therapy is safe and effective for a short term in most patients and may successfully replace treatment with insulin injection (Rafiq et al., 2008). The polymorphic enzyme cytochrome P4502C9 (CYP2C9) and 2C19 (CYP2C19) are the main enzymes that catalyze the biotransformation of sulfonylureas. Mutations in *KCNJ11*, *KCNQ1*, and *HNF1A* also affect the clinical use of sulfonylureas.

TABLE 7.1   Mutations of Genes That can Affect the PK and PD of Oral Antidiabetics

Gene	Rs Number	Alternate Names	Location	Allele	Drug Name	Phenotype
DRUG METABOLIC ENZYME CODING GENES						
CYP2C8	rs11572103	*2, Ile269Phe	Exon	T > A	Repaglinide	PK
					Pioglitazone	PK
	rs11572080 rs10509681	*3, Arg69Lys, Lys329Arg	Exon	C > T T > C	Repaglinide	PK
					Rosiglitazone	PK
					Pioglitazone	PK
					TZDs	PD
	rs1058930	*4, Ile264Met	Exon	G > C	TZDs	PD
CYP2C9	rs1799853	*2, Arg144Cys	Exon	C > T	Tolbutamide	PK
					Glibenclamide	PK
					Sulfonylureas	PD, side effects
	rs1057910	*3, 359Ile > Leu	Exon	A > C	Tolbutamide	PK
					Glibenclamide	PK
					Sulfonylureas	PD, side effects
					Nateglinide	PK, side effects
CYP2C19	rs4244285	*2, Pro227=	Exon	G > A G > C	Gliclazide	PK
	rs4986893	*3, Trp212Ter	Exon	G > A	Gliclazide	PK
DRUG TRANSPORTER CODING GENES						
ABCA1	rs2230806	Arg219Lys	Exon	C > T	Rosiglitazone	PD
	rs12208357	Arg61Cys	Exon	C > T	Metformin	PD
	rs34130495	Gly209Ser	Exon	G > A		PD
	rs34059508	Gly465Arg	Exon	G > A G > C		PD
SLC22A1	rs72552763	Met420del	Exon	GAT > -	Metformin	PD
	rs628031	Met408Val	Exon	A > G		Side effects
	rs36056065	na	Intron	GTAAGTTG > -		Side effects
	rs683369	Leu160Phe	Exon	C > G		PD
	rs2282143	Pro341Leu	Exon	C > T		PK
	rs622342	na	Intron	A > C		PD

(Continued)

TABLE 7.1   Mutations of Genes That can Affect the PK and PD of Oral Antidiabetics—cont'd

Gene	Rs Number	Alternate Names	Location	Allele	Drug Name	Phenotype
SLC22A2	rs201919874	Thr199Ile	Exon	G > A	Metformin	PK
	rs145450955	Thr201Met	Exon	G > A		PK
	rs316019	Ser270Ala	Exon	A > C		PK
SLC22A3	rs11441045	na	Intron	T > -	Metformin	PK
	rs8187717	Ala116Ser	Exon	G > T		PK
	rs8187725	Thr400Ile	Exon	C > T		PK
SLC47A1	rs2252281	na	Promoter	T > C	Metformin	PK
	rs2289669	na	Intron	G > A		PK, PD
SLC47A2	rs12943590	na	Promoter	G > A	Metformin	PK
SLC30A8	rs13266634	Arg276Trp	Exon	T > C	Metformin	PD
	rs16889462	Arg276Gln	Exon	G > A		PD

OTHER GENES

Gene	Rs Number	Alternate Names	Location	Allele	Drug Name	Phenotype
ADIPOQ	rs2241766	Gly15=	Exon	T > G	Pioglitazone	PD
	rs1501299	na	Intron	G > T	Pioglitazone	PD
					Rosiglitazone	PD
					Acarbose	PD
	rs266729	na	Upstream	C > G	Rosiglitazone	PD
ATM	rs11212617	na	Downstream	C > A	Metformin	PD
CAPN10	rs3792269	Pro200=	Exon	A > G	Metformin	PD
FMO5	rs7541245	na	Intron	C > A	Metformin	PD
GLP1R	rs367543060	Thr149Met	Exon	C > T	DPP-4 inhibitors	PD
HNF1A	na	Pro129Thr	Exon	C > A	Gliclazide	PD
	na	Glu132Lys	Exon	G > A		
	rs765432081	Arg159Trp	Exon	C > T		
	na	Arg229Pro	Exon	G > C		
	na	Trp267Arg	Exon	T > C		
	rs762703502	Pro291fsGln	Exon	- > C		
KCNJ11	rs5219	Glu23Lys	Exon	T > C	Sulfonylureas	PD
					Repaglinide	PD

TABLE 7.1 Mutations of Genes That can Affect the PK and PD of Oral Antidiabetics—cont'd

Gene	Rs Number	Alternate Names	Location	Allele	Drug Name	Phenotype
KCNQ1	rs163184	na	Intron	T > G	Sulfonylureas	PD
	rs2237892	na	Intron	C > T	Repaglinide	PD
	rs2237895	na	Intron	A > C	Repaglinide	PD
LPIN1	rs10192566	na	Intron	C > G	Rosiglitazone	PD
LPL	rs328	Ser474Ter	Exon	C > G	Pioglitazone	PD
NEUROD1	rs1801262	Ala45Thr	Exon	C > T	Repaglinide	PD
NR1I2	rs2276706	na	Intron	G > A	Repaglinide	PK
	rs3814058	na	Intron	T > C	Repaglinide	PK
PAX4	rs6467136	na	Intron	A > G	Rosiglitazone	PK
	rs114202595	Arg121Trp	Exon	G > A	Repaglinide	PD
PPARA	rs149711321		Intron	T > C	Metformin	PD
PPARG	rs1801282	Pro12Ala	Exon	C > G	Pioglitazone	PD
					Acarbose	PD
PPARGC1A	rs8192678	Gly482Ser	Exon	C > T	Rosiglitazone	PD
					Acarbose	PD
	rs2970847	Thr394=	Exon	T > C	Rosiglitazone	PD
PTPRD	rs17584499	na	Intron	C > T	Pioglitazone	PD
SP1	rs784888	na	Intron	G > C	Metformin	PK
TCF7L2	rs12255372	na	Intron	G > T	Sulfonylureas	PD
	rs7903146	na	Intron	C > T	Sulfonylureas	PD
	rs290487	na	Intron	C > T	Repaglinide	PD

na, not applicable; PD, pharmacodynamic; PK, pharmacokinetic; TZD, thiazolidinedione.

Mutations in Drug-Metabolizing Enzyme Coding Genes

CYP2C9 gene has polymorphism, and *2 (rs1799853) and *3 (rs1057910) are two common types of loss-of-function alleles. Previous study found that compared with the wild-type CYP2C9*1/*1, the tolbutamide clearance in subjects with the CYP2C9*2/*2 and CYP2C9*3/*3 was reduced by 25% and 84%, respectively (Kirchheiner et al., 2002a). For glibenclamide, the clearance was reduced by 25% and 57%, respectively (Kirchheiner et al., 2002b). Many clinical studies found that the polymorphisms of CYP2C9 were associated with the efficacy and side effects of sulfonylureas. For example, two variant allele (CYP2C9*2/*2 or *2/*3 or *3/*3) carriers in patients with T2DM ($n = 1073$) treated with sulfonylureas had a 0.5% higher reduction in glycated hemoglobin A1c (HbA1c) levels than that of *1/*1 homozygous carriers and had three- to four-fold higher probability to reach HbA1c levels <7% (Zhou et al., 2010). CYP2C9*3 genotype was found correlated with slight hypoglycemic episodes in elderly patients (>60 years old) treated with second-generation sulfonylureas more frequently than third generation drugs (Aquilante, 2010; Yoo et al., 2011). Moreover, in a study of just 20 patients with diabetes admitted to the emergency room with severe hypoglycemia during sulfonylurea treatment compared with 337 patients with T2DM and no history of severe hypoglycemia, the *3/*3 and *2/*3 were overrepresented in the hypoglycemia group (10% vs. 2.1%).

CYP2C19 is also an enzyme that catalyzes the biotransformation of sulfonylureas, and *2 (rs4244285) and *3 (rs4986893) are two common types of loss-of-function alleles of CYP2C19. CYP2C19 poor metabolizers (CYP2C19*2/*2, *2/*3, or *3/*3 genotypes) had diminished oral clearance of gliclazide (Shao et al., 2010). After single administration of 30 mg gliclazide, the $AUC_{0-\infty}$ (area under the curve) of gliclazide in CYP2C19 poor metabolizer carriers was increased by 3.4-fold compared with CYP2C19*1 homozygotes (Zhang et al., 2007). Furthermore, the half-life ($t_{1/2}$) was also prolonged from 15.1 to 44.5 h.

Mutations in Other Genes

Mutations in hepatocyte nuclear factor 1 homeobox A (HNF1A) result in progressive β-cell dysfunction with increasing treatment requirements and a higher risk of complications with age (Frayling et al., 2001). The most common mutation of HNF1A has dominant negative effects on the expression of genes involved in glucose transport and glycolysis. In a randomized trial of sulfonylureas and metformin in patients with diabetes due to HNF1A mutations (Pro129Thr, Glu132Lys, Arg159Trp/rs765432081, Arg229Pro, Trp267Arg, and Pro291fsGln/rs762703502) and T2DM, the fall in fasting plasma glucose (FPG) to gliclazide was 3.9-fold greater in patients with HNF1A mutations than their response to metformin ($p = .002$); as expected, no difference in response to gliclazide or metformin was apparent in those with T2DM (Pearson et al., 2003). This study highlighted, for the first time, the importance of genetic etiology in determining response to treatment in diabetes and has led to change in clinical management of patients with HNF1A mutations.

Polymorphisms in genes potassium channel inwardly rectifying subfamily J member 11 (KCNJ11) may control β-cell function thus lead to an increased risk of secondary failure to Sulfonylureas therapy. KCNJ11 (coding Kir6.2 subunit of KATP channel) mutations that cause a small decrease in the ATP sensitivity of heterozygous KATP channels result in neonatal diabetes alone, whereas those mutations that produce a greater reduction in ATP sensitivity are associated with additional symptoms. As the pore of the KATP channel, polymorphisms in KCNJ11 have been studied regarding their relationship with sulfonylureas response in patients with T2DM. The most widely studied polymorphism has been rs5219 (Glu23Lys) (Gloyn et al., 2001; Florez et al., 2004; Nielsen et al., 2003). It was hypothesized that the KCNJ11 rs5219 T allele may be associated with interindividual variability in the sulfonylureas response. This hypothesis was tested in a group of newly diagnosed patients with diabetes treated with sulfonylureas who were participating in the UKPDS study (Gloyn et al., 2001). In this study, the KCNJ11 rs5219 variant was not significantly associated with response to sulfonylureas therapy. In another study, Sesti et al. (2006) investigated whether the rs5219 variant was associated with an increased risk of secondary sulfonylurea failure in patients with T2DM. They found that the impairment of glibenclamide-induced insulin release was significantly ($p = .01$) worse in patients with the rs5219 T allele.

Potassium channel voltage—gated KQT-like subfamily Q member 1 (*KCNQ1*) encodes the pore-forming subunit of a voltage-gated K^+ channel (KvLQT1), and mutations in *KCNQ1* can cause the K^+ channel dysfunction. Previous studies confirmed that *KCNQ1* was expressed in pancreatic islets and insulin-secreting cell lines (Unoki et al., 2008; Yasuda et al., 2008; Ullrich et al., 2005). Many polymorphisms of *KCNQ1* have been found associated with impaired insulin secretion or impaired incretin secretion (Hu et al., 2009; Jonsson et al., 2009; Tan et al., 2009; Holmkvist et al., 2009; Mussig et al., 2009). Variation in *KCNQ1* is also correlated with therapeutic response to sulfonylureas. In a clinical study of 87 patients with T2DM who were treated with sulfonylurea in addition to metformin, rs163184 in *KCNQ1* was significantly associated with ΔFPG (before treatment FPG minus posttreatment FPG). Carriers of the TT or TG achieved significantly higher ΔFPG in comparison with patients with the GG genotype (1.58 ± 0.13 vs. 1.04 ± 0.18 mmol/L, $p = .016$) (Schroner et al., 2011).

Sodium channel nonvoltage-gated 1 β subunit (*SCNN1B*) encodes an important subunit in the epithelial sodium channel present on the apical membrane of the renal epithelial cells. Mutations in *SCNN1B* have been found association with low renin activity and hypertension (Snyder, 2002). In a pharmacogenetics study of farglitazar, rs889299 in *SCNN1B* was found significantly associated with the risk of edema ($p = 5 \times 10^{-4}$) when treated with farglitazar plus glibenclamide in patients with T2DM in Caucasians (Spraggs et al., 2007). Patients with genotype AA or AG may have increased risk of edema when compared with patients with genotype GG.

Among the T2DM-associated genes, polymorphisms in the transcription factor 7-like 2 (high mobility group box) (*TCF7L2*) gene correlate with an ~1.4-fold increased risk of T2DM in multiple populations (Pearson, 2009a). Variation in *TCF7L2* influences the initial treatment success with sulfonylurea therapy in patients with T2DM. This was observed for both single nucleotide polymorphisms (SNPs; rs12255372 and rs7903146) that were reported to be associated with diabetes risk and is an addition to the effect of dose, adherence, sex, and baseline glycemia.

MEGLITINIDES

Mechanism

Meglitinides (repaglinide and nateglinide) are a novel class of nonsulfonylurea insulin secretagogues characterized by very rapid onset and abbreviated duration of action (Holstein and Egberts, 2003). They stimulate first-phase insulin release in a glucose-sensitive manner (Holstein and Beil, 2009), theoretically reducing the risk of hypoglycemic events (Holstein and Egberts, 2003; Dornhorst, 2001; Pearson, 2009b). Most of the commonly used meglitinides are metabolized in the liver and mainly excreted through the bile, except for a small proportion of the parent compound that has been found in the urine. Many studies reported that mutations in *CYP2C9*, *CYP2C8*, *SLCO1B1*, *SLC30A8*, *NEUROD1*, *PAX4*, *KCNJ11*, *KCNQ1*, *TCF7L2*, and *NR1I2* can affect the efficacy of meglitinides.

Mutations in Drug-Metabolizing Enzyme Coding Genes

The meglitinide class drug nateglinide is metabolized by CYP2C9. Moderate dose adjustments based on *CYP2C9* genotypes may help in reducing interindividual variability in the antihyperglycemic effects of nateglinide (Kirchheiner et al., 2005). In a prospective clinical study of 26 healthy volunteers, the clearance of nateglinide was found significantly reduced in carriers of *CYP2C9*3* alleles, whereas no significant difference was found in *CYP2C9*2* carriers when compared with the wild-type carriers (Kirchheiner et al., 2004). Moreover, the AUC of nateglinide in *CYP2C9*3* homozygotes was two-fold higher than that in wild-type *CYP2C9*1* homozygotes. Carriers of the *CYP2C9*3/*3* genotype may be at a slightly higher risk of hypoglycemia compared with carriers of *CYP2C9*1*, particularly when taking nateglinide doses above 120 mg.

Repaglinide is metabolized by CYP2C8. *CYP2C8*3* (rs11572080 or rs10509681) carriers had higher clearance than that of wild-type carriers. Clinical study of healthy volunteers found that the AUC of repaglinide in subjects with the *CYP2C8*1/*3* genotype was 45% lower than that in wild-type *CYP2C8*1* homozygotes (Niemi et al., 2003).

Mutations in Drug Transporter Coding Genes

Organic anion–transporting polypeptide 1B1 (OATP1B1), encoding the solute carrier organic anion transporter family member 1B1 (*SLCO1B1*), is an influx transporter of meglitinides. In a study of healthy volunteers, the *SLCO1B1*1B* (rs2306283) was found correlated with some PK and PD parameters of meglitinides. The AUC and C_{max} of repaglinide in the individuals with the rs2306283 GG genotype were 32% ($p = .007$) and 24% lower ($p = .056$) than those in the carriers of wild-type genotype, and the mean blood glucose concentration from 0 to 7 h after repaglinide intake was 10% higher ($p = .007$). In addition, the C_{max} of nateglinide in individuals with the rs2306283 GG genotype occurred earlier than that in the carriers of wild-type genotype ($p = .004$). However, none of other PK variables of nateglinide had differences between the participants with rs2306283 GG genotype and wild type (Kalliokoski et al., 2008a). Another function mutation in *SLCO1B1* related to PK of meglitinides is *SLCO1B1*5* (rs4149056). Previous study found that carriers of rs4149056 CC genotype in healthy volunteers had a greater mean area under the plasma repaglinide concentration–time curve and larger AUC than participants with TC or TT genotypes (Kalliokoski et al., 2008b). Moreover, a SNP (rs4149015) in *SLCO1B1* was also found related to PD of repaglinide. Niemi et al. (2005) found that participants with the rs4149015 GA genotype had higher maximum decrease in blood glucose concentration and mean change in blood glucose concentration in those with the GG genotype.

Solute carrier family 30 (zinc transporter) member 8 (*SLC30A8*) encodes ion channel zinc transporter protein member 8 (ZnT-8), which is thought to be the β-cell zinc concentration regulator. *SLC30A8* rs13266634 and rs16889462 polymorphisms were associated with repaglinide therapeutic efficacy in Chinese patients with T2DM (Huang et al., 2010). Repaglinide response on fasting serum insulin and postprandial serum insulin was better in patients with rs13266634 CT + TT genotypes than those with CC genotype. Carriers of rs16889462 GA genotype showed an enhanced repaglinide efficacy on FPG, PPG (postprandial plasma glucose), and HbAlc than the individuals with the GG genotype.

Mutations in the Other Genes

Neurogenic differentiation 1 (NEUROD1) is a transcription factor necessary for the development of pancreatic islets and insulin secretion (Naya et al., 1997). *NEUROD1* heterodimerizes with basic helix—loop—helix factor E47 to form a complex named as insulin enhancer factor 1 which acts as a transcription factor of insulin gene (Massari and Murre, 2000). In patients with T2DM, carriers of *NEUROD1* rs1801262 (Ala45Thr) T allele have attenuated efficacy on FPG (-2.79 ± 2.14 vs. -0.99 ± 1.80 mmol/L) and PPG (-6.71 ± 5.90 vs. -2.54 ± 3.39 mmol/L) than those with the C allele after repaglinide treatment (Gong et al., 2012).

Paired box gene 4 (PAX4) belongs to the pax family, which plays important roles in the growth, differentiation, proliferation, and insulin secretion of pancreatic β-cells (Horikawa et al., 1997; Sosa-Pineda et al., 1997; St-Onge et al., 1997; Yamagata et al., 1996). PAX4 promotes β-cell development by binding with the pancreatic islet cell enhancer sequence elements of insulin, glucagon, and somatostatin (Smith et al., 1999; Fujitani et al., 1999). In the same study sample of *NEUROD1*, rs114202595 (Arg121Trp) in *PAX4* was also found related to efficacy of repaglinide (Gong et al., 2012). Patients with the GG genotype showed better efficacy with respect to the level of PPG than carriers of the GA genotype (-6.53 ± 6.52 vs. -2.95 ± 1.17 mmol/L).

Nuclear receptor subfamily 1 group I member 2 (*NR1I2*) encodes the pregnane X receptor/steroid and xenobiotic receptor (PXR/SXR) that is involved in the transcriptional regulation of CYP2C8 and CYP2C9 (the major metabolic enzymes of meglitinides) (Zhang et al., 2001). As a result, polymorphisms in the ligand-binding domain regions of *NR1I2* gene may influence the transcription of CYP2C8 and CYP2C9, thus affecting PK and PD of meglitinides. In a clinical PK and PD study of healthy volunteers, the combination genotypes of rs2276706 and rs3814058 were found associated with the PK of repaglinide. Carriers of the rs2276706 GG—rs3814058 CC had lower $C_{L/F}$, longer $T_{1/2}$, and higher AUC than those with rs2276706 AA—rs3814058 TT (Du et al., 2013).

TCF7L2 is a transcription factor that plays an important role in the Wnt signaling pathway. Similar to PAX4, TCF7L2 is also involved in the growth, differentiation, proliferation, and insulin secretion of pancreatic β-cells (Grant et al., 2006). In a clinical study of Chinese patients with T2DM, the rs290487 in *TCF7L2* was found associated with the efficacy of repaglinide. After treatment with repaglinide, carriers of the rs290487 TT genotypes had a significantly higher increase in fasting serum insulin and a higher decrease in triglyceride and low-density lipoprotein cholesterol (LDL-C) levels when compared with carriers of the CT or CC genotype (Yu et al., 2010).

Another two genes related to PD of meglitinides are *KCNJ11* and *KCNQ1*. Both of them were found related to the efficacy of repaglinide. For *KCNJ11*, patients with T2DM with the rs5219 GA or AA genotype showed higher levels of FPG, PPG, and HbA1c compared with patients with the GG genotype after repaglinide treatment (Yu et al., 2010). For *KCNQ1*, carriers of the rs2237892 T allele and rs2237895 C allele were more likely to have a better response to repaglinide in PPG levels and postprandial serum insulin than carriers with the rs2237892 CC and rs2237895 AA genotypes, respectively (Dai et al., 2012).

METFORMIN

Mechanism

Metformin is the initial pharmacotherapy for T2DM recommended by the guidelines of The American Diabetes Association (ADA) and European Association for the Study of Diabetes (EASD) (Campbell, 2009). Metformin's primary effect was to reduce hepatic glucose output by increasing insulin suppression of gluconeogenesis. At the molecular level, the effects of metformin are mediated via AMP-activated protein kinase (AMPK) (Zhou et al., 2001). One possible mechanism could be that metformin acts to inhibit the mitochondrial respiratory chain and thus indirectly activate AMPK by altering the cellular concentrations of ATP and AMP (Owen et al., 2000). In recent years, additional mechanisms of metformin action have been proposed that may involve cAMP, the phosphorylation of Acc1 and Acc2, mitochondrial glycerophosphate dehydrogenase and the activated duodenal AMPK (Miller et al., 2013; Fullerton et al., 2013; Madiraju et al., 2014; Duca et al., 2015). Metformin is a good substrate for the human organic cation transporter 1 (OCT1), encoded by the solute carrier family 22 member 1 (*SLC22A1*) gene, which is primarily expressed in the liver (Kimura et al., 2005). Renal excretion of metformin is mediated primarily by organic cation transporter 2 (OCT2, encoded by *SLC22A2*) and multidrug and toxin extrusion protein 1 (MATE1, encoded by *SLC47A1*) and multidrug and toxin extrusion protein 2-K (MATE2-K, encoded by *SLC47A2*) (Gong et al., 2012). Therefore, variants in OCTs and MATEs may alter the bioavailability of metformin and thus affect metformin efficacy or its side effects. In addition, mutations in or near *ATM*, *FMO5*, *CAPN10*, *KCNJ11*, *SP1*, and *PPARA* genes were also found correlated with the efficacy of metformin.

Mutations in Drug Transporter Coding Genes

OCT1 appears to play a key role in determining one of the major pharmacologic effects of metformin, which is the inhibition of hepatic gluconeogenesis. The tissue-specific action of metformin may be related to the expression of influx transporters such as OCTs that can deliver metformin intracellularly (Shu et al., 2007). There has been some exciting work on the role of *SLC22A1* variation on metformin response. In a transgenic mouse model, knockout of liver *SLC22A1* virtually abolished hepatic lactate production, supporting a key role of OCT1 in transporting metformin into the hepatocytes (Wang et al., 2003). Since the publication of the results of the United Kingdom Prospective Diabetes Study (UKPDS) in 1998, metformin has become the most widely prescribed oral agent for the treatment of T2DM. T allele of *SLC22A1* rs12208357 (Arg61Cys) polymorphism has been found to be strongly correlated with decreased OCT1 protein expression in liver tissue samples from Caucasian subjects (Nies et al., 2009). Four variants, *SLC22A1* rs12208357 (Arg61Cys), rs34130495 (Gly209Ser), rs34059508 (Gly465Arg), and rs72552763 (Met420del) have all been shown to decrease the effectiveness of metformin, as well as to increase the renal clearance of metformin (Shu et al., 2007, 2008; Tzvetkov et al., 2009; Zhou et al., 2009). However, the study results of rs12208357 and rs72552763 variants were sometimes different (Zhou et al., 2009). *SLC22A1* rs628031 (Met408Val) and rs36056065 (GTAAGTTG > -) variants were in strong linkage disequilibrium ($r^2 = 0.929$) and predisposed patients with T2DM to the side effects of metformin (Tarasova et al., 2012). In addition, *SLC22A1* rs628031 A allele carriers in patients with T2DM showed a decreased response to metformin compared with the G allele carriers in a small group of Asian subjects (Shikata et al., 2007). The Diabetes Prevention Program (DPP) found that rs683369 (Leu160Phe) in *SLC22A1* was associated with 31% risk reduction of diabetes incidence in metformin-treated participants, but not in those treated with placebo (Jablonski et al., 2010). For *SLC22A1* rs2282143 (Pro341Leu), the CC genotype is associated with increased clearance of metformin in healthy individuals when compared with the genotypes CT + TT genotypes (Yoon et al., 2013). Some variants located in the intron region could also affect metformin efficacy. One population-based cohort study in Rotterdam showed that the minor C allele at rs622342 in the *SLC22A1* gene was associated with 0.28% less reduction in HbA1c levels (Becker et al., 2009a). Additionally, the rs622342 SNP has been associated with a decreased effect on blood glucose in heterozygotes and a lack of an effect of metformin on plasma glucose in homozygotes (Graham et al., 2011).

Three polymorphisms rs201919874 (Thr199Ile), rs145450955 (Thr201Met), and rs316019 (Ser270Ala) in *SLC22A2* are associated with differences in metformin blood levels and renal excretion (Song et al., 2008). Wang et al. (2008a) found rs316019 to be associated with reduced CL_{renal} in healthy volunteers ($n = 15$), although it might not affect plasma metformin concentration. Controversially, Chen et al. (2009) found that healthy volunteers with rs316019 mutant heterozygous ($n = 9$) had higher CL_{renal} compared with the reference genotype subjects ($n = 14$). No significant difference was found in metformin peak plasma concentration.

A few studies have investigated the impacts of polymorphisms in OCT3 on metformin PK or its efficacy. Chen et al. (2010) found that *SLC22A3* rs11441045, rs8187717 (Ala116Ser), and rs8187725 (Thr400Ile) could influence metformin uptake in vitro. Tzvetkov et al. (2009) examined whether tagging SNPs of *SLC22A3* affected metformin PK in healthy volunteers; however, there was no significant association between these SNPs and CL_{renal} of metformin.

Kajiwara et al. (2009) found seven nonsynonymous variants in *SLC47A1* and *SLC47A2* (Val10Leu/rs555657341, Gly64Asp/rs77630697, Ala310Val/rs111060526, Asp328Ala/rs111060527, and Asn474Ser/rs111060528 in the *SLC47A1* gene, and Lys64Asn/rs111060529 and Gly211Val/rs111060532 in the *SLC47A2* gene) in Japanese. Except for rs555657341, all of variants mentioned above reflected a decreased transporter activity in vitro. Recently, it has been reported that two promoter variants in *SLC47A1* and *SLC47A2* showed a significant influence on metformin response. Choi et al. (2009) sequenced the basal promoter region of the *SLC47A1* gene and found that rs2252281 was associated with reduced luciferase reporter activity in vitro and in vivo, suggesting a negative influence on MATE1 expression. A follow-up study focusing on promoter variants of *SLC47A1* (rs2252281) and *SLC47A2* (rs12943590) found that the renal and secretory clearances of metformin were higher in carriers of variant *SLC47A2* who were also *SLC47A1* wild type in 57 mixed-population healthy subjects. Besides, both *SLC47A1* and *SLC47A2* genotypes were associated with altered post-metformin glucose tolerance, with variant carriers of *SLC47A1* and *SLC47A2* having an enhanced and reduced response, respectively. Consistent with these results, patients with diabetes ($n = 145$) carrying the *SLC47A1* variant showed enhanced metformin response (Stocker et al., 2013). Previously, Caucasians population—based study of patients with diabetes revealed that rs2289669 in the *SLC47A1* gene was associated with metformin efficacy (Becker et al., 2009b; Tkac et al., 2013). The decrease in HbA1c level was greater in the AA genotype compared with the GA + GG genotype after the metformin treatment. The effect of *SLC47A1* rs2289669 polymorphism on PD ($n = 202$) and PK ($n = 28$) of metformin was also evaluated in Chinese subjects and found that the AA genotype patients had a better glucose-lowering effect after 1-year follow-up. As for the PK parameters, the AA genotype patients had a higher AUC_{12h} and lower renal clearance and renal clearance by secretion (He et al., 2015).

Mutations in the Other Genes

A polymorphism named rs11212617 near ataxia telangiectasia-mutated (*ATM*) gene was found to be associated with metformin glucose-lowering effect in the first GWAS of metformin (GoDARTS, Group UDPS, WTCCC, 2011). Subsequently, few studies tried to verify this result in multiple ethnic groups, but the conclusions were controversial. Van Leeuwen et al. (2012) performed a meta-analysis of five cohorts and discovered that the rs11212617 C allele was associated with increased treatment success to metformin in patients with T2DM when compared with the A allele.

Specificity protein 1 (SP1) is a transcription factor that modulates the expression of metformin transporters. Goswami and colleagues focused on whether genetic variants in *SP1* could affect PK of metformin, and then affect its efficacy. Five variants in *SP1* (rs784892, rs2694855, rs2683511, rs10747673, and rs784888), which could modulate the expression of metformin transporters, were associated with changes in treatment HbA1c and metformin secretory clearance (Goswami et al., 2014). Population PK modeling confirmed a 24% reduction in apparent clearance in the rs784888 GG genotype carriers.

Peroxisome proliferator—activated receptor-α (PPAR-α, encoded by *PPARA*) and hepatocyte nuclear factor 4, alpha (HNF4-α, encoded by *HNF4A*) are multifunctional transcription factors and important regulators of OCT1 (Nie et al., 2005). Therefore, mutations in these two genes may affect PD of metformin through influence the transcription of OCT1. In a pharmacogenetics study of metformin, polymorphisms in both of *PPARA* and *HNF4A* were genotyped. Association analysis suggested that 17 SNPs and 6 SNPs in *PPARA* and *HNF4A*, respectively, were significantly associated with metformin efficacy (Goswami et al., 2014). The most significant variant among these SNPs was rs149711321 in *PPARA* ($p = 1 \times 10^{-5}$). The carriers of allele T of rs149711321 had decreased post-HbA1c levels compared with patients with the allele C after treatment with metformin.

Flavin-containing monooxygenase-5 (FMO5) has been confirmed that can catalyze the oxygenation of nitrogen-containing drugs, whereas metformin is a nitrogen-rich drug (Lattard et al., 2004; Breitenstein et al., 2015). As a result, mutations in *FMO5* may affect the PD of metformin. Breitenstein and colleagues recruited 258 patients with T2DM who had new metformin exposure and were included in a GWAS from Mayo Genome Consortia (Breitenstein et al., 2015; Bielinski et al., 2011). After the association analysis, rs7541245 in

FMO5 was found significantly associated with a decrease in glycemic response during metformin exposure. Allele A of rs7541245 is correlated with decreased response to metformin in patients with T2DM when compared with the allele C.

Calpain-10 (*CAPN10*), encoding the Calpain-10 protein, belongs to calpains that are important intracellular proteases in calcium-regulated signaling pathways. Previous studies suggested that Calpain-10 may affect both insulin resistance and insulin secretion (Brown et al., 2007; Ling et al., 2009). Ivan Tkac and colleagues found that rs3792269 (Pro200=) in *CAPN10* was significantly associated with less treatment success of metformin in T2DM. The reduction in HbA1c of carriers of the minor G allele was associated with a smaller reduction in HbA1c (Tkac et al., 2015).

THIAZOLIDINEDIONES

Mechanism

TZDs (pioglitazone, rosiglitazone) are PPARγ ligands that induce binding of PPARγ with one or more coactivator proteins to a PPAR response element (PPRE), promoting transactivation of a large number of target genes involved in fatty acid uptake and storage, glucose uptake, adipocyte differentiation, and adipocyte-derived cytokine production. Physiologically, TZDs increase insulin-stimulated glucose uptake into muscle, insulin suppression of hepatic glucose output, and insulin-stimulated lipolysis (Yki-Jarvinen, 2004). The major metabolizing enzyme for TZDs is CYP2C8 (Jaakkola et al., 2006; Budde et al., 2003; Cox et al., 2000). Therefore, mutations in the coding gene of these enzymes may affect the PK and PD of TZDs. Moreover, other genes reported to affect the efficacy of TZDs include *LPL, ADIPOQ, PPARG, PTPRD, ABCA1, LPIN1,* PPARGC1A, and *PAX4.*

Mutations in Drug-Metabolizing Enzyme Coding Genes

Rosiglitazone is demethylated and hydroxylated primarily through CYP2C8 in the human liver (Baldwin et al., 1999). *CYP2C8*3* is a well-known gain of function mutation in CYP2C8. In a PK study of rosiglitazone in Caucasian healthy volunteers, the mean total clearance values in carriers of *CYP2C8*3/*3* was higher than those in carriers of *1/*3* and *1/*1* (0.046 vs. 0.038 vs. 0.033, *p* = .02) (Kirchheiner et al., 2006). The clearance of desmethyl rosiglitazone in *CYP2C8*3* allele carriers was also higher than that in patients with *CYP2C8* wild type. Similar results were also found by Kirchheiner et al. (2008) in another cohort of subjects. The *CYP2C8*3* allele was also found to have opposite effects on the PK of pioglitazone in the study by Tornio et al. (2008). They found that compared with the carriers of *CYP2C8* wild type, the weight-adjusted pioglitazone AUC was 34% and 26% lower in patients with *CYP2C8*3/*3* and *1/*3*, respectively. In addition, the half-life of pioglitazone in the carriers of *CYP2C8*1/*3* (3.4 h) and *3/*3* (3.3 h) was significantly shorter than that in participants with the wild type (4.5 h). Similar results were found in the study by Kadam et al. (2013) in healthy Caucasian volunteers. They found that oral clearance of pioglitazone was substantially higher in the *CYP2C8*3* carriers than that in the wild-type carriers. In a PK study of healthy African-American volunteers, another polymorphism *CYP2C8*2* (rs11572103) was studied. The study found that pioglitazone M-III (keto) AUC_{0-48} ratio, and the M-III and M-IV (hydroxy) AUC_{0-48} ratio in the carriers of *CYP2C8*2* were significantly lower than those in participants with the *CYP2C8*1/*1* genotype (Aquilante et al., 2013). The polymorphisms in *CYP2C8* were also found related to the PD of TZDs. In a Go-DARTS study, the carriers of *CYP2C8*3* and **4* (rs1058930) showed a 0.8% higher HbA1c than patients with the wild type. Furthermore, carriers of *CYP2C8*3* and **4* were 3.8 times more likely to fail achieving treatment target compared with carriers of wild type (Abstracts of the 46th General Assembly of the European Association, 2010).

Mutations in Drug Transporter Coding Genes

The ATP-binding cassette transporter subfamily A number 1 (*ABCA1*) encodes a transmembrane protein that plays an important role in the transport of cellular cholesterol and phospholipid. Brunham et al. (2007) found that ABCA1 probably affects glucose tolerance and insulin secretion by influencing the cholesterol homeostasis in β-cells. In a pharmacogenetic study of rosiglitazone in 105 newly diagnosed Chinese patients with T2DM, three polymorphisms (rs2230806, rs2066714, and rs2230808) in *ABCA1* were genotyped. After 48 weeks of rosiglitazone treatment, rs2230806 was found significantly correlated with rosiglitazone efficacy. Treatment failure rate was 88% for rs2230806 AA genotype patients, and for GG genotype was only 52%. Meanwhile, the improvement of insulin sensitivity was larger in patients with GG genotype (Wang et al., 2008b).

Mutations in the Other Genes

Peroxisome proliferator–activated receptor-γ (PPAR-γ, encoded by *PPARG* gene), the target of TZDs, belongs to the nuclear receptor superfamily of ligand-activated transcription factors. PPAR-γ plays a role in relieving insulin resistance and in promoting adipogenesis (Lehmann et al., 1995). PPAR-γ coactivator-1α (PGC-1α, encoded by *PPARGC1A* gene) is a transcriptional coactivator of PPAR-γ. PGC-1α interacts with PPAR-γ which permits PPAR-γ interacts with multiple transcription factors. Hsieh and colleagues investigated the effects of the common polymorphisms rs1801282 (Pro12Ala) in *PPARG* and rs8192678 (Gly482Ser) in *PPARGC1A* on the response to pioglitazone in Chinese patients with T2DM. A total of 250 patients treated with pioglitazone (30 mg/day) for 24 weeks on the basis of previous medications were recruited. The rs1801282 GG and CG genotypes (26.0% vs. 13.5%) and C allele (15.6% vs. 7.3%) were significantly more frequent in pioglitazone responders than in nonresponders. The decrease in fasting glucose and HbA1c levels was significantly greater in subjects with the CG + GG carriers compared with the CC genotypes (Hsieh et al., 2010). In addition, Pei and colleagues recruited 67 Chinese patients with T2DM treated with pioglitazone to study *PPARG* rs1801282 effects on pioglitazone response. After pioglitazone treatment for 3 months, *PPARG* rs1801282 CG genotypes showed higher differential values of PPG and serum triglyceride (TG) compared with the CC genotypes (Pei et al., 2013). Moreover, Zhang and colleagues investigated whether *PPARGC1A* rs2970847 (Thr394=) and rs8192678 polymorphisms influence rosiglitazone response in Chinese patients with T2DM. Forty-one patients with different rs2970847 or rs8192678 genotypes received oral rosiglitazone (4 mg/day) for 12 consecutive weeks were enrolled in their study. The rs2970847 A allele (AA + AG) carriers showed a smaller attenuation of the PINS (postprandial serum insulin) and h-LDL levels than the GG genotype patients. rs8192678 CC genotype had a greater decrease in FPG and PINS levels compared with the CT + TT genotype (Zhang et al., 2010).

ADIPOQ (Adiponectin C1Q and collagen domain containing) encodes an adipose tissue-specific protein named adiponectin, which is expressed exclusively in differentiated adipocytes (Maeda et al., 1996). Previous studies found that adiponectin levels were negatively related to the serum insulin levels (Hotta et al., 2000; Yu et al., 2002) and insulin resistance (Weyer et al., 2001). *ADIPOQ* rs2241766 (Gly15=) has been shown to be associated with response to pioglitazone in patients with T2DM from Southern China. In this study, response was defined as "any decrease greater than (or equal to) 15%" of HbA1C%. *ADIPOQ* rs2241766 GT genotype exerted increased response to pioglitazone compared with the TT genotype (Yang et al., 2014). Another Korean group examined the effects of rosiglitazone on adiponectin and plasma glucose levels in relation with common *ADIPOQ* polymorphisms. About 166 Korean patients with T2DM treated with 12 weeks of rosiglitazone were enrolled in this study. The rs2241766 GG genotypes showed a smaller reduction in FPG and HbA1c and a smaller increase in the serum adiponectin concentration than other genotypes. The rs1501299 GG genotypes showed a less reduction in FPG than other genotypes (Kang et al., 2005). Sun and colleagues evaluated the influences of the adiponectin common allele rs2241766 and rs266729 polymorphisms on the response to rosiglitazone monotherapy in 42 Chinese patients with T2DM. They showed an attenuated rosiglitazone effect in patients with the rs266729 CG + GG heterozygote genotype on FPG, PPG, HOMA-IR (the homeostasis model assessment of insulin resistance) compared with CC homozygote genotype. However, they found an enhanced rosiglitazone effect on serum adiponectin concentrations in patients with the rs266729 CC genotype and the rs2241766 TG + GG genotype compared with other genotypes (Sun et al., 2008).

Lipoprotein lipase (LPL), synthesized and secreted by parenchyma cells, is a glycoprotein. Previous study confirmed that treatment with pioglitazone increased *LPL* gene expression in vivo (Bogacka et al., 2004). To found whether polymorphism in *LPL* would affect the efficacy of TZDs, Wang and colleagues investigated the influence of the *LPL* rs328 (Ser474Ter) on the response rate in 113 patients with diabetes treated with pioglitazone for 10 weeks. Response to pioglitazone treatment was defined as either a more than 10% relative reduction in FBG or a more than 1% decrease in HbA1c levels after 10-week treatment. Using the criteria of >10% relative reduction in FBG, response rate in the CC genotype group is significantly higher than the CG genotype group (Wang et al., 2007).

Lipin1 protein, a product of the *LPIN1* gene, is required for normal adipose tissue development and metabolism. Pioglitazone has been reported to increase the expression of human adipocyte lipin1. Thus, a study carried out in 262 South Korean patients with T2DM evaluated the effects of *LPIN1* polymorphisms on rosiglitazone response. After 12-week rosiglitazone (4 mg/day) treatment combined with previous medications, they found that *LPIN1* rs10192566 was significantly associated with rosiglitazone response. Carriers of the rs10192566 G allele (GG + GC) showed a significantly larger decrease in FPG, 2h-PPG and HbA1c than the patients with CC genotype even after multiple regression (Kang et al., 2008).

PAX4, which has been found correlated with efficacy of repaglinide, was also analyzed in pharmacogenetics studies of rosiglitazone. Chen and colleagues investigated the association of *PAX4* polymorphisms with therapeutic effect of OADs in Chinese patients with T2DM. A total of 209 newly diagnosed patients with T2DM were randomly assigned to treatment with repaglinide or rosiglitazone for 48 weeks. In the rosiglitazone cohort, *PAX4* rs6467136 GA + AA carriers showed greater decrease in 2-h glucose levels and higher cumulative attainment rates of target 2-h glucose levels than the GG homozygotes (Chen et al., 2014).

Protein tyrosine phosphatase receptor type D, encoded by the *PTPRD* gene, is a member of protein tyrosine phosphatase receptor type IIA subfamily. *PTPRD* has been found associated with T2DM in a GWAS study with the strongest association signal and the largest odds ratio (Tonks, 2006; Tsai et al., 2010). In a pharmacogenetics study of pioglitazone in Chinese patients with T2DM, patients with *PTPRD* rs17584499 CT + TT genotypes showed significantly lower differential value of PPG compared with the CC genotypes (Pei et al., 2013).

α-GLUCOSIDASE INHIBITORS

α-Glucosidase inhibitors block the enzymatic degradation of complex carbohydrates in the small intestine. These compounds lower postprandial glucose and improve glycemic control without increasing the risk for weight gain or hypoglycemia. Acarbose is one of the mostly used α-glucosidase inhibitors in T2DM therapy. In the STOP-NIDDM (study to prevent non-insulin-dependent diabetes mellitus) trial, a primary intervention study, acarbose treatment was associated with a significant lower incidence of T2DM and a halved risk of major cardiovascular events in 1429 patients with impaired fasting glucose tolerance (Chiasson et al., 2003). As acarbose acts locally in the gastrointestinal tract, its systemic bioavailability is low. Thus, it seems unlikely that transport proteins play a role in the therapeutic action of this agent. Less than 2% of an oral dose of acarbose is absorbed from the gastrointestinal tract as unchanged drug. Acarbose is metabolized exclusively within the gastrointestinal tract, primarily by intestinal microflora and to a lesser extent by digestive enzymes. Digestive enzyme preparations containing α-amylase may reduce the effect of acarbose and should not be taken concomitantly (Hiele et al., 1992). Recently, only a few of pharmacogenetics studies of α-glucosidase inhibitors have been reported. All of these studies used acarbose to treatment of T2DM.

PPARG and *PPARGC1A* are two well-known genes related to drug reaction of TZDs, and they were also found to be associated with the efficacy to T2DM during treatment with acarbose. In a pharmacogenetics study based on STOP-NIDDM trial, rs1801282 in *PPARG* and rs8192678 in *PPARGC1A* were genotyped in 770 participants. Association analysis found that the carriers of rs1801282 CG + GG genotype showed a significantly higher reduction in 2-h serum insulin levels than the subjects with the CC genotype after treated with acarbose, whereas patients with the rs8192678 TT + CT genotype showed more decrease in 2-h glucose levels compared with the carriers of CC genotype (Andrulionyte et al., 2004).

Polymorphisms in the *ADIPOQ* gene were reported to associate with the administration of TZDs in previous studies (Yu et al., 2002). One of these polymorphisms rs1501299 was also found correlated with the efficacy of acarbosein the patients with impaired glucose tolerance (IGT). Pharmacogenetics study showed that, after being treated with acarbose, 31.9% (58 of 181) patients with IGT with the GG genotype and 31.5% (46 of 146) patients with IGT with the GT genotype were progressed to T2DM, whereas in the carriers of the TT genotype, the ratio raise up to 57.1% (16 of 28) (Zacharova et al., 2005).

DPP-4 INHIBITORS

The three approved preparations of DPP-4 inhibitors, sitagliptin, vildagliptin, and saxagliptin, promote glucose homeostasis through inhibition of DPP-4, the key enzyme responsible for degradation of two intestinal glucoregulatory incretin hormones: glucagon-like peptide-1 (GLP-1) and glucose-dependent insulinotropic peptide. It is estimated that GLP-1 and glucose-dependent insulinotropic peptide are responsible for 50–60% of the total insulin secreted in response to a meal. Generally, DPP-4 inhibitors are well tolerated. Analysis of phase III clinical trials revealed gastrointestinal disturbances, headache, and urinary tract and nasopharyngeal infections as relevant adverse effects (Drucker and Nauck, 2006; Gallwitz, 2007).

Similar to the α-glucosidase inhibitors, only a few pharmacogenetics studies for DPP-4 inhibitors have been conducted. None of the genetics factors analyzed to date have been found directly related to the efficacy of DPP-4 inhibitors in the treatment of T2DM. However, some genetic study results suggest that some polymorphisms may affect the reaction of DPP-4 inhibitors. For example, GLP1 is a natural endogenous agonist of GLP1R that is mainly expressed in the pancreatic β-cells. Activated GLP1R stimulates the adenylyl cyclase pathway which leads to increased insulin synthesis and insulin release (Drucker et al., 1987). Previous study found that the rs367543060 (Thr149Met) T allele reduced GLP1R function which suggested that DPP-4 inhibitors will be less effective in patients with the rs367543060 CT or TT genotype (Beinborn et al., 2005).

CONCLUSION

Numerous genes that influence the pharmacogenetics of oral antidiabetics have been discovered to date. The number of polymorphisms that impact the therapeutic efficacy of oral antidiabetics is growing continuously. The ultimate goal of the pharmacogenetic analysis on the oral antidiabetics is to achieve accurate dosage, to prevent hypoglycemia, and to avoid the use of wrong medicines. It is our belief that continued development of pharmacogenetics will enable patients to receive personalized diabetic therapies.

References

Abstracts of the 46th General Assembly of the European Association for the Study of Diabetes (EASD). Stockholm, Sweden. September 20–24, 2010. Diabetologia 53 (Suppl. 1), 2010, S7–S533.

Andrulionyte, L., Zacharova, J., Chiasson, J.L., et al., 2004. Common polymorphisms of the PPAR-gamma2 (Pro12Ala) and PGC-1alpha (Gly482Ser) genes are associated with the conversion from impaired glucose tolerance to type 2 diabetes in the STOP-NIDDM trial. Diabetologia 47 (12), 2176–2184.

Aquilante, C.L., Wempe, M.F., Spencer, S.H., et al., 2013. Influence of CYP2C8*2 on the pharmacokinetics of pioglitazone in healthy African-American volunteers. Pharmacotherapy 33 (9), 1000–1007.

Aquilante, C.L., 2010. Sulfonylurea pharmacogenomics in type 2 diabetes: the influence of drug target and diabetes risk polymorphisms. Expert Rev. Cardiovasc. Ther. 8 (3), 359–372.

Baldwin, S.J., Clarke, S.E., Chenery, R.J., 1999. Characterization of the cytochrome P450 enzymes involved in the in vitro metabolism of rosiglitazone. Br. J. Clin. Pharmacol. 48 (3), 424–432.

Becker, M.L., Visser, L.E., van Schaik, R.H., et al., 2009a. Genetic variation in the organic cation transporter 1 is associated with metformin response in patients with diabetes mellitus. Pharmacogenomics J. 9 (4), 242–247.

Becker, M.L., Visser, L.E., van Schaik, R.H., et al., 2009b. Genetic variation in the multidrug and toxin extrusion 1 transporter protein influences the glucose-lowering effect of metformin in patients with diabetes: a preliminary study. Diabetes 58 (3), 745–749.

Beinborn, M., Worrall, C.I., McBride, E.W., et al., 2005. A human glucagon-like peptide-1 receptor polymorphism results in reduced agonist responsiveness. Regul. Pept. 130 (1–2), 1–6.

Bielinski, S.J., Chai, H.S., Pathak, J., et al., 2011. Mayo Genome Consortia: a genotype-phenotype resource for genome-wide association studies with an application to the analysis of circulating bilirubin levels. Mayo Clin. Proc. 86 (7), 606–614.

Bogacka, I., Xie, H., Bray, G.A., et al., 2004. The effect of pioglitazone on peroxisome proliferator-activated receptor-gamma target genes related to lipid storage in vivo. Diabetes Care 27 (7), 1660–1667.

Breitenstein, M.K., Wang, L., Simon, G., et al., 2015. Leveraging an electronic health record-linked biorepository to generate a metformin pharmacogenomics hypothesis. AMIA Jt. Summits Transl. Sci. Proc. 2015, 26–30.

Brown, A.E., Yeaman, S.J., Walker, M., 2007. Targeted suppression of calpain-10 expression impairs insulin-stimulated glucose uptake in cultured primary human skeletal muscle cells. Mol. Genet. Metab. 91 (4), 318–324.

Brunham, L.R., Kruit, J.K., Pape, T.D., et al., 2007. Beta-cell ABCA1 influences insulin secretion, glucose homeostasis and response to thiazolidinedione treatment. Nat. Med. 13 (3), 340–347.

Budde, K., Neumayer, H.H., Fritsche, L., et al., 2003. The pharmacokinetics of pioglitazone in patients with impaired renal function. Br. J. Clin. Pharmacol. 55 (4), 368–374.

Campbell, R.K., 2009. Type 2 diabetes: where we are today: an overview of disease burden, current treatments, and treatment strategies. J. Am. Pharm. Assoc. 2003 49 (Suppl. 1), S3–S9.

Chen, Y., Li, S., Brown, C., et al., 2009. Effect of genetic variation in the organic cation transporter 2, OCT2, on the renal elimination of metformin. Pharmacogenet. Genomics 19 (7), 497.

Chen, L., Pawlikowski, B., Schlessinger, A., et al., 2010. Role of organic cation transporter 3 (SLC22A3) and its missense variants in the pharmacologic action of metformin. Pharmacogenet. Genomics 20 (11), 687.

Chen, M., Hu, C., Zhang, R., et al., 2014. Association of PAX4 genetic variants with oral antidiabetic drugs efficacy in Chinese type 2 diabetes patients. Pharmacogenomics J.

Chiasson, J.L., Josse, R.G., Gomis, R., et al., 2003. Acarbose treatment and the risk of cardiovascular disease and hypertension in patients with impaired glucose tolerance: the STOP-NIDDM trial. JAMA 290 (4), 486–494.

Choi, J.H., Yee, S.W., Kim, M.J., et al., 2009. Identification and characterization of novel polymorphisms in the basal promoter of the human transporter, MATE1. Pharmacogenet. Genomics 19 (10), 770.

Cox, P.J., Ryan, D.A., Hollis, F.J., et al., 2000. Absorption, disposition, and metabolism of rosiglitazone, a potent thiazolidinedione insulin sensitizer, in humans. Drug Metab. Dispos. 28 (7), 772–780.

Dai, X.P., Huang, Q., Yin, J.Y., et al., 2012. KCNQ1 gene polymorphisms are associated with the therapeutic efficacy of repaglinide in Chinese type 2 diabetic patients. Clin. Exp. Pharmacol. Physiol. 39 (5), 462–468.

Danaei, G., Finucane, M.M., Lu, Y., et al., 2011. National, regional, and global trends in fasting plasma glucose and diabetes prevalence since 1980: systematic analysis of health examination surveys and epidemiological studies with 370 country-years and 2.7 million participants. Lancet 378 (9785), 31–40.

Dornhorst, A., 2001. Insulinotropic meglitinide analogues. Lancet 358 (9294), 1709–1716.

Drucker, D.J., Philippe, J., Mojsov, S., et al., 1987. Glucagon-like peptide I stimulates insulin gene expression and increases cyclic AMP levels in a rat islet cell line. Proc. Natl. Acad. Sci. USA 84 (10), 3434–3438.

Drucker, D.J., Nauck, M.A., 2006. The incretin system: glucagon-like peptide-1 receptor agonists and dipeptidyl peptidase-4 inhibitors in type 2 diabetes. Lancet 368 (9548), 1696–1705.

Du, Q.Q., Wang, Z.J., He, L., et al., 2013. PXR polymorphisms and their impact on pharmacokinetics/pharmacodynamics of repaglinide in healthy Chinese volunteers. Eur. J. Clin. Pharmacol. 69 (11), 1917–1925.

Duca, F.A., Cote, C.D., Rasmussen, B.A., et al., 2015. Metformin activates a duodenal Ampk-dependent pathway to lower hepatic glucose production in rats. Nat. Med. 21 (5), 506–511.

Florez, J.C., Burtt, N., de Bakker, P.I., et al., 2004. Haplotype structure and genotype-phenotype correlations of the sulfonylurea receptor and the islet ATP-sensitive potassium channel gene region. Diabetes 53 (5), 1360–1368.

Frayling, T.M., Evans, J.C., Bulman, M.P., et al., 2001. beta-cell genes and diabetes: molecular and clinical characterization of mutations in transcription factors. Diabetes 50 (Suppl. 1), S94–S100.

Fujitani, Y., Kajimoto, Y., Yasuda, T., et al., 1999. Identification of a portable repression domain and an E1A-responsive activation domain in Pax4: a possible role of Pax4 as a transcriptional repressor in the pancreas. Mol. Cell. Biol. 19 (12), 8281–8291.

Fullerton, M.D., Galic, S., Marcinko, K., et al., 2013. Single phosphorylation sites in Acc1 and Acc2 regulate lipid homeostasis and the insulin-sensitizing effects of metformin. Nat. Med. 19 (12), 1649–1654.

Gallwitz, B., 2007. Sitagliptin: profile of a novel DPP-4 inhibitor for the treatment of type 2 diabetes. Drugs Today (Barc) 43 (1), 13–25.

Gloyn, A.L., Hashim, Y., Ashcroft, S.J., et al., 2001. Association studies of variants in promoter and coding regions of beta-cell ATP-sensitive K-channel genes SUR1 and Kir6.2 with type 2 diabetes mellitus (UKPDS 53). Diabet. Med. 18 (3), 206–212.

GoDARTS, Group UDPS, WTCCC, 2011. Common variants near ATM are associated with glycemic response to metformin in type 2 diabetes. Nat. Genet. 43 (2), 117–120.

Gong, Z.C., Huang, Q., Dai, X.P., et al., 2012. NeuroD1 A45T and PAX4 R121W polymorphisms are associated with plasma glucose level of repaglinide monotherapy in Chinese patients with type 2 diabetes. Br. J. Clin. Pharmacol. 74 (3), 501–509.

Gong, L., Goswami, S., Giacomini, K.M., et al., 2012. Metformin pathways: pharmacokinetics and pharmacodynamics. Pharmacogenet. Genomics 22 (11), 820–827.

Goswami, S., Yee, S.W., Stocker, S., et al., 2014. Genetic variants in transcription factors are associated with the pharmacokinetics and pharmacodynamics of metformin. Clin. Pharmacol. Ther. 96 (3), 370–379.

Graham, G.G., Punt, J., Arora, M., et al., 2011. Clinical pharmacokinetics of metformin. Clin. Pharmacokinet. 50 (2), 81–98.

Grant, S.F., Thorleifsson, G., Reynisdottir, I., et al., 2006. Variant of transcription factor 7-like 2 (TCF7L2) gene confers risk of type 2 diabetes. Nat. Genet. 38 (3), 320–323.

He, R., Zhang, D., Lu, W., et al., 2015. SLC47A1 gene rs2289669 G>A variants enhance the glucose-lowering effect of metformin via delaying its excretion in Chinese type 2 diabetes patients. Diabetes Res. Clin. Pract.

Hiele, M., Ghoos, Y., Rutgeerts, P., et al., 1992. Effects of acarbose on starch hydrolysis. Study in healthy subjects, ileostomy patients, and in vitro. Dig. Dis. Sci. 37 (7), 1057–1064.

Holmkvist, J., Banasik, K., Andersen, G., et al., 2009. The type 2 diabetes associated minor allele of rs2237895 KCNQ1 associates with reduced insulin release following an oral glucose load. PLoS ONE 4 (6), e5872.

Holstein, A., Egberts, E.H., 2003. Risk of hypoglycaemia with oral antidiabetic agents in patients with type 2 diabetes. Exp. Clin. Endocrinol. Diabetes 111 (7), 405–414.

Holstein, A., Beil, W., 2009. Oral antidiabetic drug metabolism: pharmacogenomics and drug interactions. Expert Opin. Drug Metab. Toxicol. 5 (3), 225–241.

Horikawa, Y., Iwasaki, N., Hara, M., et al., 1997. Mutation in hepatocyte nuclear factor-1 beta gene (TCF2) associated with MODY. Nat. Genet. 17 (4), 384–385.

Hotta, K., Funahashi, T., Arita, Y., et al., 2000. Plasma concentrations of a novel, adipose-specific protein, adiponectin, in type 2 diabetic patients. Arterioscler. Thromb. Vasc. Biol. 20 (6), 1595–1599.

Hsieh, M.C., Lin, K.D., Tien, K.J., et al., 2010. Common polymorphisms of the peroxisome proliferator-activated receptor−γ (Pro12Ala) and peroxisome proliferator-activated receptor−γ coactivator−1 (Gly482Ser) and the response to pioglitazone in Chinese patients with type 2 diabetes mellitus. Metabolism 59 (8), 1139–1144.

Hu, C., Wang, C., Zhang, R., et al., 2009. Variations in KCNQ1 are associated with type 2 diabetes and beta cell function in a Chinese population. Diabetologia 52 (7), 1322–1325.

Huang, Q., Yin, J.Y., Dai, X.P., et al., 2010. Association analysis of SLC30A8 rs13266634 and rs16889462 polymorphisms with type 2 diabetes mellitus and repaglinide response in Chinese patients. Eur. J. Clin. Pharmacol. 66 (12), 1207–1215.

Jaakkola, T., Laitila, J., Neuvonen, P.J., et al., 2006. Pioglitazone is metabolised by CYP2C8 and CYP3A4 in vitro: potential for interactions with CYP2C8 inhibitors. Basic Clin. Pharmacol. Toxicol. 99 (1), 44–51.

Jablonski, K.A., McAteer, J.B., de Bakker, P.I., et al., 2010. Common variants in 40 genes assessed for diabetes incidence and response to metformin and lifestyle intervention in the diabetes prevention program. Diabetes 59 (10), 2672–2681.

Jonsson, A., Isomaa, B., Tuomi, T., et al., 2009. A variant in the KCNQ1 gene predicts future type 2 diabetes and mediates impaired insulin secretion. Diabetes 58 (10), 2409–2413.

Kadam, R., Bourne, D., Kompella, U., et al., 2013. Effect of cytochrome P450 2C8*3 on the population pharmacokinetics of pioglitazone in healthy Caucasian volunteers. Biol. Pharm. Bull. 36 (2), 245–251.

Kajiwara, M., Terada, T., Ogasawara, K., et al., 2009. Identification of multidrug and toxin extrusion (MATE1 and MATE2-K) variants with complete loss of transport activity. J. Human Genet. 54 (1), 40–46.

Kalliokoski, A., Backman, J.T., Neuvonen, P.J., et al., 2008a. Effects of the SLCO1B1*1B haplotype on the pharmacokinetics and pharmacodynamics of repaglinide and nateglinide. Pharmacogenet. Genomics 18 (11), 937–942.

Kalliokoski, A., Neuvonen, M., Neuvonen, P.J., et al., 2008b. Different effects of SLCO1B1 polymorphism on the pharmacokinetics and pharmacodynamics of repaglinide and nateglinide. J. Clin. Pharmacol. 48 (3), 311–321.

Kang, E.S., Park, S.Y., Kim, H.J., et al., 2005. The influence of adiponectin gene polymorphism on the rosiglitazone response in patients with type 2 diabetes. Diabetes Care 28 (5), 1139–1144.

Kang, E.S., Park, S.E., Han, S.J., et al., 2008. LPIN1 genetic variation is associated with rosiglitazone response in type 2 diabetic patients. Mol. Genet. Metab. 95 (1), 96–100.

Kimura, N., Masuda, S., Tanihara, Y., et al., 2005. Metformin is a superior substrate for renal organic cation transporter OCT2 rather than hepatic OCT1. Drug Metab. Pharmacokinet. 20 (5), 379–386.

Kirchheiner, J., Bauer, S., Meineke, I., et al., 2002a. Impact of CYP2C9 and CYP2C19 polymorphisms on tolbutamide kinetics and the insulin and glucose response in healthy volunteers. Pharmacogenetics 12 (2), 101–109.

Kirchheiner, J., Brockmoller, J., Meineke, I., et al., 2002b. Impact of CYP2C9 amino acid polymorphisms on glyburide kinetics and on the insulin and glucose response in healthy volunteers. Clin. Pharmacol. Ther. 71 (4), 286–296.

Kirchheiner, J., Meineke, I., Muller, G., et al., 2004. Influence of CYP2C9 and CYP2D6 polymorphisms on the pharmacokinetics of nateglinide in genotyped healthy volunteers. Clin. Pharmacokinet. 43 (4), 267–278.

Kirchheiner, J., Roots, I., Goldammer, M., et al., 2005. Effect of genetic polymorphisms in cytochrome p450 (CYP) 2C9 and CYP2C8 on the pharmacokinetics of oral antidiabetic drugs: clinical relevance. Clin. Pharmacokinet. 44 (12), 1209–1225.

Kirchheiner, J., Thomas, S., Bauer, S., et al., 2006. Pharmacokinetics and pharmacodynamics of rosiglitazone in relation to CYP2C8 genotype. Clin. Pharmacol. Ther. 80 (6), 657–667.

Kirchheiner, J., Meineke, I., Fuhr, U., et al., 2008. Impact of genetic polymorphisms in CYP2C8 and rosiglitazone intake on the urinary excretion of dihydroxyeicosatrienoic acids. Pharmacogenomics 9 (3), 277–288.

Kitabchi, A.E., Umpierrez, G.E., Miles, J.M., et al., 2009. Hyperglycemic crises in adult patients with diabetes. Diabetes Care 32 (7), 1335–1343.

Lattard, V., Zhang, J., Cashman, J.R., 2004. Alternative processing events in human FMO genes. Mol. Pharmacol. 65 (6), 1517–1525.

Lehmann, J.M., Moore, L.B., Smith-Oliver, T.A., et al., 1995. An antidiabetic thiazolidinedione is a high affinity ligand for peroxisome proliferator-activated receptor gamma (PPAR gamma). J. Biol. Chem. 270 (22), 12953–12956.

Ling, C., Groop, L., Guerra, S.D., et al., 2009. Calpain-10 expression is elevated in pancreatic islets from patients with type 2 diabetes. PLoS ONE 4 (8), e6558.

Madiraju, A.K., Erion, D.M., Rahimi, Y., et al., 2014. Metformin suppresses gluconeogenesis by inhibiting mitochondrial glycerophosphate dehydrogenase. Nature 510 (7506), 542–546.

Maeda, K., Okubo, K., Shimomura, I., et al., 1996. cDNA cloning and expression of a novel adipose specific collagen-like factor, apM1 (AdiPose Most abundant Gene transcript 1). Biochem. Biophys. Res. Commun. 221 (2), 286–289.

Massari, M.E., Murre, C., 2000. Helix-loop-helix proteins: regulators of transcription in eucaryotic organisms. Mol. Cell. Biol. 20 (2), 429–440.

Mathers, C.D., Loncar, D., 2006. Projections of global mortality and burden of disease from 2002 to 2030. PLoS Med. 3 (11), e442.

Miller, R.A., Chu, Q., Xie, J., et al., 2013. Biguanides suppress hepatic glucagon signalling by decreasing production of cyclic AMP. Nature 494 (7436), 256–260.

Mussig, K., Staiger, H., Machicao, F., et al., 2009. Association of type 2 diabetes candidate polymorphisms in KCNQ1 with incretin and insulin secretion. Diabetes 58 (7), 1715–1720.

Naya, F.J., Huang, H.P., Qiu, Y., et al., 1997. Diabetes, defective pancreatic morphogenesis, and abnormal enteroendocrine differentiation in BETA2/neuroD-deficient mice. Genes Dev. 11 (18), 2323–2334.

Nie, W., Sweetser, S., Rinella, M., et al., 2005. Transcriptional regulation of murine Slc22a1 (Oct1) by peroxisome proliferator agonist receptor-alpha and -gamma. Am. J. Physiol. Gastrointest. Liver Physiol. 288 (2), G207–G212.

Nielsen, E.M., Hansen, L., Carstensen, B., et al., 2003. The E23K variant of Kir6.2 associates with impaired post-OGTT serum insulin response and increased risk of type 2 diabetes. Diabetes 52 (2), 573–577.

Niemi, M., Leathart, J.B., Neuvonen, M., et al., 2003. Polymorphism in CYP2C8 is associated with reduced plasma concentrations of repaglinide. Clin. Pharmacol. Ther. 74 (4), 380–387.

Niemi, M., Backman, J.T., Kajosaari, L.I., et al., 2005. Polymorphic organic anion transporting polypeptide 1B1 is a major determinant of repaglinide pharmacokinetics. Clin. Pharmacol. Ther. 77 (6), 468–478.

Nies, A.T., Koepsell, H., Winter, S., et al., 2009. Expression of organic cation transporters OCT1 (SLC22A1) and OCT3 (SLC22A3) is affected by genetic factors and cholestasis in human liver. Hepatology 50 (4), 1227−1240.

Owen, M.R., Doran, E., Halestrap, A.P., 2000. Evidence that metformin exerts its anti-diabetic effects through inhibition of complex 1 of the mitochondrial respiratory chain. Biochem. J. 348 (Pt 3), 607−614.

Pearson, E.R., Liddell, W.G., Shepherd, M., et al., 2000. Sensitivity to sulphonylureas in patients with hepatocyte nuclear factor-1alpha gene mutations: evidence for pharmacogenetics in diabetes. Diabet Med. 17 (7), 543−545.

Pearson, E.R., Starkey, B.J., Powell, R.J., et al., 2003. Genetic cause of hyperglycaemia and response to treatment in diabetes. Lancet 362 (9392), 1275−1281.

Pearson, E.R., 2009a. Translating TCF7L2: from gene to function. Diabetologia 52 (7), 1227−1230.

Pearson, E.R., 2009b. Pharmacogenetics and future strategies in treating hyperglycaemia in diabetes. Front. Biosci. Landmark Ed. 14, 4348−4362.

Pei, Q., Huang, Q., Yang, G-p, et al., 2013. PPAR-γ2 and PTPRD gene polymorphisms influence type 2 diabetes patients' response to pioglitazone in China. Acta Pharmacol. Sin. 34 (2), 255−261.

Rafiq, M., Flanagan, S.E., Patch, A.M., et al., 2008. Effective treatment with oral sulfonylureas in patients with diabetes due to sulfonylurea receptor 1 (SUR1) mutations. Diabetes Care 31 (2), 204−209.

Schroner, Z., Dobrikova, M., Klimcakova, L., et al., 2011. Variation in KCNQ1 is associated with therapeutic response to sulphonylureas. Med. Sci. Monit. 17 (7), Cr392−396.

Sesti, G., Laratta, E., Cardellini, M., et al., 2006. The E23K variant of KCNJ11 encoding the pancreatic beta-cell adenosine 5'-triphosphate-sensitive potassium channel subunit Kir6.2 is associated with an increased risk of secondary failure to sulfonylurea in patients with type 2 diabetes. J. Clin. Endocrinol. Metab. 91 (6), 2334−2339.

Shao, H., Ren, X.M., Liu, N.F., et al., 2010. Influence of CYP2C9 and CYP2C19 genetic polymorphisms on pharmacokinetics and pharmacodynamics of gliclazide in healthy Chinese Han volunteers. J. Clin. Pharm. Ther. 35 (3), 351−360.

Shi, Y., Hu, F.B., 2014. The global implications of diabetes and cancer. Lancet 383 (9933), 1947−1948.

Shikata, E., Yamamoto, R., Takane, H., et al., 2007. Human organic cation transporter (OCT1 and OCT2) gene polymorphisms and therapeutic effects of metformin. J. Human Genet. 52 (2), 117−122.

Shu, Y., Sheardown, S.A., Brown, C., et al., 2007. Effect of genetic variation in the organic cation transporter 1 (OCT1) on metformin action. J. Clin. Invest. 117 (5), 1422−1431.

Shu, Y., Brown, C., Castro, R.A., et al., 2008. Effect of genetic variation in the organic cation transporter 1, OCT1, on metformin pharmacokinetics. Clin. Pharmacol. Ther. 83 (2), 273−280.

Smith, S.B., Ee, H.C., Conners, J.R., et al., 1999. Paired-homeodomain transcription factor PAX4 acts as a transcriptional repressor in early pancreatic development. Mol. Cell. Biol. 19 (12), 8272−8280.

Snyder, P.M., 2002. The epithelial Na$^+$ channel: cell surface insertion and retrieval in Na+ homeostasis and hypertension. Endocr. Rev. 23 (2), 258−275.

Song, I.S., Shin, H.J., Shim, E.J., et al., 2008. Genetic variants of the organic cation transporter 2 influence the disposition of metformin. Clin. Pharmacol. Ther. 84 (5), 559−562.

Sosa-Pineda, B., Chowdhury, K., Torres, M., et al., 1997. The Pax4 gene is essential for differentiation of insulin-producing beta cells in the mammalian pancreas. Nature 386 (6623), 399−402.

Spraggs, C., McCarthy, A., McCarthy, L., et al., 2007. Genetic variants in the epithelial sodium channel associate with oedema in type 2 diabetic patients receiving the peroxisome proliferator-activated receptor gamma agonist farglitazar. Pharmacogenet. Genomics 17 (12), 1065−1076.

Stocker, S.L., Morrissey, K.M., Yee, S.W., et al., 2013. The effect of novel promoter variants in MATE1 and MATE2 on the pharmacokinetics and pharmacodynamics of metformin. Clin. Pharmacol. Ther. 93 (2), 186−194.

St-Onge, L., Sosa-Pineda, B., Chowdhury, K., et al., 1997. Pax6 is required for differentiation of glucagon-producing alpha-cells in mouse pancreas. Nature 387 (6631), 406−409.

Sun, H., Gong, Z.C., Yin, J.Y., et al., 2008. The association of adiponectin allele 45T/G and -11377C/G polymorphisms with type 2 diabetes and rosiglitazone response in Chinese patients. Br. J. Clin. Pharmacol. 65 (6), 917−926.

Tan, J.T., Nurbaya, S., Gardner, D., et al., 2009. Genetic variation in KCNQ1 associates with fasting glucose and beta-cell function: a study of 3,734 subjects comprising three ethnicities living in Singapore. Diabetes 58 (6), 1445−1449.

Tarasova, L., Kalnina, I., Geldnere, K., et al., 2012. Association of genetic variation in the organic cation transporters OCT1, OCT2 and multidrug and toxin extrusion 1 transporter protein genes with the gastrointestinal side effects and lower BMI in metformin-treated type 2 diabetes patients. Pharmacogenet. Genomics 22 (9), 659−666.

Tkac, I., Klimcakova, L., Javorsky, M., et al., 2013. Pharmacogenomic association between a variant in SLC47A1 gene and therapeutic response to metformin in type 2 diabetes. Diabetes Obes. Metab. 15 (2), 189−191.

Tkac, I., Javorsky, M., Klimcakova, L., et al., 2015. A pharmacogenetic association between a variation in calpain 10 (CAPN10) gene and the response to metformin treatment in patients with type 2 diabetes. Eur. J. Clin. Pharmacol. 71 (1), 59−63.

Tonks, N.K., 2006. Protein tyrosine phosphatases: from genes, to function, to disease. Nat. Rev. Mol. Cell Biol. 7 (11), 833−846.

Tornio, A., Niemi, M., Neuvonen, P.J., et al., 2008. Trimethoprim and the CYP2C8*3 allele have opposite effects on the pharmacokinetics of pioglitazone. Drug Metab. Dispos. 36 (1), 73−80.

Tsai, F.J., Yang, C.F., Chen, C.C., et al., 2010. A genome-wide association study identifies susceptibility variants for type 2 diabetes in Han Chinese. PLoS Genet. 6 (2), e1000847.

Tzvetkov, M., Vormfelde, S., Balen, D., et al., 2009. The effects of genetic polymorphisms in the organic cation trans-porters OCT1, OCT2, and OCT3 on the renal clearance of metformin. Clin. Pharmacol. Ther. 86 (3), 299−306.

Ullrich, S., Su, J., Ranta, F., et al., 2005. Effects of I(Ks) channel inhibitors in insulin-secreting INS-1 cells. Pflugers Arch. 451 (3), 428−436.

Unoki, H., Takahashi, A., Kawaguchi, T., et al., 2008. SNPs in KCNQ1 are associated with susceptibility to type 2 diabetes in East Asian and European populations. Nat. Genet. 40 (9), 1098−1102.

Van Leeuwen, N., Nijpels, G., Becker, M., et al., 2012. A gene variant near ATM is significantly associated with met-formin treatment response in type 2 diabetes: a replication and meta-analysis of five cohorts. Diabetologia 55 (7), 1971−1977.

Wang, D.S., Kusuhara, H., Kato, Y., et al., 2003. Involvement of organic cation transporter 1 in the lactic acidosis caused by metformin. Mol. Pharmacol. 63 (4), 844−848.

Wang, G., Wang, X., Zhang, Q., et al., 2007. Response to pioglitazone treatment is associated with the lipoprotein lipase S447X variant in subjects with type 2 diabetes mellitus. Int. J. Clin. Pract. 61 (4), 552−557.

Wang, Z.-J., Yin, O.Q., Tomlinson, B., et al., 2008a. OCT2 polymorphisms and in-vivo renal functional consequence: studies with metformin and cimetidine. Pharmacogenetics Genomics 18 (7), 637−645.

Wang, J., Bao, Y.-Q., Hu, C., et al., 2008b. Effects of ABCA1 variants on rosiglitazone monotherapy in newly diag-nosed type 2 diabetes patients. Acta Pharmacol. Sin. 29 (2), 252−258.

Weyer, C., Funahashi, T., Tanaka, S., et al., 2001. Hypoadiponectinemia in obesity and type 2 diabetes: close associ-ation with insulin resistance and hyperinsulinemia. J. Clin. Endocrinol. Metab. 86 (5), 1930−1935.

Yamagata, K., Furuta, H., Oda, N., et al., 1996. Mutations in the hepatocyte nuclear factor-4alpha gene in maturity-onset diabetes of the young (MODY1). Nature 384 (6608), 458−460.

Yang, H., Ye, E., Si, G., et al., 2014. Adiponectin gene polymorphism rs2241766 T/G is associated with response to pioglitazone treatment in type 2 diabetic patients from Southern China. PLoS ONE.

Yasuda, K., Miyake, K., Horikawa, Y., et al., 2008. Variants in KCNQ1 are associated with susceptibility to type 2 diabetes mellitus. Nat. Genet. 40 (9), 1092−1097.

Yki-Jarvinen, H., 2004. Thiazolidinediones. N. Engl. J. Med. 351 (11), 1106−1118.

Yoo, H.D., Kim, M.S., Cho, H.Y., et al., 2011. Population pharmacokinetic analysis of glimepiride with CYP2C9 ge-netic polymorphism in healthy Korean subjects. Eur. J. Clin. Pharmacol. 67 (9), 889−898.

Yoon, H., Cho, H.-Y., Yoo, H.-D., et al., 2013. Influences of organic cation transporter polymorphisms on the popu-lation pharmacokinetics of metformin in healthy subjects. AAPS J. 15 (2), 571−580.

Yu, J.G., Javorschi, S., Hevener, A.L., et al., 2002. The effect of thiazolidinediones on plasma adiponectin levels in normal, obese, and type 2 diabetic subjects. Diabetes 51 (10), 2968−2974.

Yu, M., Xu, X.J., Yin, J.Y., et al., 2010. KCNJ11 Lys23Glu and TCF7L2 rs290487(C/T) polymorphisms affect therapeu-tic efficacy of repaglinide in Chinese patients with type 2 diabetes. Clin. Pharmacol. Ther. 87 (3), 330−335.

Zacharova, J., Chiasson, J.L., Laakso, M., 2005. The common polymorphisms (single nucleotide polymorphism [SNP] +45 and SNP +276) of the adiponectin gene predict the conversion from impaired glucose tolerance to type 2 diabetes: the STOP-NIDDM trial. Diabetes 54 (3), 893−899.

Zhang, J., Kuehl, P., Green, E.D., et al., 2001. The human pregnane X receptor: genomic structure and identification and functional characterization of natural allelic variants. Pharmacogenetics 11 (7), 555−572.

Zhang, Y., Si, D., Chen, X., et al., 2007. Influence of CYP2C9 and CYP2C19 genetic polymorphisms on pharmacoki-netics of gliclazide MR in Chinese subjects. Br. J. Clin. Pharmacol. 64 (1), 67−74.

Zhang, K.H., Huang, Q., Dai, X.P., et al., 2010. Effects of the peroxisome proliferator activated receptor-γ Coactivator-1α (PGC-1α) Thr394Thr and Gly482Ser polymorphisms on rosiglitazone response in Chinese patients with type 2 diabetes mellitus. J. Clin. Pharmacol. 50 (9), 1022–1030.

Zhou, G., Myers, R., Li, Y., et al., 2001. Role of AMP-activated protein kinase in mechanism of metformin action. J. Clin. Invest. 108 (8), 1167–1174.

Zhou, K., Donnelly, L.A., Kimber, C.H., et al., 2009. Reduced-function SLC22A1 polymorphisms encoding organic cation transporter 1 and glycemic response to metformin: a GoDARTS study. Diabetes 58 (6), 1434–1439.

Zhou, K., Donnelly, L., Burch, L., et al., 2010. Loss-of-function CYP2C9 variants improve therapeutic response to sulfonylureas in type 2 diabetes: a Go-DARTS study. Clin. Pharmacol. Ther. 87 (1), 52–56.

8

Hepatic Drug Metabolism in Pediatric Patients

E.H.J. Krekels[1], J.E. Rower[2], J.E. Constance[2],
C.A.J. Knibbe[1,3], C.M.T. Sherwin[2]

[1]Leiden University, Leiden, The Netherlands; [2]University of Utah, Salt Lake City, UT, United States; [3]St. Antonius Hospital, Nieuwegein, The Netherlands

OUTLINE

Ontogeny of Hepatic Drug Metabolism   181

Ontogeny of Intrinsic Hepatic Clearance   184
   Ontogeny of Hepatic CYP Enzymes   184
     CYP1A   184
     CYP2A   186
     CYP2B   187
     CYP2C   187
     CYP2D   188
     CYP2E   188
     CYP3A   189

Ontogeny of Hepatic UGT Enzymes   190

Ontogeny of Hepatic Blood Flow   194

Ontogeny of Plasma Protein Binding   195

Ontogeny of Hepatic Drug Transporters   196

Conclusion   196

References   197

ONTOGENY OF HEPATIC DRUG METABOLISM

Generally, drug clearance is the pharmacokinetic parameter used to determine drug dosing regimens. This is because the rate of drug elimination from the body determines the dose or dosing rate necessary to reach therapeutic target concentrations. Drugs can be eliminated from the body as unchanged (parent) drug, after enzymatic biotransformation, or a combination of these. Enzymatic drug metabolism occurs at various sites in the body, including the liver, kidneys, gastrointestinal mucosa, and the lungs. As the enzymes of drug metabolism have a central role in the elimination of many drugs, the maturational profile (ontogeny) of these enzymes can be clinically relevant. Moreover, oral drug bioavailability, prodrug activation, and/or the formation of potentially toxic metabolites are directly related to enzymatic biotransformation for specific drugs. Understanding the ontogeny of metabolic processes during childhood is therefore imperative to establish rational pediatric drug dosing recommendations and for sound clinical judgment regarding the use of certain drugs in young children.

The liver has the largest capacity for xenobiotic biotransformation, making this the most relevant organ for metabolic drug clearance. Hepatic drug metabolism occurs in hepatocytes, which comprise 70–85% of an adult's liver mass. As illustrated in Fig. 8.1, hepatic metabolic drug clearance is, to varying degrees, dependent on (1) intrinsic clearance, (2) hepatic blood flow and perfusion, (3) plasma protein binding, and (4) active transport processes in the hepatocytes.

Intrinsic clearance is the maximum clearance capacity in the absence of rate-limiting factors, such as blood flow and perfusion or plasma protein binding. Intrinsic clearance is largely defined by enzyme expression and activity per unit of liver. For children, developmental changes in posttranslational modifications of drug-metabolizing enzymes (Barbier et al., 2000a; Basu et al., 2003; Mackenzie, 1990), or the lipid composition of the membranes that enzymes reside in (Castuma and Brenner, 1989), may influence the correlation between enzyme expression and enzyme activity. Moreover, in addition to relative enzyme expression and activity per unit of liver, absolute intrinsic metabolic clearance is also influenced by liver size.

Absolute liver weight increases 10-fold during childhood, from ~130 g in neonates to 1300 g in 15-year olds (Valentin, 2001). Relative liver weight peaks in infants (<12 months

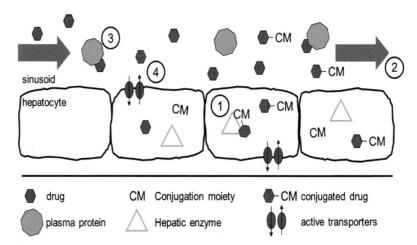

FIGURE 8.1 Schematic representation of the determinants of hepatic metabolic clearance. (1) Intrinsic clearance, (2) hepatic blood flow and perfusion, (3) plasma protein binding, and (4) active transport processes of the hepatocytes. *Adapted from Krekels, E.H.J., Danhof, M., Tibboel, D., Knibbe, C.A.J., 2012a. Ontogeny of hepatic glucuronidation; methods and results. Curr. Drug Metab. 13 (6), 728e743.*

old) at 4% of the total bodyweight and then decreases to 2−2.7% of the total bodyweight in adults (Noda et al., 1997). Exact measures of the amount of drug-metabolizing enzymes per unit of human liver are difficult to obtain experimentally, and few data are available in children. Nonetheless, available data suggest that maturation accounts for only 10% of the interindividual variability in reported enzyme amounts per gram of liver (Barter et al., 2008). However, the change in relative abundance of specific isoenzymes as a function of age can have a significant impact on the intrinsic clearance of isoenzyme-specific substrates. Stated simply, doubling the expression of an isoenzyme present at relatively low amounts may cause dramatic changes in intrinsic metabolic clearance for substrates of that isoenzyme, without significantly impacting the total amount of enzyme per gram of liver.

Liver volume is a critical factor for liver transplantation and, consequently, much data describing developmental changes in liver volume during childhood are available. As with liver weight, liver volume corresponds with enzymatic capacity, and therefore, total hepatic metabolic intrinsic clearance. Various equations defining liver volume as a function of age, bodyweight, height, or body surface area (BSA) have been proposed. The largest meta-analysis of data obtained in children and adults of different races, revealed BSA (in m^2) to be the most predictive covariate for describing liver volume (LV; in liters) during childhood, according to Eq. (8.1) (Johnson et al., 2005):

$$LV = 0.722 \cdot BSA^{1.176} \qquad (8.1)$$

The extent to which plasma protein binding and liver blood flow and perfusion influence intrinsic clearance depends on the drug extraction ratio. For drugs with a low hepatic extraction ratio, only the unbound fraction of the drug is metabolized. Therefore, plasma protein binding is the rate-limiting factor for the hepatic metabolic clearance of these drugs. On the other hand, the metabolic clearance of drugs with a high extraction ratio is not limited to the unbound fraction, causing blood flow and perfusion to become the more important determinant of hepatic metabolic clearance. Additionally, active influx or efflux of drug via transport mechanisms within hepatocellular membranes can significantly affect the intracellular concentration of drugs. This alters plasma clearance by changing the concentration of drug available for metabolism.

The following is a review of the current knowledge concerning maturational changes in mechanisms of hepatic drug clearance. As drug clearance is multifactorial, and there is often high variability among these contributing factors, collecting in vivo data reflecting specific facets of hepatic maturation is challenging. It follows that defining the ontogeny of a specific process in the absence of other contributing factors may be more practical using in vitro methodology. For instance, measuring enzyme activity using an in vitro method can provide a more accurate and robust reflection of in vivo intrinsic clearance capacity for a specific isoenzyme. These in vitro studies typically determine enzyme activity by measuring substrate depletion or metabolite formation with a compound selective for a specific isoenzyme of interest, using isolated hepatocytes, liver homogenates, or microsomal preparations. Though one must keep in mind the limitations and context of each study type, the presented findings can be utilized to understand the clinical impact of ontogeny on therapeutic interventions in the child.

ONTOGENY OF INTRINSIC HEPATIC CLEARANCE

The next two sections discuss the ontogeny of xenobiotic-metabolizing enzymes in the cytochrome P450 (CYP) and uridine 5′-diphospho-glucuronosyltransferase (UGT) families. Changes in the expression and activity of CYP and UGT enzymes drive the developmental changes in intrinsic clearance for the vast majority of prescribed drugs that undergo metabolism. The ontogeny of drug-metabolizing enzymes is studied on different levels, from gene expression to phenotypic activity. Evidence of developmental changes can be measured based on mRNA transcription, enzyme expression, in vitro enzyme activity, or in vivo drug clearance. As with any experimental paradigm, the results on enzyme ontogeny need to be interpreted within the context of the methodological approach used to procure the data.

For example, in vivo studies assaying drug clearance from plasma will not exclusively determine say, the maturational trajectory of hepatic activity related to a certain isoenzyme but would rather reflect a composite of factors contributing to clearance. Therefore, the inherent complexity of drug metabolism can present unique challenges to isolating the enzyme's ontogeny from that of the other factors. Finally, improvements in the accuracy and precision of experimental techniques over time can make comparisons across studies difficult or inappropriate. Therefore, the reader is urged to consider the limitations of these studies when interpreting their results.

Ontogeny of Hepatic CYP Enzymes

The majority of drug metabolism involves the CYP superfamily of enzymes, which are responsible for the phase 1 oxidative metabolism for a plethora of lipophilic drugs (Alcorn and McNamara, 2002). These enzymes are categorized into several subfamilies based on genetic sequence homology, with subfamilies 1, 2, and 3 playing the most important role in drug metabolism (Nelson et al., 1996). As a family, CYP substrate specificity is broad. CYPs are responsible for the metabolism of both endogenous and exogenous compounds; however, individual CYP isoforms demonstrate distinct substrate specificities (Guengerich, 1994). Some of the prototypical substrates, inducers, and inhibitors of CYP isoenzymes are provided in Table 8.1.

Due to the wide variety of drugs metabolized by CYP enzymes, their ontogeny has generally been well studied. The maturation of CYP isoenzymes is a highly variable process, but adult levels of activity are largely achieved by the completion of the first year of life. Age is often the primary predictor for the development of enzyme activity at the population level, although there may be correlations with other factors including bodyweight, diet, and genetic polymorphisms. Even after accounting for these factors, interindividual variability in the expression and/or activity of CYP enzymes may still be high. The increase in relative expression of CYP enzyme as a function of age is described in Fig. 8.2, using a model-based approach built upon current experimental data (Abduljalil et al., 2014).

CYP1A

CYP1A2 is the major hepatic isoform of the human CYP1A subfamily (Shimada et al., 1994). Studies suggest negligible to no detectable CYP1A2 mRNA or protein expression/activity during gestation (Hakkola et al., 1994). Postnatally, CYP1A2 is the last major CYP enzyme to fully mature (Berthou et al., 1988; Sonnier and Cresteil, 1998). CYP1A2 expression is not detectable

TABLE 8.1 Overview of Substrates, Inhibitors, and Inducers of CYP Enzymes

CYP Isoform	Substrates	Inhibitors	Inducers	References
1A2	Caffeine Naproxen Theophylline Antidepressants Antipsychotics	Fluoroquinolones	Tobacco Omeprazole	Batty et al. (1995), Brosen et al. (1993), Fontana et al. (1999), Granfors et al. (2004), Kobayashi et al. (1998), Lake et al. (1998), Parsons and Neims (1978), and Rost et al. (1992)
2A6	Valproic Acid Nicotine (Cotinine) Anesthetics	Methoxsalen Tranylcypromine Tryptamine	Dexamethasone	Bagdas et al. (2014), Onica et al. (2007), and Zhang et al. (2001)
2B6	Efavirenz Nevirapine Antidepressants Anesthetics	Clopidigrel Ticlopidine	Rifampicin Anticonvulsants	Chang et al. (1997), Ducharme et al. (1997), and Nishiya et al. (2008)
2C8	Statins Chemotherapeutics Antidiabetics	Gemfibrozil Trimethoprim Thizaolidinediones	Rifampicin	Backman et al. (2002), Niemi et al. (2004), and Sahi et al. (2003)
2C9	Warfarin NSAIDs Sulfonylureas Angiotensin Blockers	Antifungals		Back et al. (1988), Blum et al. (1991), Hynninen et al. (2007), and Kaukonen et al. (1998)
2C19	Clopidogrel Antidepressants Antiepileptics Proton Pump Inhibitors	Ketoconazole Proton pump inhibitors		Andersson et al. (1990), Emoto et al. (2004), and Raucy et al. (2002)
2D6	Antidepressants Analgesics Antipsychotics Beta-blockers	Antidepressants		Brynne et al. (1999) and Kotlyar et al. (2005)
2E1	Anesthetics Chlorzoxazone Acetaminophen	Disulfiram Nicotine	Ethanol Nicotine	Kharasch et al. (1993) and Raucy et al. (1989)
3A	Chemotherapeutics Antiinfectives Benzodiazepines	HIV protease inhibitors Macrolide antibiotics Azole antifungals	Barbiturates Nevirapine Efavirenz	Engels et al. (2004), Hammond and Fry (1990), Hariparsad et al. (2004), Havlir et al. (1995), Kantola et al. (1998), Kehrer et al. (2002), Kivisto et al. (1997), von Bahr et al. (1998), von Moltke et al. (1998), and Wang et al. (1997)

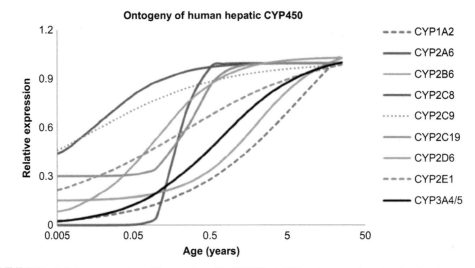

FIGURE 8.2   Relative expression of human hepatic CYP450 at different ages using simulated ontogeny profiles based on best-fit equations determined by Abduljalil et al. (2014).

until at least 1 month of age and reaches full maturity between 1 and 3 years of age (Ratanasavanh et al., 1991; Sonnier and Cresteil, 1998; Tanaka, 1998; Tateishi et al., 1997).

Both in vitro and in vivo findings agree that total demethylation of the CYP1A2 substrate caffeine increases exponentially with increasing postnatal age in the first 6 months of life (Carrier et al., 1988; Pons et al., 1988). Additionally, caffeine clearance was found to be linearly dependent on gestational age (Carrier et al., 1988). A population pharmacokinetic study of theophylline in neonates reported increased bodyweight-corrected theophylline clearance was associated with increased postnatal age, per CYP1A2 maturation (Kim et al., 2013). This is in agreement with an earlier study that found hepatic clearance of theophylline to increase with increasing age (Björkman, 2005).

Several other factors may also affect CYP1A2 enzyme expression and activity. CYP1A2, for instance, develops at a higher rate in infants fed with formula compared with those who are breast-fed (Blake et al., 2006). Additionally, there are clinically relevant CYP1A2 polymorphisms known to alter activity in adults, which may also have consequence for children who carry these variants. Specifically, the CYP1A2*1F allele is associated with reduced enzyme activity (Laika et al., 2009), whereas the CYP1A2*1D allele is associated with increased activity (Uslu et al., 2010).

CYP2A

CYP2A enzymes comprise a small portion of total hepatic CYP expression in adults, with CYP2A6 representing the primary isoform. CYP2A6 activity has yet to be demonstrated in fetal liver tissue (Hakkola et al., 1994; Maenpaa et al., 1993), and little is known about the development of this enzyme immediately following birth, but immunochemical assays suggest that enzyme expression reaches adult values within the first year of life (Tateishi et al., 1997).

CYP2A6 polymorphisms, rather than age, are thought to play the most important role in determining individual clearance of cotinine (the primary metabolite of nicotine), as children with reduced function alleles had longer cotinine half-lives than those with wild-type CYP2A6 (Dempsey et al., 2013; Zhu et al., 2013). Although the half-life of the CYP2A6 substrate nicotine was found to be three- to fourfold longer in newborns when compared with adults, this study did not find a corresponding difference between neonates and adults in the elimination half-life of cotinine, which is also metabolized by CYP2A6 (Dempsey et al., 2000).

CYP2B

CYP2B6 is the predominant isoform for hepatic drug metabolism in the CYP2B family, yet even when fully matured CYP2B6 is expressed at very low levels relative to other CYP enzymes (Shimada et al., 1994). In fetal livers, CYP2B6 mRNA or protein has not been detected (Hakkola et al., 1994; Maenpaa et al., 1993). Little is known about the ontogeny of this enzyme after birth; however, greater expression of 2B6 in infants older than 1 year compared with those younger than 1 year of age, suggests that complete maturation takes at least 1 year (Tateishi et al., 1997).

Clinical pediatric studies of the CYP2B6 substrate efavirenz demonstrate that clearance of this drug increases with age and/or bodyweight after birth, reaching 90% of adult clearance at 9 months of age (Salem et al., 2014). Additionally, the *CYP2B6-G516T* polymorphism was found to alter the clearance of efavirenz (Kwara et al., 2008; Viljoen et al., 2011). The *G/G* genotype was associated with a higher rate of clearance for efavirenz in children younger than 5 years compared with older children, but this was not the case for children with the *G/T* or *T/T* genotype (Saitoh et al., 2007). These data suggest that polymorphic variants influence patterns of CYP maturation.

CYP2C

CYP2C enzymes comprise approximately 20% of the CYP450 content in the human adult liver (Shimada et al., 1994) and metabolize a diverse set of substrates with little overlap between CYP2C isoforms. CYP2C8, CYP2C9, and CYP2C19 are the principal isoforms expressed (Goldstein and de Morais, 1994; Shimada et al., 1994). Low levels of CYP2C mRNA and protein have been observed in fetal livers (Hakkola et al., 1994; Maenpaa et al., 1993; Ratanasavanh et al., 1991; Treluyer et al., 1998). However, studies using fetal and neonatal hepatic microsomal preparations did not detect CYP2C activity (Cresteil et al., 1985; Pasanen et al., 1987).

CYP2C mRNA levels increase rapidly after birth, reaching adult values within the first month of life, largely due to the synthesis of CYP2C9 mRNA (Ratanasavanh et al., 1991; Treluyer et al., 1996; Treluyer et al., 1998). Similarly, postnatal protein expression increases rapidly, reaching one-third of typical adult CYP2C levels by the first month, without further large increases until ~9 months to 1 year of age (Treluyer et al., 1996, 1998). The trends in mRNA and protein expression are supported by CYP2C activity assessments. CYP2C activity is limited in newborns <8 days old, but then increases to ~50% of adult activity levels within the first month of life, and reaches adult levels at ~1 year of age (Treluyer et al., 1996).

Combined, these data suggest that the in vivo activity of this enzyme subfamily matures quickly and may reach peak activity levels in children greater than those observed in adults. Clinical data with CYP2C8 substrates are limited, as few CYP2C8-metabolized drugs are prescribed in pediatric patients. However, among adults and children from ages 0.8—23 years, the half-life of the chemotherapeutic, paclitaxel, was found to be similar, supporting a relatively rapid postnatal expression profile for CYP2C8 (Gelderblom et al., 2003; Horton et al., 2007).

CYP2C9 is the most abundant CYP2C isoform. Pharmacokinetic studies of the CYP2C9 substrate, valproic acid demonstrated that weight-normalized clearance was slower in neonates when compared with children and young adults (Gal et al., 1988). More specifically, weight-normalized valproic acid clearance increases after birth, peaking at values greater than those observed in adults during early childhood, prior to decreasing to adult values that are attained at around 10 years of age (Ogungbenro and Aarons, 2014). Other studies found this effect on valproic acid metabolism to be strongly correlated with bodyweight rather than age (Correa et al., 2008; Jankovic et al., 2010). However, this finding is not consistent across all studies. For instance, among children between 1 and 16 years of age, both factors were found to be significantly associated with valproic acid clearance (Juarez-Olguin et al., 2011). Treatment success with a well-known CYP2C9 substrate, warfarin, is improved when the presence of CYP2C9 activity reducing polymorphisms are accounted for, including *CYP2C9*2* and *3 in Caucasians, and *5, *6, *8, and *11 in African-Americans. However, the ontogeny of these CYP2C9 polymorphic variants is not well understood.

A review of proton pump inhibitor use, all CYP2C19 substrates, in young children provides evidence of a general trend toward decreasing drug half-lives in these children as they age through the first 6−12 months of life. Additionally, genetic variation in *CYP2C19* was found to contribute to differences in pantoprazole elimination, with the *2 allele reducing elimination, while the *17 allele appeared to increase drug clearance (Ward and Kearns, 2013).

CYP2D

Though CYP2D6 constitutes only 2% of the total hepatic CYP450 expression, it is responsible for the metabolism of many currently used therapeutics (Shimada et al., 1994). CYP2D6 mRNA has been observed in the fetal liver as early as 12 weeks of gestation; however, detectable levels of fetal protein or enzyme activity have not been observed (Hakkola et al., 1994; Ladona et al., 1991; Shimada et al., 1996; Treluyer et al., 1991). Postnatally, CYP2D6 expression and activity increase, with mRNA expression increasing to values two- to three-fold higher than that of adults within the first month (Treluyer et al., 1991). No differences in enzyme expression were observed between infants older or younger than 1 year of age, suggesting that maturation of CYP2D6 expression is completed within the first year of life (Tateishi et al., 1997).

The urinary recovery ratio of dextromethorphan to its CYP2D6 metabolite, dextrophan, did not change with postnatal age between 0.5 and 12 months (Blake et al., 2007), suggesting rapid maturation of this enzyme, as described in vitro. However, CYP2D6 genotype is significantly associated with differences in dextromethorphan metabolism (Blake et al., 2007) and this, rather than maturation, may best explain variation in CYP2D6 mediated metabolism in children.

CYP2E

CYP2E1 is the predominant enzyme in the CYP2E family and comprises ∼7% of total CYP abundance in adults (Shimada et al., 1994). Several studies have demonstrated that fetal CYP2E1 mRNA and protein levels are below limits of detection (Hakkola et al., 1994; Jones et al., 1992; Komori et al., 1989; Shimada et al., 1996; Vieira et al., 1996), although low prenatal levels of CYP2E1 mRNA and activity have been reported (Carpenter et al., 1996). Postnatal expression and activity of CYP2E1 increase rapidly within the first days of life, independent of gestational age and fully mature to adult levels within the first year (Vieira et al., 1996). Minimal pharmacokinetic data on CYP2E1-specific substrates are available in the pediatric population, as many drugs with CYP2E1-mediated metabolism are also metabolized by other enzymes. One study suggests that the CYP2E1-specific metabolism of acetaminophen is significantly associated with both postnatal age and weight in neonates <1 month old (Cook et al., 2016).

CYP3A

CYP3A is the most abundant CYP subfamily. It represents nearly 30% of the total liver CYP abundance in adults and is responsible for the metabolism of ~50% of currently marketed therapeutics (Shimada et al., 1994). Primary members of this subfamily are CYP3A4, CYP3A5, and CYP3A7.

CYP3A4 mRNA expression is below detectable limits in embryonic liver tissue at 6−12 weeks of gestation (Schuetz et al., 1994), but low mRNA levels of about 10% of adult levels have been found in fetal liver tissue at <30 weeks gestational age (Lacroix et al., 1997). CYP3A4 mRNA increases rapidly after birth, and reaches 50% of adult levels within 6−12 months of age (de Wildt et al., 2000), with some studies suggesting that the increase to this level occurs within the first postnatal week (Lacroix et al., 1997). After birth, enzyme activity reaches 30−40% of adult levels within the first 3 months and adult levels are achieved after 1 year (Ratanasavanh et al., 1991; Stevens et al., 2003). Moreover, in vitro production of CYP3A4/5 metabolites of amprenavir was decreased in neonatal microsomes, when compared with microsomes derived from infants or adults (Treluyer et al., 2003).

CYP3A5 mRNA has been detected in embryonic liver (Schuetz et al., 1994), while protein was detected only in ~10% of fetal livers (Hakkola et al., 2001; Wrighton et al., 1990). Hepatic protein expression of CYP3A5 was detected in approximately half of children and adolescents younger than 19 years, whereas CYP3A5 protein was found in a quarter of adult liver tissue (Wrighton et al., 1990), demonstrating CYP3A5 protein expression, and thus, activity to be highly variable at all stages of life.

At birth, when CYP3A4 expression is low, CYP3A7 represents about 30% of fetal liver CYP enzymes (Kitada and Kamataki, 1994; Shimada et al., 1996). Postnatal factors, however, cause a rapid reduction in CYP3A7 expression and activity, accompanied by a corresponding rise in CYP3A4 expression and activity. Indeed, CYP3A7 expression peaks 1 week after birth, before rapidly decreasing through the first year of life (Lacroix et al., 1997; Tateishi et al., 1997). Although CYP3A7 mRNA is present in most adult livers, these levels are more than 10 times lower than those observed in fetal livers (Lacroix et al., 1997).

Due to the many drugs that are metabolized by CYP3A isoforms, CYP3A substrate pharmacokinetics have been relatively well characterized in neonates and young children. The clearance of midazolam, a prominent CYP3A4/5 probe substrate, is typically lower in neonates compared with children (Burtin et al., 1994; de Wildt et al., 2002; Lee et al., 1999) but demonstrates wide interindividual variability (Altamimi et al., 2014). One summary analysis described a sigmoidal increase in allometrically weight-normalized midazolam clearance as a function of postmenstrual age, plateauing after ~2 years (Anderson and Larsson, 2010). The clearance of cisapride was also found to increase with postconceptional age in neonates (Kearns et al., 2003). As another example, age and CYP3A5 polymorphic status (*CYP3A5*3*) were factors associated with a need to reduce tacrolimus dosage among pediatric kidney transplant patients (de Wildt et al., 2011).

Ontogeny of Hepatic UGT Enzymes

UGTs are high-capacity, low-affinity enzymes that are responsible for glucuronidation in phase 2 metabolism. UGTs are mainly expressed in the cytosol of hepatocytes, although they have also been found to be expressed extra-hepatically in both adults and fetuses (Court et al., 2012; Cubitt et al., 2009; Nakamura et al., 2008; Ohno and Nakajin, 2009; Tukey and Strassburg, 2000). In addition to drugs and other xenobiotics, these enzymes also conjugate endogenous compounds like bilirubin and steroid hormones (Tukey and Strassburg, 2000).

In humans, there are 19 functional UGTs divided into three families, namely UGT1A, UGT2A, and UGT2B (Mackenzie et al., 2005). Similar to CYP enzymes, substrate specificities of the UGTs are broad, but in contrast, the specificities often overlap. The result is that one isoform may glucuronidate a wide range of compounds and that one compound may be metabolized by multiple UGT isoforms. As a result, few substrates exist which can be used to study a unique UGT isoenzyme. An overview of currently known UGT substrates is provided in Table 8.2.

Generally, UGT expression and activity is significantly reduced in early life, but the maturation patterns differ greatly between various UGT isoenzymes. The clinical impact of the reduced glucuronidation capacity in neonates first became apparent in the mid-20th century, when babies treated with chloramphenicol started to develop gray baby syndrome resulting from drug accumulation (Vest, 1958). Clinical investigations in neonates revealed a build-up of unglucuronidated chloramphenicol in the blood and a reduced recovery of the glucuronide metabolite in urine. Glucuronide recovery patterns for chloramphenicol reached adult values around the age of 3 months. For preterm born babies, the metabolite recovery was lower and the maturation slower (Vest, 1958).

In contrast to the extreme toxic consequences related to the inability to glucuronidate and eliminate chloramphenicol, many UGT substrates are not exclusively metabolized by UGT enzymes. For such drugs, a limited glucuronidation capacity in early life can be compensated for by metabolism or elimination via other pathways. This can manifest as a lower fraction of drug being glucuronidated in children compared with adults. Sulfotransferases are, for instance, known to be expressed at higher levels in neonatal liver when compared with adult (Richard et al., 2001), leading to increased sulfation of typical UGT substrates like acetaminophen in neonates (Alam et al., 1977; Levy et al., 1975; Miller et al., 1976). Additionally, unchanged renal excretion of parent compound may also increase to compensate for decreased glucuronidation capacity, although renal function itself is also still developing in neonates.

Prior to 20 weeks gestation, no mRNA transcripts of the UGT enzymes 1A1, 1A3, 1A4, 1A5, 1A6, 1A7, 1A8, 1A9, 1A10, 2B4, 2B7, 2B10, and 2B15 are detectable in fetal livers (Strassburg et al., 2002). However, in pooled liver samples of fetuses aged between 22 and 40 weeks, transcripts can be detected for UGT1A1, 1A4, 1A6, 1A9, 2A2, 2A3, 2B4, 2B7, 2B10, 2B11, 2B15, and 2B17 (Court et al., 2012). Most transcript levels in hepatic tissue samples at this developmental age are considerably lower than adult values, except for UGT2B4 for which

TABLE 8.2 Overview of Reported Substrate Specificities of Known UGT Substrates

UGT Isoform	General Substrate	Isoform-Specific Substrate	References
1A1	Acetaminophen 1-Naphthol Thyroxine 4-Methylumbelliferone Carvediol	Bilirubin SN-38 (irinotecan metabolite)	Bosma et al. (1994), Court et al. (2001), Iyer et al. (1998), Kato et al. (2008), Takekuma et al. (2006), and Uchaipichat et al. (2004)
1A3	1-Naphthol 4-Methylumbelliferone Thyroxine	R-lorazepam	Court (2005), Kato et al. (2008), and Uchaipichat et al. (2004)
1A4	Valproic acid	Trifluoperazine Lamotrigine Imipramine	Argikar and Remmel, (2009), Benedetti et al. (2005), Court (2005), and Miyagi and Collier (2007)
1A6	Acetaminophen 1-Naphthol Valproic acid 4-Methylumbelliferone Chloramphenicol	Serotonin	Chen et al. (2010), Court et al. (2001), Ethell et al. (2003), Krishnaswamy et al. (2003), and Uchaipichat et al. (2004)
1A7	1-Naphthol 4-Methylumbelliferone		Uchaipichat et al. (2004)
1A8	1-Naphthol 4-Methylumbelliferone Valproic acid		Argikar and Remmel (2009) and Uchaipichat et al. (2004)
1A9	Acetaminophen 4-Methylumbelliferone Valproic acid 1-Naphthol Indomethacin Propofol R-Oxazepam Chloramphenicol		Chen et al. (2010), Court (2005), Court et al. (2001, 2002), Ethell et al. (2003), Mano et al. (2007), and Uchaipichat et al. (2004)
1A10	1-Naphthol 4-Methylumbelliferone Valproic acid Estrone		Argikar and Remmel (2009), Kallionpää et al. (2015), and Uchaipichat et al. (2004)
2B4	Androsterone Carvediol		Takekuma et al. (2006) and Turgeon et al. (2001)
2B7	1-Naphthol 4-Methylumbelliferone Valproic acid Indomethacin Testosterone Androsterone Estradiol Lorazepam Carbamazepine	Morphine Zidovudine	Argikar and Remmel (2009), Barbier et al. (2000b), Chen et al. (2010), Chung et al. (2008), Coffman et al. (1997, 1998), Court et al. (2002, 2003), Innocenti et al. (2001), Kallionpää et al. (2015), Mano et al. (2007), Staines et al. (2004), Takekuma et al. (2006), Turgeon et al. (2001), and Uchaipichat et al. (2004)

(Continued)

TABLE 8.2   Overview of Reported Substrate Specificities of Known UGT Substrates—cont'd

UGT Isoform	General Substrate	Isoform-Specific Substrate	References
2B10	R-oxazepam Epirubicin Carvediol Chloramphenicol Estrone Amitriptyline Imipramine Clomipramine Trimipramine		Zhou et al. (2010)
2B11	4-Methylumbelliferone 1-Naphthol 4-Nitrophenol 4-Hydroxy-esterone 4-Hydroxybiphenylmethol Estriol 2-Aminophenol 2-Hydroxyesteriol		Ohno et al. (2004)
2B15	4-Methylumbelliferone Testosterone	S-oxazepam S-lorazepam	Chung et al. (2008), Court (2005), He et al. (2009), Turgeon et al. (2001), and Uchaipichat et al. (2004)
2B17	4-Methylumbelliferone Testosterone Dihydrotestosterone Androsterone		Turgeon et al. (2001) and Uchaipichat et al. (2004)
2B28	Eugenol 1-Naphthol 4-Methylumbelliferone Testosterone		Levesque et al. (1997)

expression levels are already more than half of the adult values (Court et al., 2012). By 6 months postnatal age, transcripts of UGT1A1, 1A3, 1A4, 1A6, 2B7, 2B10, and 2B15 are present at adult values, but transcript levels of UGT1A9 and 2B4 remain lower than in adults (Strassburg et al., 2002). Transcript levels reach adult values around the age of 1.5 years for UGT1A9, while UGT2B4 has a longer maturational profile that extends beyond 2 years of age to achieve adult mRNA levels (Strassburg et al., 2002).

For UGT1A1 and 1A6, good agreement exists across mRNA transcript, protein expression, and enzymatic activity levels, having all reached equivalency with adult values by the age of 6 months (Miyagi and Collier, 2011; Strassburg et al., 2002). In contrast, adult levels of protein expression for UGT1A9 have been reported to be achieved within the first half year of life, but assessment of UGT1A9 mRNA transcript seemed to indicate a longer maturational timeframe (Miyagi et al., 2012). UGT2B7 expression levels are reported to have reached adult values by the age of 7 months by some (Strassburg et al., 2002), while other reports suggest age-dependent increases reaching adult values by the age of 12–17 years (Zaya et al., 2006). Nonetheless, good correlation exists between enzyme expression and in vitro glucuronidation activity for UGT2B7 (Kwara et al., 2009; Zaya et al., 2006).

Using a model-based approach, the expression patterns of four UGT isoenzymes throughout childhood have been constructed based on current, yet limited, experimental data (Abduljalil et al., 2014). These profiles are presented in Fig. 8.3.

In vitro glucuronidation of 4-methylumbelliferone and trifluoperazine reaches adult values around the age of 1.5 years (Miyagi and Collier, 2007), while in vitro glucuronidation activity across a series of 18 endogenous and exogenous compounds, all substrates of UGT isoenzymes, demonstrated that by the age of 2 years activity toward these drugs had not reached adult values, with the glucuronidation of some compounds 40-fold lower than adults at that age (Strassburg et al., 2002). However, this does not seem to reflect general maturation patterns of in vivo glucuronidation clearance of a wide range of different UGT substrates well. These conflicting findings could result from protocols for activity studies with microsomes not being optimized to yield accurate results for UGT-mediated metabolism (Engtrakul et al., 2005).

In the 1980s, glucuronidation of bilirubin and 2-aminophenol in microsomes or liver homogenates revealed fetal and neonatal activity to be between 1% and 6% of adult values (Coughtrie et al., 1988; Leakey et al., 1987; Onishi et al., 1979), with adult values being reached 2–3 months postpartum in both term and preterm neonates (Coughtrie et al., 1988; Onishi et al., 1979). More detailed studies revealed bilirubin glucuronidation to be at 0.1% of adult activity in fetuses between 17 and 30 weeks of gestation, increasing slowly to 1% toward the end of gestation. Irrespective of whether birth is term or preterm, the event initiates rapid increases in bilirubin glucuronidation, reaching adult values after 14 weeks (Kawade and Onishi, 1981), a pattern that is similar for other UGT substrates (Burchell et al., 1989). The glucuronidation of testosterone, 1-naphthol (Coughtrie et al., 1988;

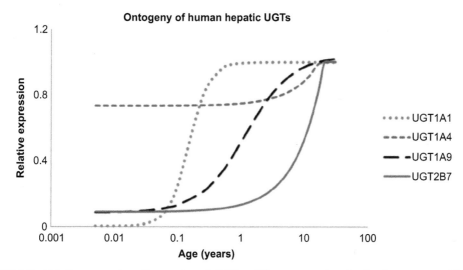

FIGURE 8.3   Relative expression of human hepatic UGT at different ages using simulated ontogeny profiles based on best-fit equations determined by Abduljalil et al. (2014).

Leakey et al., 1987), androsterone, estrone, 2-aminophenol, 4-nitrophenol (Leakey et al., 1987), acetaminophen (Rollins et al., 1979), and morphine (Pacifici et al., 1982) is also absent or low in fetuses and neonates, with glucuronidation capacity for the first two compounds reaching adult values around the age of 1 year (Coughtrie et al., 1988).

It was observed that overall weight-corrected acetaminophen and salicylamide clearance differed only slightly between early life and adulthood. However, it was the ratio of recovered glucuronide and sulfate metabolite to parent compound in urine that changed with age. For instance, in neonates, sulfated metabolites predominate, whereas among children 12 years and older, the recovered ratios were similar to adults, and favored the glucuronide metabolites (Alam et al., 1977; Levy et al., 1975; Miller et al., 1976). When looking at the glucuronidation pathway of acetaminophen in particular, absolute glucuronidation clearance increases linearly with bodyweight in term and preterm neonates and infants (Krekels et al., 2015).

Morphine and zidovudine are both mainly metabolized by UGT2B7 (Barbier et al., 2000b; Coffman et al., 1997; Court et al., 2003) and as they are prescribed regularly in the pediatric population, the maturation of their clearance has been studied extensively. The UGT2B7-mediated glucuronidation is significantly reduced at birth, but still detectable even in preterm neonates as young as 24 weeks (Barrett et al., 1996; Choonara et al., 1990; Hartley et al., 1994). Clearance of both drugs increases rapidly in the first 2 weeks after birth (Boucher et al., 1993; Knibbe et al., 2009; Krekels et al., 2012c; Mirochnick et al., 1999) followed by a prolonged slower increase (Bouwmeester et al., 2003; Capparelli et al., 2003; Choonara et al., 1989; McRorie et al., 1992). Despite decreased glucuronidation capacity, sulfation and unchanged renal excretion of morphine is relatively low even in the very young (Barrett et al., 1996; Choonara et al., 1990), suggesting that maturational increases in morphine clearance can be mostly attributed to increases in the glucuronidation capacity. Different studies identified different age or bodyweight-based descriptions for the maturation patterns of morphine and zidovudine clearance, but generally glucuronidation is thought to increase with gestational or postnatal age and/or bodyweight (Boucher et al., 1993; Bouwmeester et al., 2003; Choonara et al., 1989, 1992; Hartley et al., 1994; Lynn et al., 2000; McRorie et al., 1992; Saarenmaa et al., 2000). When age-based descriptors of the maturation patterns are used, maturation is found to be slower in preterm neonates compared with term neonates (Mirochnick et al., 1999). Expressed per kilogram bodyweight or scaled allometrically, adult clearance values are reached in the first months of life (Anand et al., 2008; Bouwmeester et al., 2004; McRorie et al., 1992; Mirochnick et al., 1999), but as children are still gaining weight, absolute clearance values increase over a much longer time.

ONTOGENY OF HEPATIC BLOOD FLOW

In adults, typical hepatic blood flow is 1.35 L/min in females and 1.5 L/min in males, but how these values change in children under normal physiological conditions is unknown and, especially in the very young, difficult to measure directly.

Propofol and other high extraction ratio drugs are sometimes used as an in vivo probe to investigate hepatic blood flow. Indeed, after completion of enzyme maturation, changes in clearance for high extraction ratio drugs can be assumed to mainly reflect changes in hepatic blood flow. Caution is therefore warranted when deriving maturation patterns in hepatic blood flow from drug plasma clearances before enzyme maturation is completed, because the extraction ratio may be reduced as well.

Maturation of the enzymes involved in propofol metabolism appears to be completed around the age of 2 years (Peeters et al., 2010), suggesting that propofol clearance reflects hepatic blood flow above that age. In this higher age-range linear or allometric increases with bodyweight have been reported for propofol clearance (Kataria et al., 1994; Peeters et al., 2010), while other work describes complex multidirectional changes in the clearance of propofol over the entire human age range (Wang et al., 2010). In neonates, propofol clearance was found to be low and increase with age (Allegaert et al., 2007, 2008), but it is unknown how well these findings reflect hepatic blood flow as glucuronidation capacity is likely rate limiting in this population.

For calculations that require hepatic blood flow values to derive in vivo clearance from in vitro data in young children, generally one of the following assumptions is made: (1) hepatic blood flow per gram of liver is the same in children and adults (Edginton et al., 2006a), (2) the percentage of cardiac output directed to the liver remains constant with age (Edginton et al., 2006a,b), and (3) hepatic blood flow is proportional to metabolic rate/BSA (Björkman, 2005).

ONTOGENY OF PLASMA PROTEIN BINDING

Plasma protein binding is generally reduced in children compared with adults, leading to increased proportions of unbound drug. This in turn influences hepatic clearance, particularly of drugs with low-to-intermediate extraction ratios. The increase in unbound drug fractions in children can be mainly attributed to lower concentrations of serum albumin and alpha-1-glycoprotein (AGP). Neonates and young infants have albumin and AGP levels that are 20% and 60% lower than adults, respectively; although AGP levels vary considerably under various pathophysiological conditions. The constitutive concentrations of both plasma proteins increase linearly with age until adulthood (McNamara and Alcorn, 2002).

In addition to differences in plasma protein abundance, distinct differences in binding affinity of drugs for plasma proteins have been demonstrated between adults and neonates (Windorfer et al., 1974). These differences generally reduce plasma protein binding further in early life. Moreover, drugs bound to neonatal serum proteins appear to be more vulnerable to displacement by endogenous compounds like bilirubin and free fatty acids, both of which are present in higher concentrations in neonates compared with adults (Fredholm et al., 1975; Windorfer et al., 1974).

Nevertheless, the clinical importance of increased free drug will be minimal for drugs that are typically <90% bound (Fredholm et al., 1975). For example, morphine and zidovudine are bound for only 38% and 23%, respectively, in adults (Luzier and Morse, 1993; Olsen, 1975; Quevedo et al., 2008), and the impact of age-related changes in unbound drug fractions on the hepatic metabolic clearance of both drugs has been shown to be marginal in the first three years of life (Krekels et al., 2012b). In contrast, a clinically relevant increase in clearance is observed for micafungin in neonates. Micafungin is very highly protein bound (>99%), and the increased hepatocyte uptake and subsequent biliary elimination among neonates may be due to an elevated free fraction of this drug (Yanni et al., 2011).

ONTOGENY OF HEPATIC DRUG TRANSPORTERS

Transporters facilitate the movement of drug from blood into the hepatocyte, as well as the removal of drug from the hepatocyte into the bile. Human hepatocytes express a variety of transporters from the ATP-binding cassette (ABC) and solute carrier (SLC) superfamilies. The arrangement of transporters at the membranes of hepatocytes allow vectorial transport of drugs into the hepatocyte and/or into the bile canaliculus for elimination. The organic anion transporting polypeptide (OATP) and organic cation transporter (OCT) families, both SLCs, are largely involved with flux of drugs across the basolateral membrane from blood into hepatocyte. Members of the ABC family (efflux only) such as the multidrug resistance—associated protein 2 (MRP2), breast cancer resistance protein (BCRP), and P-glycoprotein (P-gp) expressed on the canalicular/apical membrane of the hepatocytes are the major transporters responsible for biliary excretion of drugs or drug metabolites (Ho and Kim, 2005). Although there is considerable evidence on the influence of drug transporters on hepatic clearance in adults, these data are limited in pediatric populations. As such, information on the ontogeny of these transporters is limited. Furthermore, in vitro studies are hampered by the lack of transporter-specific probes, and the difficulty in relating mRNA transcripts to transporter activity (Brouwer et al., 2015).

Available data on the ontogeny of a few hepatic transporters, including BCRP (Prasad et al., 2013; Yanni et al., 2011), MRP3 (Yanni et al., 2011), and P-gp (Prasad et al., 2014; Tang et al., 2007), suggest that expression levels remain constant from childhood to adulthood. For instance, the expression of MRP2 does not show age-dependent differences after the age of 7 years (Deo et al., 2012). However before that age, a bi-phasic age-related change in expression was observed, with a peak around 1 year of age (Tang et al., 2007). Reports on OATP1B1 and OATP1B3 ontogeny have conflicting results. For both OATP1B1 and OATP1B3, expression has been reported to be low in the first years of life, and to increase age dependently after the age of 6 years (Thomson et al., 2014). However, others have reported the expression of both proteins to be at adult values in neonates, without age-related changes in expression levels in later childhood (Prasad et al., 2014; Yanni et al., 2011).

A number of drugs that have been used to treat children are known to be actively transported into or out of the liver. These include tacrolimus (P-gp), morphine (OCT1, OATP1B1, P-gp, MRP2, and MRP3), pravastatin (OATP1B1, OATP2B1, OATP1B3, P-gp, and MRP2), atorvastatin (OATP1B1), bosentan (OATP1B1, OATP1B3 and possibly OATP2B1), ondansetron (OCT1), metformin (OCT1), cimetidine (OCT2), and tramadol (OCT1). However, the extent to which maturation of the transporters influences overall hepatic metabolic clearance of these drugs is unknown.

CONCLUSION

Many factors contribute to the extent to which drugs are metabolized by the liver, with the primary determinants being enzyme expression and activity. Additionally, hepatic blood flow and perfusion, plasma protein binding, and hepatic drug transporters also influence hepatic drug metabolism. In young children, these processes are dynamic and highly variable between individuals in the first few months to years of life.

For the development of drug dosing regimens, understanding the net effect of developmental changes on total plasma clearance is critical. Although the data discussed in this chapter can be used to understand general trends in the ontogeny of hepatic clearance, a careful assessment of total drug clearance is needed to understand the clinical impact of these developmental changes for a specific drug. A detailed understanding of maturational changes in all determinants of drug clearance and their influence on total clearance are required to best derive empirical dosing regimens for drugs that have not previously been used in children. As knowledge of maturational processes and drug metabolism is far from complete, new approaches are needed to better characterize the maturation of specific isoenzymes and other determinants of hepatic metabolism.

References

Abduljalil, K., Jamei, M., Rostami-Hodjegan, A., Johnson, T.N., May 2014. Changes in individual drug-independent system parameters during virtual paediatric pharmacokinetic trials: introducing time-varying physiology into a paediatric PBPK model. AAPS J. 16 (3), 568–576.

Alam, S.N., Roberts, R.J., Fischer, L.J., 1977. Age-related differences in salicylamide and acetaminophen conjugation in man. J. Pediatr. 90, 130–135.

Alcorn, J., McNamara, P.J., 2002. Ontogeny of hepatic and renal systemic clearance pathways in infants: part I. Clin. Pharmacokinet. 41, 959–998.

Allegaert, K., Peeters, M.Y., Verbesselt, R., Tibboel, D., Naulaers, G., de Hoon, J.N., Knibbe, C.A., 2007. Inter-individual variability in propofol pharmacokinetics in preterm and term neonates. Br. J. Anaesth. 99, 864–870.

Allegaert, K., Vancraeynest, J., Rayyan, M., de Hoon, J., Cossey, V., Naulaers, G., Verbesselt, R., 2008. Urinary propofol metabolites in early life after single intravenous bolus. Br. J. Anaesth. 101, 827–831.

Altamimi, M.I., Sammons, H., Choonara, I., 2014. Inter-individual variation in midazolam clearance in children. Arch. Dis. Childhood 100, 95–100.

Anand, K.J., Anderson, B.J., Holford, N.H., Hall, R.W., Young, T., Shephard, B., et al., 2008. Morphine pharmacokinetics and pharmacodynamics in preterm and term neonates: secondary results from the NEOPAIN trial. Br. J. Anaesth. 101, 680–689.

Anderson, B.J., Larsson, P., 2010. A maturation model for midazolam clearance. Paediatr. Anaesth. 21 (3), 302–308.

Andersson, T., Cederberg, C., Edvardsson, G., Heggelund, A., Lundborg, P., 1990. Effect of omeprazole treatment on diazepam plasma levels in slow versus normal rapid metabolizers of omeprazole. Clin. Pharmacol. Ther. 47 (1), 79–85.

Argikar, U.A., Remmel, R.P., 2009. Effect of aging on glucuronidation of valproic acid in human liver microsomes and the role of UDP-glucuronosyltransferase UGT1A4, UGT1A8, and UGT1A10. Drug Metab. Dispos. 37, 229–236.

Back, D.J., Tjia, J.F., Karbwang, J., Colbert, J., 1988. In vitro inhibition studies of tolbutamide hydroxylase activity of human liver microsomes by azoles, sulphonamides and quinolines. Br. J. Clin. Pharmacol. 26 (1), 23–29.

Backman, J.T., Kyrklund, C., Neuvonen, M., Neuvonen, P.J., 2002. Gemfibrozil greatly increases plasma concentrations of cerivastatin. Clin. Pharmacol. Ther. 72 (6), 685–691.

Bagdas, D., Muldoon, P.P., Zhu, A.Z., Tyndale, R.F., Damaj, M.I., 2014. Effects of methoxsalen, a CYP2A5/6 inhibitor, on nicotine dependence behaviors in mice. Neuropharmacology 85, 67–72.

Barbier, O., Girard, C., Breton, R., Belanger, A., Hum, D.W., 2000a. N-glycosylation and residue 96 are involved in the functional properties of UDP-glucuronosyltransferase enzymes. Biochemistry 39, 11540–11552.

Barbier, O., Turgeon, D., Girard, C., Green, M.D., Tephly, T.R., Hum, D.W., Belanger, A., 2000b. 3′-azido-3′-deoxy-thimidine (AZT) is glucuronidated by human UDP-glucuronosyltransferase 2B7 (UGT2B7). Drug Metab. Dispos. 28, 497–502.

Barrett, D.A., Barker, D.P., Rutter, N., Pawula, M., Shaw, P.N., 1996. Morphine, morphine-6-glucuronide and morphine-3-glucuronide pharmacokinetics in newborn infants receiving diamorphine infusions. Br. J. Clin. Pharmacol. 41, 531–537.

Barter, Z.E., Chowdry, J.E., Harlow, J.R., Snawder, J.E., Lipscomb, J.C., Rostami-Hodjegan, A., 2008. Covariation of human microsomal protein per gram of liver with age: absence of influence of operator and sample storage may justify interlaboratory data pooling. Drug Metab. Dispos. 36, 2405–2409.

Basu, N.K., Kole, L., Owens, I.S., 2003. Evidence for phosphorylation requirement for human bilirubin UDP-glucuronosyltransferase (UGT1A1) activity. Biochem. Biophys. Res. Commun. 303, 98–104.

Batty, K.T., Davis, T.M., Ilett, K.F., Dusci, L.J., Langton, S.R., 1995. The effect of ciprofloxacin on theophylline pharmacokinetics in healthy subjects. Br. J. Clin. Pharmacol. 39, 305–311.

Benedetti, M.S., Whomsley, R., Baltes, E., Tonner, F., 2005. Alteration of thyroid hormone homeostasis by antiepileptic drugs in humans: involvement of glucuronosyltransferase induction. Eur. J. Clin. Pharmacol. 61, 863–872.

Berthou, F., Ratanasavanh, D., Alix, D., Carlhant, D., Riche, C., Guillouzo, A., 1988. Caffeine and theophylline metabolism in newborn and adult human hepatocytes; comparison with adult rat hepatocytes. Biochem. Pharmacol. 37, 3691–3700.

Björkman, S., 2005. Prediction of drug disposition in infants and children by means of physiologically based pharmacokinetic (PBPK) modelling: theophylline and midazolam as model drugs. Br. J. Clin. Pharmacol. 59 (6), 691–704.

Blake, M.J., Abdel-Rahman, S.M., Pearce, R.E., Leeder, J.S., Kearns, G.L., 2006. Effect of diet on the development of drug metabolism by cytochrome P-450 enzymes in healthy infants. Pediatr. Res. 60, 717–723.

Blake, M.J., Gaedigk, A., Pearce, R.E., Bomgaars, L.R., Christensen, M.L., Stowe, C., et al., 2007. Ontogeny of dextromethorphan O- and N-demethylation in the first year of life. Clin. Pharmacol. Ther. 81, 510–516.

Blum, R.A., Wilton, J.H., Hilligoss, D.M., Gardner, M.J., Henry, E.B., Harrison, N.J., Schentag, J.J., 1991. Effect of fluconazole on the disposition of phenytoin. Clin. Pharmacol. Ther. 49 (4), 420–425.

Bosma, P.J., Seppen, J., Goldhoorn, B., Bakker, C., Oude Elferink, R.P., Chowdhury, J.R., et al., 1994. Bilirubin UDP-glucuronosyltransferase 1 is the only relevant bilirubin glucuronidating isoform in man. J. Biol. Chem. 269, 17960–17964.

Boucher, F.D., Modlin, J.F., Weller, S., Ruff, A., Mirochnick, M., Pelton, S., et al., 1993. Phase I evaluation of zidovudine administered to infants exposed at birth to the human immunodeficiency virus. J. Pediatr. 122, 137–144.

Bouwmeester, N.J., van den Anker, J.N., Hop, W.C., Anand, K.J., Tibboel, D., 2003. Age- and therapy-related effects on morphine requirements and plasma concentrations of morphine and its metabolites in postoperative infants. Br. J. Anaesth. 90, 642–652.

Bouwmeester, N.J., Anderson, B.J., Tibboel, D., Holford, N.H., 2004. Developmental pharmacokinetics of morphine and its metabolites in neonates, infants and young children. Br. J. Anaesth. 92, 208–217.

Brosen, K., Skjelbo, E., Rasmussen, B.B., Poulsen, H.E., Loft, S., 1993. Fluvoxamine is a potent inhibitor of cytochrome P4501A2. Biochem. Pharmacol. 45, 1211–1214.

Brouwer, K.L.R., Aleksunes, L.M., Brandys, B., Giacoia, G.P., Knipp, G., Lukacova, V., et al., 2015. Human ontogeny of drug transporters: review and recommendations of the pediatric transporter working group. Clin. Pharmacol. Ther.

Brynne, N., Svanstrom, C., Aberg-Wistedt, A., Hallen, B., Bertilsson, L., 1999. Fluoxetine inhibits the metabolism of tolterodine-pharmacokinetic implications and proposed clinical relevance. Br. J. Clin. Pharmacol. 48 (4), 553–563.

Burchell, B., Coughtrie, M., Jackson, M., Harding, D., Fournel-Gigleux, S., Leakey, J., Hume, R., 1989. Development of human liver UDP-glucuronosyltransferases. Dev. Pharmacol. Ther. 13 (2–4), 70–77.

Burtin, P., Jacqz-Aigrain, E., Girard, P., Lenclen, R., Magny, J.F., Betremieux, P., et al., 1994. Population pharmacokinetics of midazolam in neonates. Clin. Pharmacol. Ther. 56, 615–625.

Capparelli, E.V., Englund, J.A., Connor, J.D., Spector, S.A., McKinney, R.E., Palumbo, P., Baker, C.J., 2003. Population pharmacokinetics and pharmacodynamics of zidovudine in HIV-infected infants and children. J. Clin. Pharmacol. 43, 133–140.

Carpenter, S.P., Lasker, J.M., Raucy, J.L., 1996. Expression, induction, and catalytic activity of the ethanol-inducible cytochrome P450 (CYP2E1) in human fetal liver and hepatocytes. Mol. Pharmacol. 49, 260–268.

Carrier, O., Pons, G., Rey, E., Richard, M.O., Moran, C., Badoual, J., Olive, G., 1988. Maturation of caffeine metabolic pathways in infancy. Clin. Pharmacol. Ther. 44, 145–151.

Castuma, C.E., Brenner, R.R., 1989. The influence of fatty acid unsaturation and physical properties of microsomal membrane phospholipids on UDP-glucuronyltransferase activity. Biochem. J. 258, 723–731.

Chang, T.K., Yu, L., Maurel, P., Waxman, D.J., 1997. Enhanced cyclophosphamide and ifosfamide activation in primary human hepatocyte cultures: response to cytochrome P-450 inducers and autoinduction by oxazaphosphorines. Cancer Res. 57 (10), 1946–1954.

Chen, M., LeDuc, B., Kerr, S., Howe, D., Williams, D.A., 2010. Identification of human UGT2B7 as the major isoform involved in the O-glucuronidation of chloramphenicol. Drug Metab. Dispos. 38, 368–375.

Choonara, I.A., McKay, P., Hain, R., Rane, A., 1989. Morphine metabolism in children. Br. J. Clin. Pharmacol. 28, 599–604.

Choonara, I., Ekbom, Y., Lindstrom, B., Rane, A., 1990. Morphine sulphation in children. Br. J. Clin. Pharmacol. 30, 897–900.

Choonara, I., Lawrence, A., Michalkiewicz, A., Bowhay, A., Ratcliffe, J., 1992. Morphine metabolism in neonates and infants. Br. J. Clin. Pharmacol. 34, 434–437.

Chung, J.Y., Cho, J.Y., Yu, K.S., Kim, J.R., Lim, K.S., Sohn, D.R., et al., 2008. Pharmacokinetic and pharmacodynamic interaction of lorazepam and valproic acid in relation to UGT2B7 genetic polymorphism in healthy subjects. Clin. Pharmacol. Ther. 83, 595–600.

Coffman, B.L., Rios, G.R., King, C.D., Tephly, T.R., 1997. Human UGT2B7 catalyzes morphine glucuronidation. Drug Metab. Dispos. 25, 1–4.

Coffman, B.L., King, C.D., Rios, G.R., Tephly, T.R., 1998. The glucuronidation of opioids, other xenobiotics, and androgens by human UGT2B7Y(268) and UGT2B7H(268). Drug Metab. Dispos. 26, 73–77.

Cook, S.F., Stockmann, C., Samiee-Zafarghandy, S., King, A.D., Deutsch, N., Williams, E.F., Wilkins, D.G., Sherwin, C.M., van den Anker, J.N., May 21, 2016. Neonatal maturation of paracetamol (acetaminophen) glucuronidation, sulfation, and oxidation based on a parent-metabolite population pharmacokinetic model. Clin. Pharmacokinet.

Correa, T., Rodriguez, I., Romano, S., 2008. Population pharmacokinetics of valproate in Mexican children with epilepsy. Biopharm. Drug Dispos. 29, 511–520.

Coughtrie, M.W., Burchell, B., Leakey, J.E., Hume, R., 1988. The inadequacy of perinatal glucuronidation: immunoblot analysis of the developmental expression of individual UDP-glucuronosyltransferase isoenzymes in rat and human liver microsomes. Mol. Pharmacol. 34, 729–735.

Court, M., Duan, S.X., Von Moltke, L.L., Greenblatt, D.J., Patten, C.J., Miners, J.O., Mackenzie, P.I., 2001. Interindividual variability in acetaminophen glucuronidation by human liver microsomes: identification of relevant acetaminophen UDP-glucuronosyltransferase isoforms. J. Pharmacol. Exp. Ther. 299, 998–1006.

Court, M., Duan, S.X., Guillemette, C., Journault, K., Krishnaswamy, S., Von Moltke, L.L., Greenblatt, D.J., 2002. Stereoselective conjugation of oxazepam by human UDP-glucuronosyltransferases (UGTs): S-oxazepam is glucuronidated by UGT2B15, while R-oxazepam is glucuronidated by UGT2B7 and UGT1A9. Drug Metab. Dispos. 30, 1257–1265.

Court, M., Krishnaswamy, S., Hao, Q., Duan, S.X., Patten, C.J., Von Moltke, L.L., Greenblatt, D.J., 2003. Evaluation of 3′-azido-3′-deoxythymidine, morphine, and codeine as probe substrates for UDP-glucuronosyltransferase 2B7 (UGT2B7) in human liver microsomes: specificity and influence of the UGT2B7*2 polymorphism. Drug Metab. Dispos. 31, 1125–1133.

Court, M.H., Zhang, X., Ding, X., Yee, K.K., Hesse, L.M., Finel, M., 2012. Quantitative distribution of mRNAs encoding the 19 human UDP-glucuronosyltransferase enzymes in 26 adult and 3 fetal tissues. Xenobiotica; Fate Foreign Compounds Biol. Syst. 42 (3), 266–277.

Court, M., 2005. Isoform-selective probe substrates for in vitro studies of human UDP-glucuronosyltransferases. Methods Enzymol. 400, 104–116.

Cresteil, T., Beaune, P., Kremers, P., Celier, C., Guengerich, F.P., Leroux, J.P., 1985. Immunoquantification of epoxide hydrolase and cytochrome P-450 isozymes in fetal and adult human liver microsomes. Eur. J. Biochem. 151, 345–350.

Cubitt, H.E., Houston, J.B., Galetin, A., 2009. Relative importance of intestinal and hepatic glucuronidation-impact on the prediction of drug clearance. Pharm. Res. 26, 1073–1083.

De Wildt, S.N., Kearns, G.L., Leeder, J.S., van den Anker, J.N., 2000. Cytochrome P450 3A: ontogeny and drug disposition. Clin. Pharmacokinet. 37, 485–505.

De Wildt, S.N., Kearns, G.L., Hop, W.C., Murry, D.J., Abdel-Rahman, S.M., van den Anker, J.N., 2002. Pharmacokinetics and metabolism of oral midazolam in preterm infants. Br. J. Clin. Pharmacol. 53, 390–392.

De Wildt, S.N., van Schaik, R.H., Soldin, O.P., Soldin, S.J., Brojeni, P.Y., van der Heiden, I.P., et al., 2011. The interactions of age, genetics, and disease severity on tacrolimus dosing requirements after pediatric kidney and liver transplantation. Eur. J. Clin. Pharmacol. 67, 1231–1241.

Dempsey, D., Jacob III, P., Benowitz, N.L., 2000. Nicotine metabolism and elimination kinetics in newborns. Clin. Pharmacol. Ther. 67, 458–465.

Dempsey, D.A., Sambol, N.C., Jacob 3rd, P., Hoffmann, E., Tyndale, R.F., Fuentes-Afflick, E., Benowitz, N.L., 2013. CYP2A6 genotype but not age determines cotinine half-life in infants and children. Clin. Pharmacol. Ther. 94, 400–406.

Deo, A.K., Prasad, B., Balogh, L., Lai, Y., Unadkat, J.D., 2012. Interindividual variability in hepatic expression of the multidrug resistance-associated protein 2 (MRP2/ABCC2): quantification by liquid chromatography/tandem mass spectrometry. Drug Metab. Disposition: Biol. Fate Chemicals 40 (5), 852–855.

Ducharme, M.P., Bernstein, M.L., Granvil, C.P., Gehrcke, B., Wainer, I.W., 1997. Phenytoin-induced alteration in the N-dechloroethylation of ifosfamide stereoisomers. Cancer Chemother. Pharmacol. 40 (6), 531–533.

Edginton, A.N., Schmitt, W., Voith, B., Willmann, S., 2006a. A mechanistic approach for the scaling of clearance in children. Clin. Pharmacokinet. 45, 683–704.

Edginton, A.N., Schmitt, W., Willmann, S., 2006b. Development and evaluation of a generic physiologically based pharmacokinetic model for children. Clin. Pharmacokinet. 45, 1013–1034.

Emoto, C., Murase, S., Sawada, Y., Jones, B.C., Iwasaki, K., 2004. In vitro inhibitory effect of 1-aminobenzotriazole on drug oxidations catalyzed by human cytochrome P450 enzymes: a comparison with SKF-525A and ketoconazole. Drug Metab. Pharmacokinet. 18 (5), 287–295.

Engels, F.K., Ten Tije, A.J., Baker, S.D., Lee, C.K., Loos, W.J., Vulto, A.G., et al., 2004. Effect of cytochrome P450 3A4 inhibition on the pharmacokinetics of docetaxel. Clin. Pharmacol. Ther. 75 (5), 448–454.

Engtrakul, J.J., Foti, R.S., Strelevitz, T.J., Fisher, M.B., 2005. Altered AZT (3′-azido-3′-deoxythymidine) glucuronidation kinetics in liver microsomes as an explanation for underprediction of in vivo clearance: comparison to hepatocytes and effect of incubation environment. Drug Metab. Dispos. 33, 1621–1627.

Ethell, B.T., Anderson, G.D., Burchell, B., 2003. The effect of valproic acid on drug and steroid glucuronidation by expressed human UDP-glucuronosyltransferases. Biochem. Pharmacol. 65, 1441–1449.

Fontana, R.J., Lown, K.S., Paine, M.F., Fortlage, L., Santella, R.M., Felton, J.S., et al., 1999. Effects of a chargrilled meat diet on expression of CYP3A, CYP1A, and P-glycoprotein levels in healthy volunteers. Gastroenterology 117, 89–98.

Fredholm, B., Rane, A., Persson, B., 1975. Diphenylhydantoin binding to proteins in plasma and its dependence on free fatty acid and bilirubin concentration in dogs and newborn infants. Pediat. Res. 9, 26–30.

Gal, P., Oles, K.S., Gilman, J.T., Weaver, R., 1988. Valproic acid efficacy, toxicity, and pharmacokinetics in neonates with intractable seizures. Neurology 38, 467–471.

Gelderblom, H., Baker, S.D., Zhao, M., Verweij, J., Sparreboom, A., 2003. Distribution of paclitaxel in plasma and cerebrospinal fluid. Anticancer Drugs 14, 365–368.

Goldstein, J.A., de Morais, S.M., 1994. Biochemistry and molecular biology of the human CYP2C subfamily. Pharmacogenetics 4, 285–299.

Granfors, M.T., Backman, J.T., Neuvonen, M., Neuvonen, P.J., 2004. Ciprofloxacin greatly increases concentrations and hypotensive effect of tizanidine by inhibiting its cytochrome P450 1A2-mediated presystemic metabolism. Clin. Pharmacol. Ther. 76, 598–606.

Guengerich, F.P., 1994. Catalytic selectivity of human cytochrome P450 enzymes: relevance to drug metabolism and toxicity. Toxicol. Lett. 70 (2), 133–138.

Hakkola, J., Pasanen, M., Purkunen, R., Saarikoski, S., Pelkonen, O., Maenpaa, J., et al., 1994. Expression of xenobiotic-metabolizing cytochrome P450 forms in human adult and fetal liver. Biochem. Pharmacol. 48, 59–64.

Hakkola, J., Raunio, H., Purkunen, R., Saarikoski, S., Vahakangas, K., Pelkonen, O., et al., 2001. Cytochrome P450 3A expression in the human fetal liver: evidence that CYP3A5 is expressed in only a limited number of fetal livers. Biol. Neonate 80, 193–201.

Hammond, A.H., Fry, J.R., 1990. The in vivo induction of rat hepatic cytochrome P450-dependent enzyme activities and their maintenance in culture. Biochem. Pharmacol. 40 (3), 637–642.

Hariparsad, N., Nallani, S.C., Sane, R.S., Buckley, D.J., Buckley, A.R., Desai, P.B., 2004. Induction of CYP3A4 by efavirenz in primary human hepatocytes: comparison with rifampin and phenobarbital. J. Clin. Pharmacol. 44 (11), 1273–1281.

Hartley, R., Green, M., Quinn, M.W., Rushforth, J.A., Levene, M.I., 1994. Development of morphine glucuronidation in premature neonates. Biol. Neonate 66, 1–9.

Havlir, D., Cheeseman, S.H., McLaughlin, M., Murphy, R., Erice, A., Spector, S.A., et al., 1995. High-dose nevirapine: safety, pharmacokinetics, and antiviral effect in patients with human immunodeficiency virus infection. J. Infect. Dis. 171 (3), 537–545.

He, X., Hesse, L.M., Hazarika, S., Masse, G., Harmatz, J.S., Greenblatt, D.J., Court, M.H., 2009. Evidence for oxazepam as an in vivo probe of UGT2B15: oxazepam clearance is reduced by UGT2B15 D85Y polymorphism but unaffected by UGT2B17 deletion. Br. J. Clin. Pharmacol. 68, 721–730.

Ho, R.H., Kim, R.B., 2005. Transporters and drug therapy: implications for drug disposition and disease. Clin. Pharmacol. Ther. 78 (3), 260–277.

Horton, T.M., Ames, M.M., Reid, J.M., Krailo, M.D., Pendergrass, T., Mosher, R., et al., 2007. A phase 1 and pharmacokinetic clinical trial of paclitaxel for the treatment of refractory leukemia in children: a children's oncology group study. Pediatr. Blood Cancer 50, 788–792.

Hynninen, V.V., Olkkola, K.T., Leino, K., Lundgren, S., Neuvonen, P.J., Rane, A., et al., 2007. Effect of voriconazole on the pharmacokinetics of diclofenac. Fundam. Clin. Pharmacol. 21 (6), 651–656.

Innocenti, F., Iyer, L., Ramirez, J., Green, M.D., Ratain, M.J., 2001. Epirubicin glucuronidation is catalyzed by human UDP-glucuronosyltransferase 2B7. Drug Metab. Dispos. 29, 686–692.

Iyer, L., King, C.D., Whitington, P.F., Green, M.D., Roy, S.K., Tephly, T.R., et al., 1998. Genetic predisposition to the metabolism of irinotecan (CPT-11). Role of uridine diphosphate glucuronosyltransferase isoform 1A1 in the glucuronidation of its active metabolite (SN-38) in human liver microsomes. J. Clin. Invest. 101, 847–854.

Jankovic, S.M., Milovanovic, J.R., Jankovic, S., 2010. Factors influencing valproate pharmacokinetics in children and adults. Int. J. Clin. Pharmacol. Ther. 48, 767–775.

Johnson, T.N., Tucker, G.T., Tanner, M.S., Rostami-Hodjegan, A., 2005. Changes in liver volume from birth to adulthood: a meta-analysis. Liver Transpl. 11, 1481–1493.

Jones, S.M., Boobis, A.R., Moore, G.E., Stanier, P.M., 1992. Expression of CYP2E1 during human fetal development: methylation of the CYP2E1 gene in human fetal and adult liver samples. Biochem. Pharmacol. 43, 1876–1879.

Juarez-Olguin, H., Lugo-Goytia, G., Flores-Murrieta, F., Ruiz-Garcia, M., Lares Asseff, I., Flores Perez, J., 2011. Effect of treatment and additional disease on pharmacokinetic of valproic acid in children with epilepsy. Rev. Invest. Clin. 62, 516–523.

Kallionpää, R.A., Järvinen, E., Finel, M., 2015. Glucuronidation of estrone and 16α-hydroxyestrone by human UGT enzymes; the key roles of UGT1A10 and UGT2B7. J. Steroid Biochem. Mol. Biol.

Kantola, T., Kivisto, K.T., Neuvonen, P.J., 1998. Effect of itraconazole on the pharmacokinetics of atorvastatin. Clin. Pharmacol. Ther. 64 (1), 58–65.

Kataria, B.K., Ved, S.A., Nicodemus, H.F., Hoy, G.R., Lea, D., Dubois, M.Y., et al., 1994. The pharmacokinetics of propofol in children using three different data analysis approaches. Anesthesiology 80, 104–122.

Kato, Y., Ikushiro, S., Emi, Y., Tamaki, S., Suzuki, H., Sakaki, T., et al., 2008. Hepatic UDP-glucuronosyltransferases responsible for glucuronidation of thyroxine in humans. Drug Metab. Dispos. 36, 51–55.

Kaukonen, K.M., Olkkola, K.T., Neuvonen, P.J., 1998. Fluconazole but not itraconazole decreases the metabolism of losartan to E-3174. Eur. J. Clin. Pharmacol. 53 (6), 445–449.

Kawade, N., Onishi, S., 1981. The prenatal and postnatal development of UDP-glucuronyltransferase activity towards bilirubin and the effect of premature birth on this activity in the human liver. Biochem. J. 196, 257–260.

Kearns, G.L., Robinson, P.K., Wilson, J.T., Wilson-Costello, D., Knight, G.R., Ward, R.M., van den Anker, J.N., 2003. Cisapride disposition in neonates and infants: in vivo reflection of cytochrome P450 3A4 ontogeny. Clin. Pharmacol. Ther. 74, 312–325.

Kehrer, D.F., Mathijssen, R.H., Verweij, J., de Bruijn, P., Sparreboom, A., 2002. Modulation of irinotecan metabolism by ketoconazole. J. Clin. Oncol. 20 (14), 3122–3129.

Kharasch, E.D., Thummel, K.E., Mhyre, J., Lillibridge, J.H., 1993. Single-dose disulfiram inhibition of chlorzoxazone metabolism: a clinical probe for P450 2E1. Clin. Pharmacol. Ther. 53 (6), 643–650.

Kim, S.E., Kim, B.H., Lee, S., Sohn, J.A., Kim, H.S., Cho, J.Y., et al., 2013. Population pharmacokinetics of theophylline in premature Korean infants. Ther. Drug Monit. 35, 338–344.

Kitada, M., Kamataki, T., 1994. Cytochrome P450 in human fetal liver: significance and fetal-specific expression. Drug Metab. Rev. 26, 305–323.

Kivisto, K.T., Lamberg, T.S., Kantola, T., Neuvonen, P.J., 1997. Plasma buspirone concentrations are greatly increased by erythromycin and itraconazole. Clin. Pharmacol. Ther. 62 (3), 348–354.

Knibbe, C.A., Krekels, E.H., van den Anker, J.N., DeJongh, J., Santen, G.W., van Dijk, M., et al., 2009. Morphine glucuronidation in preterm neonates, infants and children younger than 3 years. Clin. Pharmacokinet. 48, 371–385.

Kobayashi, K., Nakajima, M., Chiba, K., Yamamoto, T., Tani, M., Ishizaki, T., Kuroiwa, Y., 1998. Inhibitory effects of antiarrhythmic drugs on phenacetin O-deethylation catalysed by human CYP1A2. Br. J. Clin. Pharmacol. 45, 361–368.

Komori, M., Nishio, K., Fujitani, T., Ohi, H., Kitada, M., Mima, S., et al., 1989. Isolation of a new human fetal liver cytochrome P450 cDNA clone: evidence for expression of a limited number of forms of cytochrome P450 in human fetal livers. Arch. Biochem. Biophys. 272, 219–225.

Kotlyar, M., Brauer, L.H., Tracy, T.S., Hatsukami, D.K., Harris, J., Bronars, C.A., Adson, D.E., 2005. Inhibition of CYP2D6 activity by bupropion. J. Clin. Psychopharmacol. 25 (3), 226–229.

Krekels, E.H.J., Danhof, M., Tibboel, D., Knibbe, C.A.J., 2012a. Ontogeny of hepatic glucuronidation; methods and results. Curr. Drug Metab. 13 (6), 728–743.

Krekels, E.H.J., Johnson, T.N., den Hoedt, S.M., Rostami-Hodjegan, A., Danhof, M., Tibboel, D., Knibbe, C.A.J., 2012b. From pediatric covariate model to semiphysiological function for maturation: Part II-sensitivity to physiological and physicochemical properties. CPT: Pharmacometrics Syst. Pharmacol. 1, e10.

Krekels, E.H.J., Neely, M., Panoilia, E., Tibboel, D., Capparelli, E., Danhof, M., et al., 2012c. From pediatric covariate model to semiphysiological function for maturation: Part I—extrapolation of a covariate model from morphine to zidovudine. CPT: Pharmacometrics Syst. Pharmacol.

Krekels, E.H.J., van Ham, S., Allegaert, K., de Hoon, J., Tibboel, D., Danhof, M., Knibbe, C.A.J., 2015. Developmental changes rather than repeated administration drive paracetamol glucuronidation in neonates and infants. Eur. J. Clin. Pharmacol.

Krishnaswamy, S., Duan, S.X., Von Moltke, L.L., Greenblatt, D.J., Court, M.H., 2003. Validation of serotonin (5-hydroxtryptamine) as an in vitro substrate probe for human UDP-glucuronosyltransferase (UGT) 1A6. Drug Metab. Dispos. 31, 133–139.

Kwara, A., Lartey, M., Sagoe, K.W., Xexemeku, F., Kenu, E., Oliver-Commey, J., et al., 2008. Pharmacokinetics of efavirenz when co-administered with rifampin in TB/HIV co-infected patients: pharmacogenetic effect of CYP2B6 variation. J. Clin. Pharmacol. 48 (9), 1032–1040.

Kwara, A., Lartey, M., Boamah, I., Rezk, N.L., Oliver-Commey, J., Kenu, E., et al., 2009. Interindividual variability in pharmacokinetics of generic nucleoside reverse transcriptase inhibitors in TB/HIV-coinfected Ghanaian patients: UGT2B7*1c is associated with faster zidovudine clearance and glucuronidation. J. Clin. Pharmacol. 49, 1079–1090.

Lacroix, D., Sonnier, M., Moncion, A., Cheron, G., Cresteil, T., 1997. Expression of CYP3A in the human liver—evidence that the shift between CYP3A7 and CYP3A4 occurs immediately after birth. Eur. J. Biochem. 247, 625–634.

Ladona, M.G., Lindstrom, B., Thyr, C., Dun-Ren, P., Rane, A., 1991. Differential foetal development of the O- and N-demethylation of codeine and dextromethorphan in man. Br. J. Clin. Pharmacol. 32, 295–302.

Laika, B., Leucht, S., Heres, S., Schneider, H., Steimer, W., 2009. Pharmacogenetics and olanzapine treatment: CYP1A2*1F and serotonergic polymorphisms influence therapeutic outcome. Pharmacogenomic. J. 10, 20–29.

Lake, B.G., Tredger, J.M., Renwick, A.B., Barton, P.T., Price, R.J., 1998. 3,3′-Diindolylmethane induces CYP1A2 in cultured precision-cut human liver slices. Xenobiotica 28 (8), 803–811.

Leakey, J.E., Hume, R., Burchell, B., 1987. Development of multiple activities of UDP-glucuronyltransferase in human liver. Biochem. J. 243, 859–861.

Lee, T.C., Charles, B.G., Harte, G.J., Gray, P.H., Steer, P.A., Flenady, V.J., 1999. Population pharmacokinetic modeling in very premature infants receiving midazolam during mechanical ventilation: midazolam neonatal pharmacokinetics. Anesthesiology 90, 451–457.

Levesque, E., Beaulieu, M., Green, M.D., Tephly, T.R., Belanger, A., Hum, D.W., 1997. Isolation and characterization of UGT2B15(Y85): a UDP-glucuronosyltransferase encoded by a polymorphic gene. Pharmacogenetics 7, 317–325.

Levy, G., Khanna, N.N., Soda, D.M., Tsuzuki, O., Stern, L., 1975. Pharmacokinetics of acetaminophen in the human neonate: formation of acetaminophen glucuronide and sulfate in relation to plasma bilirubin concentration and D-glucaric acid excretion. Pediatrics 55, 818–825.

Luzier, A., Morse, G.D., 1993. Intravascular distribution of zidovudine: role of plasma proteins and whole blood components. Antivir. Res. 21, 267–280.

Lynn, A.M., Nespeca, M.K., Bratton, S.L., Shen, D.D., 2000. Intravenous morphine in postoperative infants: intermittent bolus dosing versus targeted continuous infusions. Pain 88, 89–95.

Mackenzie, P.I., Bock, K.W., Burchell, B., Guillemette, C., Ikushiro, S., Iyanagi, T., et al., 2005. Nomenclature update for the mammalian UDP glycosyltransferase (UGT) gene superfamily. Pharmacogenet. Genomics 15, 677–685.

Mackenzie, P.I., 1990. The effect of N-linked glycosylation on the substrate preferences of UDP glucuronosyltransferases. Biochem. Biophys. Res. Commun. 166, 1293–1299.

Maenpaa, J., Pelkonen, O., Cresteil, T., Rane, A., 1993. The role of cytochrome P450 3A (CYP3A) isoform(s) in oxidative metabolism of testosterone and benzphetamine in human adult and fetal liver. J. Steroid Biochem. Mol. Biol. 44 (1), 61–67.

Mano, Y., Usui, T., Kamimura, H., 2007. Contribution of UDP-glucuronosyltransferases 1A9 and 2B7 to the glucuronidation of indomethacin in the human liver. Eur. J. Clin. Pharmacol. 63, 289–296.

McNamara, P.J., Alcorn, J., 2002. Protein binding predictions in infants. AAPS Pharm. Sci. 4, E4.

McRorie, T.I., Lynn, A.M., Nespeca, M.K., Opheim, K.E., Slattery, J.T., 1992. The maturation of morphine clearance and metabolism. Am. J. Dis. Child 146, 972–976.

Miller, R.P., Roberts, R.J., Fischer, L.J., 1976. Acetaminophen elimination kinetics in neonates, children, and adults. Clin. Pharmacol. Ther. 19, 284–294.

Mirochnick, M., Capparelli, E., Connor, J., 1999. Pharmacokinetics of zidovudine in infants: a population analysis across studies. Clin. Pharmacol. Ther. 66, 16–24.

Miyagi, S.J., Collier, A.C., 2007. Pediatric development of glucuronidation: the ontogeny of hepatic UGT1A4. Drug Metab. Dispos. 35, 1587–1592.

Miyagi, S.J., Collier, A.C., 2011. The development of UDP-glucuronosyltransferases 1A1 and 1A6 in the pediatric liver. Drug Metab. Dispos. 39 (5), 912–919.

Miyagi, S.J., Milne, A.M., Coughtrie, M.W.H., Collier, A.C., 2012. Neonatal development of hepatic UGT1A9: implications of pediatric pharmacokinetics. Drug Metab. Dispos. 40 (7), 1321–1327.

Nakamura, A., Nakajima, M., Yamanaka, H., Fujiwara, R., Yokoi, T., 2008. Expression of UGT1A and UGT2B mRNA in human normal tissues and various cell lines. Drug Metab. Dispos. 36, 1461–1464.

Nelson, D.R., Koymans, L., Kamataki, T., Stegeman, J.J., Feyereisen, R., Waxman, D.J., et al., 1996. P450 superfamily: update on new sequences, gene mapping, accession numbers and nomenclature. Pharmacogenetics 6 (1), 1–42.

Niemi, M., Kajosaari, L.I., Neuvonen, M., Backman, J.T., Neuvonen, P.J., 2004. The CYP2C8 inhibitor trimethoprim increases the plasma concentrations of repaglinide in healthy subjects. Br. J. Clin. Pharmacol. 57 (4), 441–447.

Nishiya, Y., Hagihara, K., Ito, T., Tajima, M., Miura, S., Kurihara, A., et al., 2008. Mechanism-based inhibition of human cytochrome P450 2B6 by ticlopidine, clopidogrel, and the thiolactone metabolite of prasugrel. Drug Metab. Dispos. 37 (3), 589–593.

Noda, T., Todani, T., Watanabe, Y., Yamamoto, S., 1997. Liver volume in children measured by computed tomography. Pediatr. Radiol. 27 (3), 250–252.

Ogungbenro, K., Aarons, L., 2014. A physiologically based pharmacokinetic model for valproic acid in adults and children. Eur. J. Pharm. Sci. 63, 45–52.

Ohno, S., Nakajin, S., 2009. Determination of mRNA expression of human UDP-glucuronosyltransferases and application for localization in various human tissues by real-time reverse transcriptase-polymerase chain reaction. Drug Metab. Dispos. 37, 32–40.

Ohno, A., Saito, Y., Hanioka, N., Jinno, H., Saeki, M., Ando, M., et al., 2004. Involvement of human hepatic UGT1A1, UGT2B4, and UGT2B7 in the glucuronidation of carvedilol. Drug Metab. Dispos. 32, 235–239.

Olsen, G.D., 1975. Morphine binding to human plasma proteins. Clin. Pharmacol. Ther. 17, 31–35.

Onica, T., Nichols, K., Larin, M., Ng, L., Maslen, A., Dvorak, Z., et al., 2007. Dexamethasone-mediated up-regulation of human CYP2A6 involves the glucocorticoid receptor and increased binding of hepatic nuclear factor 4 alpha to the proximal promoter. Mol. Pharmacol. 73 (2), 451–460.

Onishi, S., Kawade, N., Itoh, S., Isobe, K., Sugiyama, S., 1979. Postnatal development of uridine diphosphate glucuronyltransferase activity towards bilirubin and 2-aminophenol in human liver. Biochem. J. 184, 705–707.

Pacifici, G.M., Sawe, J., Kager, L., Rane, A., 1982. Morphine glucuronidation in human fetal and adult liver. Eur. J. Clin. Pharmacol. 22, 553–558.

Parsons, W.D., Neims, A.H., 1978. Effect of smoking on caffeine clearance. Clin. Pharmacol. Ther. 24, 40–45.

Pasanen, M., Pelkonen, O., Kauppila, A., Park, S.S., Friedman, F.K., Gelboin, H.V., 1987. Characterization of human fetal hepatic cytochrome P-450-associated 7-ethoxyresorufin O-deethylase and aryl hydrocarbon hydroxylase activities by monoclonal antibodies. Dev. Pharmacol. Ther. 10, 125–132.

Peeters, M.Y., Allegaert, K., Blussé van Oud-Alblas, H.J., Cella, M., Tibboel, D., Danhof, M., Knibbe, C.A., 2010. Prediction of propofol clearance in children from an allometric model developed in rats, children and adults versus a 0.75 fixed-exponent allometric model. Clin. Pharmacokinet. 49, 269–275.

Pons, G., Blais, J.C., Rey, E., Plissonnier, M., Richard, M.O., Carrier, O., et al., 1988. Maturation of caffeine N-demethylation in infancy: a study using the 13CO2 breath test. Pediatr. Res. 23, 632–636.

Prasad, B., Lai, Y., Lin, Y., Unadkat, J.D., 2013. Interindividual variability in the hepatic expression of the human breast cancer resistance protein (BCRP/ABCG2): effect of age, sex, and genotype. J. Pharm. Sci. 102 (3), 787–793.

Prasad, B., Evers, R., Gupta, A., Hop, C.E.C.A., Salphati, L., Shukla, S., et al., 2014. Interindividual variability in hepatic organic anion-transporting polypeptides and P-glycoprotein (ABCB1) protein expression: quantification by liquid chromatography tandem mass spectroscopy and influence of genotype, age, and sex. Drug Metab. Dispos. 42 (1), 78–88.

Quevedo, M.A., Ribone, S.R., Moroni, G.N., Brinon, M.C., 2008. Binding to human serum albumin of zidovudine (AZT) and novel AZT derivatives. Experimental and theoretical analyses. Bioorg. Med. Chem. 16, 2779–2790.

Ratanasavanh, D., Beaune, P., Morel, F., Flinois, J.P., Guengerich, F.P., Guillouzo, A., 1991. Intralobular distribution and quantitation of cytochrome P-450 enzymes in human liver as a function of age. Hepatology 13, 1142–1151.

Raucy, J.L., Lasker, J.M., Lieber, C.S., Black, M., 1989. Acetaminophen activation by human liver cytochromes P450IIE1 and P450IA2. Arch. Biochem. Biophys. 271 (2), 270–283.

Raucy, J.L., Mueller, L., Duan, K., Allen, S.W., Strom, S., Lasker, J.M., 2002. Expression and induction of CYP2C P450 enzymes in primary cultures of human hepatocytes. J. Pharmacol. Exp. Ther. 302 (2), 475–482.

Richard, K., Hume, R., Kaptein, E., Stanley, E.L., Visser, T.J., Coughtrie, M.W., 2001. Sulfation of thyroid hormone and dopamine during human development: ontogeny of phenol sulfotransferases and arylsulfatase in liver, lung, and brain. J. Clin. Endocrinol. Metab. 86 (6), 2734–2742.

Rollins, D.E., von Bahr, C., Glaumann, H., Moldeus, P., Rane, A., 1979. Acetaminophen: potentially toxic metabolite formed by human fetal and adult liver microsomes and isolated fetal liver cells. Science 205, 1414–1416.

Rost, K.L., Brosicke, H., Brockmoller, J., Scheffler, M., Helge, H., Roots, I., 1992. Increase of cytochrome P450IA2 activity by omeprazole: evidence by the 13C-[N-3-methyl]-caffeine breath test in poor and extensive metabolizers of S-mephenytoin. Clin. Pharmacol. Ther. 52, 170–180.

Saarenmaa, E., Neuvonen, P.J., Rosenberg, P., Fellman, V., 2000. Morphine clearance and effects in newborn infants in relation to gestational age. Clin. Pharmacol. Ther. 68, 160–166.

Sahi, J., Black, C.B., Hamilton, G.A., Zheng, X., Jolley, S., Rose, K.A., et al., 2003. Comparative effects of thiazolidinediones on in vitro P450 enzyme induction and inhibition. Drug Metab. Dispos. 31 (4), 439–446.

Saitoh, A., Fletcher, C.V., Brundage, R., Alvero, C., Fenton, T., Hsia, K., Spector, S.A., 2007. Efavirenz pharmacokinetics in HIV-1-infected children are associated with CYP2B6-G516T polymorphism. J. Acquir. Immune Defic. Syndr. 45, 280–285.

Salem, A.H., Fletcher, C.V., Brundage, R.C., 2014. Pharmacometric characterization of efavirenz developmental pharmacokinetics and pharmacogenetics in HIV-infected children. Antimicrob. Agents Chemother. 58 (1), 136–143.

Schuetz, J.D., Beach, D.L., Guzelian, P.S., 1994. Selective expression of cytochrome P450 CYP3A mRNAs in embryonic and adult human liver. Pharmacogenetics 4, 11–20.

Shimada, T., Yamazaki, H., Mimura, M., Inui, Y., Guengerich, F.P., 1994. Interindividual variations in human liver cytochrome P-450 enzymes involved in the oxidation of drugs, carcinogens and toxic chemicals: studies with liver microsomes of 30 Japanese and 30 Caucasians. J. Pharmacol. Exp. Ther. 270 (1), 414–423.

Shimada, T., Yamazaki, H., Mimura, M., Wakamiya, N., Ueng, Y.F., Guengerich, F.P., Inui, Y., 1996. Characterization of microsomal cytochrome P450 enzymes involved in the oxidation of xenobiotic chemicals in human fetal liver and adult lungs. Drug Metab. Dispos. 24 (5), 515–522.

Sonnier, M., Cresteil, T., 1998. Delayed ontogenesis of CYP1A2 in the human liver. Eur. J. Biochem. 251, 893–898.

Staines, A.G., Coughtrie, M.W., Burchell, B., 2004. N-glucuronidation of carbamazepine in human tissues is mediated by UGT2B7. J. Pharmacol. Exp. Ther. 311, 1131–1137.

Stevens, J.C., Hines, R.N., Gu, C., Koukouritaki, S.B., Manro, J.R., Tandler, P.J., Zaya, M.J., 2003. Developmental expression of the major human hepatic CYP3A enzymes. J. Pharmacol. Exp. Ther. 307, 573–582.

Strassburg, C.P., Strassburg, A., Kneip, S., Barut, A., Tukey, R.H., Rodeck, B., Manns, M.P., 2002. Developmental aspects of human hepatic drug glucuronidation in young children and adults. Gut 50, 259–265.

Takekuma, Y., Takenaka, T., Kiyokawa, M., Yamazaki, K., Okamoto, H., Kitabatake, A., et al., 2006. Contribution of polymorphisms in UDP-glucuronosyltransferase and CYP2D6 to the individual variation in disposition of carvedilol. J. Pharm. Pharm. Sci. 9, 101–112.

Tanaka, E., 1998. In vivo age-related changes in hepatic drug-oxidizing capacity in humans. J. Clincal Pharm. Ther. 23, 247–255.

Tang, L., Hines, R.N., Schuetz, E.G., Meibohm, B., 2007. Age-associated protein expression of P-glycoprotein (MDR1/P-gp) and MRP2 in human pediatric liver. Clin. Pharmacol. Ther. 81 (Suppl. 1), S101.

Tateishi, T., Nakura, H., Asoh, M., Watanabe, M., Tanaka, M., Kumai, T., et al., 1997. A comparison of hepatic cytochrome P450 protein expression between infancy and postinfancy. Life Sci. 61, 2567–2574.

Thomson, M.M., Hines, R.N., Schuetz, E.G., Meibohm, B., 2014. Age-associated expression of OATP1B1 and OATP1B3 in human pediatric liver. AAPS J. W4301. Suppl. 2.

Treluyer, J.M., Jacqz-Aigrain, E., Alvarez, F., Cresteil, T., 1991. Expression of CYP2D6 in developing human liver. Eur. J. Biochem. 202, 583—588.

Treluyer, J.M., Cheron, G., Sonnier, M., Cresteil, T., 1996. Cytochrome P-450 expression in sudden infant death syndrome. Biochem. Pharmacol. 52, 497—504.

Treluyer, J.M., Gueret, G., Cheron, G., Sonnier, M., Cresteil, T., 1998. Developmental expression of CYP2C and CYP2C-dependent activities in the human liver: in-vivo/in-vitro correlation and inducibility. Pharmacogenetics 7, 441—452.

Treluyer, J.M., Bowers, G., Cazali, N., Sonnier, M., Rey, E., Pons, G., Cresteil, T., 2003. Oxidative metabolism of amprenavir in the human liver. Effect of the CYP3A maturation. Drug Metab. Dispos. 31, 275—281.

Tukey, R.H., Strassburg, C.P., 2000. Human UDP-glucuronosyltransferases: metabolism, expression, and disease. Annu. Rev. Pharmacol. Toxicol. 40, 581—616.

Turgeon, D., Carrier, J.S., Levesque, E., Hum, D.W., Belanger, A., 2001. Relative enzymatic activity, protein stability, and tissue distribution of human steroid-metabolizing UGT2B subfamily members. Endocrinology 142, 778—787.

Uchaipichat, V., Mackenzie, P.I., Guo, X.H., Gardner-Stephen, D., Galetin, A., Houston, J.B., Miners, J.O., 2004. Human udp-glucuronosyltransferases: isoform selectivity and kinetics of 4-methylumbelliferone and 1-naphthol glucuronidation, effects of organic solvents, and inhibition by diclofenac and probenecid. Drug Metab. Dispos. 32, 413—423.

Uslu, A., Ogus, C., Ozdemir, T., Bilgen, T., Tosun, O., Keser, I., 2010. The effect of CYP1A2 gene polymorphisms on theophylline metabolism and chronic obstructive pulmonary disease in Turkish patients. BMB Rep. 43, 530—534.

Valentin, J., 2001. Basic Anatomical and Physiological Data for Use in Radiological Protection: Reference Values. ICRP Publication, p. 89.

Vest, M., 1958. Insufficient glucuronide formation in the newborn and its relationship to the pathogenesis of icterus neonatorum. Arch. Dis. Child 33, 473—476.

Vieira, I., Sonnier, M., Cresteil, T., 1996. Developmental expression of CYP2E1 in the human liver. Hypermethylation control of gene expression during the neonatal period. Eur. J. Biochem. 238, 476—483.

Viljoen, M., Karlsson, M.O., Meyers, T.M., Gous, H., Dandara, C., Rheeders, M., 2011. Influence of CYP2B6 516G>T polymorphism and interoccasion variability (IOV) on the population pharmacokinetics of efavirenz in HIV-infected South African children. Eur. J. Clin. Pharmacol. 68, 339—347.

Von Bahr, C., Steiner, E., Koike, Y., Gabrielsson, J., 1998. Time course of enzyme induction in humans: effect of pentobarbital on nortriptyline metabolism. Clin. Pharmacol. Ther. 64 (1), 18—26.

Von Moltke, L.L., Greenblatt, D.J., Grassi, J.M., Granda, B.W., Duan, S.X., Fogelman, S.M., et al., 1998. Protease inhibitors as inhibitors of human cytochromes P450: high risk associated with ritonavir. J. Clin. Pharmacol. 38 (2), 106—111.

Wang, R.W., Newton, D.J., Scheri, T.D., Lu, A.Y., 1997. Human cytochrome P450 3A4-catalyzed testosterone 6 beta-hydroxylation and erythromycin N-demethylation. Competition during catalysis. Drug Metab. Dispos. 25 (4), 502—507.

Wang, C., Peeters, M.Y.M., Allegaert, K., Tibboel, D., Danhof, M., Knibbe, C.A.J., 2010. Scaling clearance of propofol from preterm neonates to adults using an allometric model with a bodyweight-dependent maturational exponent. PAGE 19.

Ward, R.M., Kearns, G.L., 2013. Proton pump inhibitors in pediatrics : mechanism of action, pharmacokinetics, pharmacogenetics, and pharmacodynamics. Paediatric Drugs 15, 119—131.

Windorfer, A., Kuenzer, W., Urbanek, R., 1974. The influence of age on the activity of acetylsalicylic acid-esterase and protein-salicylate binding. Eur. J. Clin. Pharmacol. 7 (3), 227—231.

Wrighton, S.A., Brian, W.R., Sari, M.A., Iwasaki, M., Guengerich, F.P., Raucy, J.L., et al., 1990. Studies on the expression and metabolic capabilities of human liver cytochrome P450IIIA5 (HLp3). Mol. Pharmacol. 38, 207—213.

Yanni, S.B., Smith, P.B., Benjamin, D.K., Augustijns, P.F., Thakker, D.R., Annaert, P.P., 2011. Higher clearance of micafungin in neonates compared with adults: role of age-dependent micafungin serum binding. Biopharm. Drug Dispos. 32 (4), 222—232.

Zaya, M.J., Hines, R.N., Stevens, J.C., 2006. Epirubicin glucuronidation and UGT2B7 developmental expression. Drug Metab. Dispos. 34.

Zhang, W., Kilicarslan, T., Tyndale, R.F., Sellers, E.M., 2001. Evaluation of methoxsalen, tranylcypromine, and trypt-amine as specific and selective CYP2A6 inhibitors in vitro. Drug Metab. Dispos. 29 (6), 897–902.

Zhou, D., Guo, J., Linnenbach, A.J., Booth-Genthe, C.L., Grimm, S.W., 2010. Role of human UGT2B10 in N-glucuronidation of tricyclic antidepressants, amitriptyline, imipramine, clomipramine, and trimipramine. Drug Metab. Dispos. 38, 863–870.

Zhu, A.Z., Renner, C.C., Hatsukami, D.K., Swan, G.E., Lerman, C., Benowitz, N.L., Tyndale, R.F., 2013. The ability of plasma cotinine to predict nicotine and carcinogen exposure is altered by differences in CYP2A6: the influence of genetics, race, and sex. Cancer Epidemiol. Biomarkers Prev. 22, 708–718.

Drug Metabolism in Pregnancy

J.E. Moscovitz, L. Gorczyca, L.M. Aleksunes

Rutgers University, Piscataway, NJ, United States

OUTLINE

Introduction	208	Nuclear Receptors	220
Physiological Adaptations During Pregnancy	208	Hormonal Regulation	221
Hemodynamics, Hematology, and		Estrogen	221
Hemodilution	209	Progesterone	225
Respiratory	209	Placental Lactogen/Prolactin/Growth	
Renal Blood Flow and Filtration	210	Hormone	226
Gastrointestinal Function	210	Cortisol	227
Hepatic Phase I Enzymes	210	Extrahepatic Regulation	230
Cytochrome P450 Enzymes	210		
Carboxylesterase and Paraoxanase		Case Example: Bile Acid Metabolism	
Enzymes	214	and Transport	230
		Phase I	231
Hepatic Phase II Enzymes	215	Phase II	231
Ugts	215	Transport	232
Gsts	217	Transcription Factors	232
Sults	217	Translational Implications	233
Hepatic Transporters	218	Conclusion and Future Directions	234
Solute Carrier (SLC) Transporters	218	References	234
ATP-Binding Cassette Transporters	218		

INTRODUCTION

Pregnancy is a period of high nutritional demand. As such, the body adapts to enhance the absorption and retention of nutrients and promote the excretion of waste, all with the intent of promoting the growth and development of the fetus. These alterations include physiological changes such as slowing of gastrointestinal transit, reduced plasma albumin concentration, and enhanced hepatic and renal blood flow along with increased glomerular filtration. In addition to these adaptations, the body also regulates the expression and function of metabolizing enzymes and membrane transporters in response to pregnancy. This is critical not only in nutrient disposition but can also alter how tissues such as the liver metabolize drugs and endogenous chemicals such as bile acids and lipids.

During pregnancy, it is estimated that 35–64% of pregnant women are prescribed medications (other than vitamins and minerals) (Daw et al., 2011). There are a number of critical disorders that require new or continued pharmacotherapy during gestation. These include gestational diabetes, psychiatric disorders, seizure diseases, and cancer to name a few. As a consequence of pregnancy, the disposition of these medications can be significantly altered leading to exaggerated or insufficient pharmacotherapy, negatively affecting a woman's overall health. Requisite to predicting the molecular changes in drug metabolism (phase I and phase II) and transport during pregnancy is understanding how the expression and function of these proteins change over gestation. A number of enzymes, carriers, and export pumps are expressed within the liver, and their regulation has been tied to hormones that are elevated during pregnancy.

This chapter highlights the adaptive regulation of physiological and molecular pathways that influence drug disposition in pregnancy. Attention is placed on the roles of individual hormones and nuclear receptors that mediate molecular and biochemical changes in metabolism and transport during pregnancy. Clinical data from pregnant women typically reflect the overall changes in a drug's pharmacokinetics; interpretation of the mechanism can be limited by difficulties in determining the exact contribution of changes in particular enzymes or transporters. Likewise, mice and rats have been used to delineate altered drug disposition pathways in the maternal liver using mRNA profiling, protein expression, and ex vivo functional assays. Although these data are useful and provide the most comprehensive understanding of adaptive regulation, there are a number of differences between human and rodent pregnancies. Of note, rodent pregnancies last ∼19–20 days compared with 266 days in humans. Likewise, the exact hormones that change, as well as the magnitude and timing of change, can differ between species. Nonetheless, data generated from pregnant rodents can be used to compliment clinical findings and candidate hormone studies using primary human hepatocytes.

PHYSIOLOGICAL ADAPTATIONS DURING PREGNANCY

Throughout pregnancy, numerous maternal physiological and anatomical changes occur that alter the uterus and allow for the development of the placenta and fetus. These alterations include an increase in glomerular filtration rate, renal blood flow, and portal vein blood flow, which in turn affect pharmacokinetic determinants such as plasma volume, oral absorption, and plasma protein binding among others. Additionally, changes in the expression and activity of maternal hepatic drug-metabolizing enzymes and transporters contribute to altered pharmacokinetics.

Hemodynamics, Hematology, and Hemodilution

A number of hemodynamic changes have been described in women during pregnancy. Using echocardiography, the cardiac output has been demonstrated to increase up to 60% in the second and third trimester when compared with nonpregnant women (Clark et al., 1989; Rubler et al., 1977). This enhanced cardiac output results from elevations in both stroke volume and heart rate. Subsequent analysis has revealed reductions in systemic and peripheral vascular resistance, pulmonary vascular resistance, and colloid oncotic pressure in women during pregnancy compared with the postpartum period (Clark et al., 1989).

Doppler ultrasonography has demonstrated that the portal venous blood flow and total liver blood flow are increased significantly in pregnant women after 28 weeks of gestation (Nakai et al., 2002). By comparison, the hepatic arterial blood flow remains unchanged during pregnancy. Similar results have been determined by monitoring serial clearance of indocyanine green at different time points in pregnancy (Robson et al., 1990). Although indocyanine green is a substrate of hepatic organic anion-type transporters (Chen et al., 2000), the extraction ratio of this dye (0.74) did not change across gestation, which supports its use as a liver blood flow probe. An alternative interpretation may involve potential adaptive regulation of transporters that balance physiological changes in blood flow.

The circulating blood supply increases steadily throughout pregnancy and approaches maximal increases ($\sim$35–45%) by 30 weeks of gestation (Bader et al., 1955; Hytten and Paintin, 1963; Peck and Arias, 1979; Pritchard, 1965). Higher blood volume results from both greater amounts of plasma and red blood cells. The composition of blood across pregnancy is also altered with a notable decline in the concentration of plasma proteins such as albumin (Perucca and Crema, 1982). As a result of having less albumin in the circulation, the free fraction of drugs with narrow therapeutic indexes, such as valproic acid, phenytoin, and diazepam, can increase (Koerner et al., 1989; Riva et al., 1984).

Respiratory

There are a number of changes in respiratory anatomy and pulmonary function during pregnancy. Notably, pregnant women often complain of a stuffy nose that results from mucosal hypersecretion and edema due to elevated estradiol levels. Though the enlarged uterus pushes up on the diaphragm, breathing is not impaired. However, a number of changes in pulmonary function parameters have been noted during pregnancy. Throughout the second half of pregnancy, there is a progressive decline in expiratory reserve volume (up to 40%) and residual volume (up to 20%) without changes in total lung capacity, forced vital capacity, or peak flow rates (Baldwin et al., 1977; Elkus and Popovich, 1992). By contrast, tidal volume is enhanced from 450 to 700 mL as a result of increased respiratory drive and rib cage volume displacement (Elkus and Popovich, 1992). In addition, oxygen consumption at rest is enhanced by 30–40 mL/min in pregnant women (Pernoll et al., 1975).

Renal Blood Flow and Filtration

In response to pregnancy, renal blood flow and glomerular filtration rate are increased by 30—50% (Davison and Dunlop, 1980; Dunlop, 1981). Both parameters begin to rise in the first trimester, peak early in the second trimester, and are sustained through the remainder of gestation. Studies have suggested that progesterone is natriuretic and thus, increases in this hormone throughout pregnancy may be responsible for the enhanced urine output (Barron and Lindheimer, 1984). Likewise, elevations in aldosterone during pregnancy have been proposed as a mechanism for enhanced sodium reabsorption and prevention of excessive sodium filtration (Barron and Lindheimer, 1984).

Gastrointestinal Function

Pregnancy-related hormones, including progesterone, have been associated with a delay in gastric emptying and extended transit time in the intestinal tract. As a result, the bioavailability of drugs can be altered leading to shifts in the maximal concentrations and time to peak levels following oral administration (Parry et al., 1970). For example, pregnant women at 8—12 weeks of gestation exhibit lower maximal concentrations of acetaminophen and greater times to maximum concentrations compared with nonpregnant controls (Levy et al., 1994). Likewise, nausea and vomiting during early and late pregnancy can also alter drug absorption in intestines.

HEPATIC PHASE I ENZYMES

Cytochrome P450 Enzymes

Significant research across species has aimed to describe cytochrome P450 (CYP)/Cyp regulation during pregnancy (Table 9.1). Just under half of the 102 total mouse Cyp isoforms are enriched in the liver. In a large scale profiling of metabolic enzymes in maternal mouse livers between gestation days 7.5 and 19, Shuster et al. (2013) found a general downregulation of many important hepatic Cyp enzymes mRNA. Exceptions to this trend included the Cyp2d40, Cyp3a16, Cyp3a41 and 3a44, and Cyp17a1 genes, which were elevated in livers from pregnant mice (Shuster et al., 2013). There are several instances in which mouse and rat data have demonstrated similar directional changes (up- or downregulated) in Cyp mRNA and protein expression, such as the repression of Cyp1a2 and Cyp2e1, in dams from both species (Fortin et al., 2013; He et al., 2005, 2007; Koh et al., 2011; Walker et al., 2011). However, these widely used rodent models also exhibit conflicting data with regards to the regulation of bile acid—metabolizing enzymes, including Cyp7a1, 7b1, 8b1, and 27a1, during pregnancy (Aleksunes et al., 2012; Milona et al., 2010; Shuster et al., 2013; Zhu et al., 2013). Thus, when studying bile acid homeostasis during pregnancy, care should be taken in choosing the appropriate animal model.

Isoforms of the Cyp2 family, including 2c37 and 2c50, as well as Cyp3a11 were variably downregulated between gestation days 7 and 17 in pregnant mice (Fortin et al., 2013). The Cyp3a family was further examined during gestation in another study. Testosterone 6β

TABLE 9.1   Phase I Metabolism in Maternal Rodent Livers[a]

Enzyme	Mouse	Rat	Activity	References
CYTOCHROME P450s				
Cyp1a2	↓(M)	↓(P)	↓[b]	Fortin et al. (2013), He et al. (2005), Koh et al. (2011), and Walker et al. (2011)
Cyp2a1		↓(M)		He et al. (2007)
Cyp2a5	↔(M)			Koh et al. (2011)
Cyp2b1		↓(P)		He et al. (2005)
Cyp2b2		↓(P)		He et al. (2005)
Cyp2b9	↓(M)			Shuster et al. (2013)
Cyp2b10	↓↑(M)			Aleksunes et al. (2012), Fortin et al. (2013), and Koh et al. (2011)
Cyp2b13	↓(M)			Shuster et al. (2013)
Cyp2c6		↓(P)		He et al. (2005)
Cyp2c11		↓(M)		He et al. (2007)
Cyp2c37	↓(M)	↑(M)		Fortin et al. (2013), He et al. (2007), Koh et al. (2011), and Shuster et al. (2013)
Cyp2c50	↓(M)			Fortin et al. (2013) and Shuster et al. (2013)
Cyp2c54	↓(M)			Fortin et al. (2013) and Shuster et al. (2013)
Cyp2c55	↓(M)			Shuster et al. (2013)
Cyp2d			↑[c]	Topletz et al. (2013)
Cyp2d22/Cyp2d2	↓↑(M)	↓(M)		Fortin et al. (2013), He et al. (2007), Koh et al. (2011), Shuster et al. (2013), and Topletz et al. (2013)
Cyp2d9	↓↔(M)			Shuster et al. (2013) and Topletz et al. (2013)
Cyp2d10	↔(M)			Shuster et al. (2013) and Topletz et al. (2013)
Cyp2d11	↑(M)			Topletz et al. (2013)
Cyp2d13	↓(M)			Shuster et al. (2013)
Cyp2d23		↓(M)		He et al. (2007)
Cyp2d26	↔↑(M)			Shuster et al. (2013) and Topletz et al. (2013)
Cyp2d34	↓(M)			Shuster et al. (2013)
Cyp2d40	↑(M)			Ning et al. (2015), Shuster et al. (2013), and Topletz et al. (2013)
Cyp2e1	↓(M)	↓(M,P)		He et al. (2005, 2007) and Koh et al. (2011)
Cyp3a11	↓(M)			Aleksunes et al. (2012), Fortin et al. (2013), Koh et al. (2011), and Zhang et al. (2008)
Cyp3a13	↔↑(M)			Fortin et al. (2013) and Zhang et al. (2008)

(Continued)

TABLE 9.1   Phase I Metabolism in Maternal Rodent Livers[a]—cont'd

Enzyme	Mouse	Rat	Activity	References
Cyp3a16	↑(M)			Shuster et al. (2013) and Zhang et al. (2008)
Cyp3a25	↓(M)			Zhang et al. (2008)
Cyp3a41a/b	↑(M)			Koh et al. (2011), Shuster et al. (2013), and Zhang et al. (2008)
Cyp3a44	↑(M)			Shuster et al. (2013) and Zhang et al. (2008)
Cyp4a1		↓(P)		He et al. (2005)
Cyp4a12a/b	↓(M)			Shuster et al. (2013)
Cyp4a14	↓(M)			Aleksunes et al. (2012) and Shuster et al. (2013)
Cyp4a31	↑(M)			Shuster et al. (2013)
Cyp4f15	↓(M)			Shuster et al. (2013)
Cyp7a1	↑(M)	↔(M,P)		Aleksunes et al. (2012), Milona et al. (2010), and Zhu et al. (2013)
Cyp7b1	↔↑(M)	↔(M)		Aleksunes et al. (2012), Shuster et al. (2013), and Zhu et al. (2013)
Cyp8b1	↔↑(M)	↓(M)		Aleksunes et al. (2012), Milona et al. (2010), Shuster et al. (2013), and Zhu et al. (2013)
Cyp17a1	↑(M)			Shuster et al. (2013)
Cyp26a1	↑(M)		↑[d]	Shuster et al. (2013) and Topletz et al. (2013)
Cyp27a1	↓(M,P)	↔(M)		Aleksunes et al. (2012) and Zhu et al. (2013)
Cyp39a1	↓(M,P)			Aleksunes et al. (2012) and Shuster et al. (2013)
CARBOXYLESTERASES				
Ces1c	↔(M)			Fortin et al. (2013)
Ces1d	↓(M)			Fortin et al. (2013)
Ces1e	↔(M)			Fortin et al. (2013)
Ces1g	↔(M)			Fortin et al. (2013)
Ces2a	↓(M)			Fortin et al. (2013)
Ces2c	↔(M)			Fortin et al. (2013)
Ces2e	↔(M)			Fortin et al. (2013)
PARAOXONASES				
Pon1	↔(M)		↓[e]	Fortin et al. (2013)

[a]*Expression or activity compared with female, nonpregnant liver levels. mRNA expression (M), protein expression (P), and substrate activity are noted. ↑ denotes upregulation, ↓ denotes downregulation, and ↔ denotes no change.*
[b]*Substrate tested: caffeine, methoxyresorufin, and O-demethylation.*
[c]*Substrate tested: dextromethorphan as indicator.*
[d]*Substrate tested: atRA as indicator.*
[e]*Substrate tested: paraoxon, chlorpyrifos oxon.*

hydroxylation (an indicator of Cyp3a activity) was increased in S9 fractions prepared from livers of pregnant mice on gestation days 15 and 19 when compared with preparations from nonpregnant mice (Zhang et al., 2008). The authors of this study observed an overall enhancement of Cyp3a activity in maternal livers likely due to increases in Cyp3a16, 3a41, and 3a44 transcripts. By contrast, Cyp3a11, 3a13, and 3a25 exhibited reduced mRNA expression in pregnant mice. This differential pattern of gene expression was confirmed in a subsequent publication (Shuster et al., 2013).

Because of the inability to directly measure hepatic mRNA and protein expression in human pregnancies, changes to CYP enzyme activity have been inferred from alterations in the clearance of prototypical substrates in pregnant women (Table 9.2). Two of the earliest studies of human CYP activity in pregnancy occurred in 1983 and 1997, when different research groups observed increased metabolism of known specific CYP2D6 substrates metoprolol (Hogstedt et al., 1983) and dextromethorphan (Wadelius et al., 1997). In 2005, a study spanning multiple trimesters was performed in 25 pregnant patients and measured caffeine clearance, dextromethorphan O-, and N-demethylation as indicators of CYP1A2, 2D6, and 3A function, respectively (Tracy et al., 2005). The authors found decreased CYP1A2 activity but increased CYP2D6 and 3A activity throughout gestation, albeit at varying degrees in the different trimesters. In a later study, enhanced clearance of the hepatic CYP3A substrate midazolam was confirmed in a small patient population (13 women) at 28–32 weeks of gestation (Hebert et al., 2008). Data from these various patient-based studies are being applied to physiologically based pharmacokinetic models to predict disposition of key metabolic CYP enzymes to better select drug dosages for pregnant women. Models that have been created thus far address changes to CYP1A2, CYP2B6, CYP2C9, CYP2C19, CYP2D6, and CYP3A4 metabolism during pregnancy (Gaohua et al., 2012; Ke et al., 2013, 2014; Quinney et al., 2012). Care should be taken when extrapolating prototypical substrate data to a specific CYP isoform, as multiple isoforms, enzymes, as well as transporters and other physiological changes may contribute to observed differences in the disposition of a particular drug during pregnancy.

In addition to studies using probe substrates, the altered pharmacokinetic profiles of a number of psychiatric medications have been attributed to changes in CYP-mediated metabolism during pregnancy. The antidepressant fluoxetine is often prescribed to pregnant women. Fluoxetine is metabolized to norfluoxetine, an active metabolite, by CYP2D6 demethylation. Pharmacokinetic analysis has revealed that the ratio of norfluoxetine-to-fluoxetine is increased over twofold in late pregnancy, which may be due to enhanced CYP2D6 metabolism (Heikkinen et al., 2003; Sit et al., 2010). Similarly, enhanced metabolism of citalopram and sertraline antidepressants during pregnancy has been observed in pregnant women

TABLE 9.2 Functional Changes in Activity of CYPs in Maternal Human Liver

Enzyme	Change	Clinical Pharmacokinetics	References
CYP1A2	Decrease	Caffeine	Tracy et al. (2005)
CYP2D6[a]	Increase	Dextromethorphan O-demethylation	Tracy et al. (2005) and Wadelius et al. (1997)
CYP3A	Increase	Dextromethorphan N-demethylation, midazolam	Hebert et al. (2008) and Tracy et al. (2005)

[a]Genotype specific—poor metabolizers excluded.

(Sit et al., 2008). The interaction between pregnancy and CYP2D6 genotype has also been investigated in women prescribed paroxetine for major depression (Ververs et al., 2009). In women who were extensive or ultra-rapid CYP2D6 metabolizers, pregnancy decreased circulating paroxetine concentrations, whereas levels increased in poor and intermediate metabolizers (Ververs et al., 2009). In situations where levels of antidepressant concentrations are reduced in pregnant women, it may be critical to assess patient symptoms and consider increases in dose.

Recently, humanized mice have been generated to help study the mechanisms behind alterations in human-relevant drug metabolism during pregnancy. One particular method for creating a humanized mouse is producing a transgenic mouse line by microinjection of DNA into a fertilized egg. In this model, the transgene will subsequently be incorporated into the mouse genome. Work completed by one research group using this transgenic mouse model suggests that increased clearance of CYP2D6 substrates in pregnancy could be due to repression of the transcription factor small heterodimer partner (SHP). This event led to potentiation of hepatic nuclear factor 4-alpha recruitment to the *CYP2D6* promoter region (Koh et al., 2014a,b). The authors have also shown that subcutaneous injection of transgenic mice with 10 mg/kg 17α-ethinylestradiol for 5 days, a model of maternal cholestasis, attenuated the induction of CYP2D6 enzymatic activity observed in normal pregnancy (Pan and Jeong, 2015). An earlier study showed upregulation of the mouse homolog of CYP2D6, Cyp2d22, and overall Cyp2d activity in pregnancy (Topletz et al., 2013), similar to reports observed in humans. It is worthwhile to note that other groups have reported conflicting data in the same FVB strain in addition to C57BL/6 mice that show a decrease in Cyp2d22 mRNA in pregnant mice (Fortin et al., 2013; Koh et al., 2011; Shuster et al., 2013) and Cyp2d2 in pregnant rats (He et al., 2007).

Carboxylesterase and Paraoxanase Enzymes

The expression of liver carboxylesterase (Ces) enzymes throughout gestation has been explored in mice (Table 9.1). Many of these enzymes play critical roles in the hepatic metabolism of pesticides, particularly organophosphate pesticides. Organophosphate pesticides are environmentally persistent, and metabolites have been detected in blood and urine samples from pregnant women in the United States (Woodruff et al., 2011). In mice, Ces2a mRNA expression was significantly reduced by 50% up to gestation day 14 (Fortin et al., 2013). Although Ces1d and 1e showed early decreases in expression, neither change was sustained across multiple gestational time points. Though expression and activity profiles of organophosphate metabolism throughout gestation have not been determined in rats, studies have shown that dosing pregnant rats (gestation days 14–18) with the organophosphate pesticide chlorpyrifos reduces Ces activity in the maternal liver (Lassiter et al., 1998). It is interesting to note that for paraoxanase 1 (Pon1), activity studies in pregnant mice were conducted in parallel to mRNA profiling. Although no significant changes were observed in hepatic Pon1 mRNA expression, a 43% and 37% reduction in serum Pon1 activity toward substrates paraoxon and chlorpyrifos oxon, respectively, occurred on gestation day 14 (Fortin et al., 2013). Thus, it is important to be mindful that hepatic expression level data do not always correlate with overall enzyme activity, and vice versa.

Oseltamivir is an antiviral drug that is administered as a prodrug and requires cleavage by Ces enzymes to oseltamivir carboxylate (Shi et al., 2006). Pharmacokinetic studies have demonstrated that blood levels of the active carboxylate metabolite of oseltamivir were reduced in pregnant women due to enhanced clearance and volume of distribution (Beigi et al., 2011). A subsequent population pharmacokinetic study with a larger sample size confirmed a 30% reduction in the systemic exposure of oseltamivir carboxylate during pregnancy (Pillai et al., 2015). The fact that the pharmacokinetic profile of oseltamivir was unchanged led the authors to propose that CES1 activity was not altered during pregnancy and that enhanced excretion into urine may be due to changes in glomerular filtration and renal secretion (Beigi et al., 2011).

HEPATIC PHASE II ENZYMES

Phase II enzyme families including the UDP-glucuronosyltransferases (Ugts), glutathione S-transferases (Gsts), and sulfotransferases (Sults) conjugate endobiotics and xenobiotics with cofactors such as glucuronic acid, glutathione, or sulfate, respectively, to enhance their excretion. Conjugated metabolites tend to be less pharmacologically active and more polar than parent compounds, which prevents their diffusion across cellular membranes and facilitates their transporter-mediated excretion into bile (Xu et al., 2005). Early studies looking to understand adaptive molecular signaling during pregnancy examined expression profiles of genes encoding phases I and II drug-metabolizing enzymes in pregnant rats treated with pharmacological activators of nuclear receptors, namely phenobarbital and pregnenolone-16 alpha-carbonitrile (Ejiri et al., 2005a,b). However, the data gathered from these studies need to be interpreted cautiously, as the gene expression profiles were generated in response to potent agonists, rather than focusing on pregnancy-related changes. Only recently have gene and protein expression of phase II enzymes throughout gestation been explored in pregnant mice and rats (Table 9.3).

Ugts

Ugt enzymes are responsible for the glucuronidation and elimination of various chemicals, drugs, and toxins. To examine the expression of conjugation enzymes and their potential regulatory transcription factors during pregnancy, Wen et al. (2013) utilized time-matched virgin and pregnant mice and found a significant and global down-regulation of Ugt mRNA expression during mid-to-late gestation (gestation days 11−17) (Wen et al., 2013). Interestingly, Ugt1a5 was the only member of the Ugt family to be significantly induced, with an mRNA increase of 50−100% during gestation when compared with virgin controls. It was suggested that elevated estradiol levels during pregnancy may be one of the factors responsible for Ugt1a5 induction, since estradiol can directly stimulate Ugt1a5 transcription (Chen et al., 2009). Although protein levels of Ugt1a1, 1a9, and 2b34 remained unaltered during gestation, protein expression of Ugt1a6 decreased in pregnant mice by 40% (Wen et al., 2013). A corresponding reduction of in vitro glucuronidation of bisphenol A in S9 fractions obtained from pregnant mouse livers was comparable with changes reported in microsomes generated from pregnant rat livers, indicating conserved adaptive responses in glucuronidation between species during pregnancy (Matsumoto et al., 2002; Wen et al., 2013).

TABLE 9.3   Phase II Metabolism in Maternal Rodent Livers[a]

Enzyme	Mouse	Rat	References
UDP-GLUCURONOSYLTRANSFERASES			
Ugt1a1	↓↔(M,P)	↔↓(M,P)	Luquita et al. (2001) and Wen et al. (2013)
Ugt1a5	↑(M)	↔↓(M,P)	Luquita et al. (2001) and Wen et al. (2013)
Ugt1a6	↓(M,P)	↔↓(M,P)	Luquita et al. (2001) and Wen et al. (2013)
Ugt1a9	↓↔(M,P)		Wen et al. (2013)
Ugt2a3	↓(M)		Wen et al. (2013)
Ugt2b1	↓(M)	↔↓(M,P)	Luquita et al. (2001) and Wen et al. (2013)
Ugt2b5	↔(M)		Wen et al. (2013)
Ugt2b34	↓↔(M,P)		Wen et al. (2013)
Ugt2b35	↓(M)		Wen et al. (2013)
SULFOTRANSFERASES			
Sult1a1	↑(M,P)	↓(M)	Wen et al. (2013)
Sult1c2		↓(M)	He et al. (2007)
Sult1d1	↓(M)		Shuster et al. (2013) and Wen et al. (2013)
Sult2a1	↑↔(M,P)		Wen et al. (2013)
Sult2a2	↑↔(M,P)		Wen et al. (2013)
Sult3a1	↑(M)		Wen et al. (2013)
GLUTATHIONE S-TRANSFERASES			
Gsta1	↓↔(M,P)		Wen et al. (2013)
Gsta2		↓(M)	He et al. (2007)
Gsta4	↓↔(M,P)		Wen et al. (2013)
Gstm2	↑(M)		Wen et al. (2013)
Gstm3		↓(M)	He et al. (2007)
Gstp1	↓(M)		Wen et al. (2013)
Gstt1		↓(M)	He et al. (2007)
Gstt2		↓(M)	He et al. (2007)

[a]*Expression or activity compared with female nonpregnant liver levels. mRNA expression (M) and protein expression (P) are noted. Data were not available for substrate activity. ↑ denotes upregulation, ↓ denotes downregulation, and ↔ denotes no change.*

Similar to mice, pregnant rats exhibit a down-regulation of microsomal protein levels of all Ugt1 isoforms as well as Ugt2b1 on gestation days 19 and 20 (Luquita et al., 2001). Accordingly, glucuronidation rates for *p*-nitrophenol, bilirubin, and ethynylestradiol were all decreased in UDP-*N*-acetylglucosamine-activated microsomes, similar to the reduction observed in other rodent models (Luquita et al., 2001; Matsumoto et al., 2002; Wen et al., 2013). Interestingly, no change in the mRNA expression of Ugt1 isoforms was observed, suggesting that these enzymes may be regulated posttranscriptionally in pregnant rats or that changes in transcription occurred at earlier time points. Altogether, a general pattern of reduction of Ugt1 and Ugt2 family expression occurs in the liver during pregnancy.

Clinically, evidence suggests that increases in glucuronidation during pregnancy can alter the pharmacokinetics of medications. For example, the clearance of the antiepileptic drug lamotrigine is increased significantly in the second and third trimester (Tran et al., 2002) with maximal clearance observed at 32 gestational weeks (de Haan et al., 2004; Pennell et al., 2004). Clearance of lamotrigine returns to baseline levels by 3 weeks after parturition (Fotopoulou et al., 2009). A pharmacokinetic investigation has demonstrated that the plasma ratio of lamotrigine-2-N-glucuronide to lamotrigine is 175% higher in the third trimester (Ohman et al., 2008). This elevation has been attributed to increases in UGT expression and activity (Chen et al., 2009), although roles for altered distribution and renal clearance have also been proposed (Reimers et al., 2011). Increases in the frequency of seizures have been noted during pregnancy and attributed to altered pharmacokinetics of antiepileptic drugs (Reisinger et al., 2013), leading to the development of pregnancy-specific treatment guidelines that include dose escalations (Sabers, 2012).

Gsts

Gst enzymes serve to protect cellular macromolecules against products of oxidative stress and electrophiles by conjugating compounds with glutathione and enhancing their excretion. In addition to identifying alterations in Ugt family expression, one study examined the effect of pregnancy on hepatic Gst expression and found a similar trend of phase II enzyme downregulation in livers of pregnant mice (Wen et al., 2013). Specifically, Gstp1 mRNA decreased on gestation day 7, whereas Gsta1 and Gsta4 mRNAs were reduced from gestation days 14−17 in maternal mouse livers. Interestingly, during early gestation (day 7), the expression levels of Gstm2 mRNA increased before returning to control levels during mid-to-late gestation (Wen et al., 2013). Likewise, investigation of the expression of Gsts in maternal rat livers revealed the same trend of Gst down-regulation during late gestation as mRNA levels of Gstb2, t1, t2, and m3 all declined (He et al., 2007). The parallels between the expression of phase II enzymes in different rodent species are encouraging for the extrapolation of results between studies and may have potential for translating to humans.

Sults

Important in hormone metabolism and regulation, Sults are cytosolic enzymes that exhibit gender-specific expression patterns regulated by the presence or absence of certain sex hormones. As a result, Sults are also affected by hormonal changes that occur throughout pregnancy. Our laboratory has demonstrated the induction of Sult1a1, 2a1, 2a2, and 3a1 mRNAs between 100% and 500% in maternal mouse livers at various stages of gestation (Wen et al., 2013). Conversely, during late stages of pregnancy, mRNA expression of Sult1d1 diminished by 40−60%. Consistent with the up-regulation of its mRNA, Sult1a1 exhibited a corresponding increase in protein expression, which correlated to enhanced functional activity in the sulfation of acetaminophen. Acetaminophen-sulfate formation in liver S9 fractions increased by 20–40% on gestation days 14 and 17, signifying greater enzymatic activity of Sult1a1. Remarkably, investigation of Sult expression in a pregnant rat model revealed potential species differences, such that Sult1a1 and Sult1c2 mRNA were down-regulated on gestation day 19 (He et al., 2007). Although these two Sult isoforms were reduced in pregnant rat livers, no data were provided to determine whether these changes altered protein expression or function.

Taken together, regulation of phase II enzyme expression during pregnancy is fairly complex and governed by a variety of signaling mechanisms. It is becoming more apparent that sex-specific hormone secretion plays a significant role in regulating phase II enzymes. Sex divergent expression of phase II drug metabolizing enzymes, such as Ugt1a1, 1a5, and 2b1, in livers is observed in response to differential levels of growth hormone secretion between males and females (Buckley and Klaassen, 2009).

HEPATIC TRANSPORTERS

Although some data in humans regarding the activity of phases I and II enzymes during pregnancy exist, little to no data has been specifically generated quantifying changes in hepatic transporter expression or function. Nonetheless, several key studies have been completed in rodents aimed at characterizing gestation-specific regulation of hepatic transport systems (Table 9.4).

Solute Carrier (SLC) Transporters

The liver highly expresses several important xenobiotic, organic anion, and cation uptake transporters. These include the organic anion transporter (OAT), organic cation transporter (OCT), and organic anion transporting polypeptide (OATP) families. These transporters mediate the uptake of numerous different classes of drugs into hepatocytes, including antibiotics, antidepressants, antifungals, antivirals, diuretics, and statins. In addition, they absorb important endogenous compounds, such as pregnancy hormones and their conjugates including estrone-3-sulfate (OATP1A2, OATP1B1, OAT2) and estradiol 17β-glucuronide (OATP1B1, OATP1B3) (reviewed in Klaassen and Aleksunes, 2010). Only the mRNA of Oat2 has been shown to be up-regulated during pregnancy in mice (Aleksunes et al., 2012). In agreement among rodent models, the Na^+-taurocholate-cotransporting polypeptide (Ntcp), Oatp1a4, and Oatp1b2 transporters were repressed in pregnancy (Aleksunes et al., 2012; Shuster et al., 2013; Zhu et al., 2013). Though the overall suppression of hepatic uptake may protect the liver from exposure to toxic substances in the blood during pregnancy, translational in vitro studies need to be completed to determine if this adaptive response also occurs in the human liver during pregnancy.

ATP-Binding Cassette Transporters

In hepatocytes, ATP-binding cassette (ABC) transporters localize to the sinusoidal (basolateral) membrane, where they pump substrates back into the blood, or to the canalicular

TABLE 9.4 Transporters in Maternal Rodent Livers[a]

Transporter	Mouse	Rat	References
UPTAKE TRANSPORTERS			
Slc10a1/Ntcp	↓(M,P)	↓(M)	Aleksunes et al. (2012), Milona et al. (2010), Shuster et al. (2013), and Zhu et al. (2013)
Slc17a1/Npt1	↓(M)		Shuster et al. (2013)
Slc22a1/Oct1	↓(M,P)		Aleksunes et al. (2012) and Lee et al. (2013)
Slc22a7/Oat2	↑(M)		Aleksunes et al. (2012)
Slc29a1/Ent1	↓(M)		Aleksunes et al. (2012)
Slc47a1/Mate1	↓↔(M,P)		Aleksunes et al. (2012), Lee et al. (2013), Shuster et al. (2013)
Slco1a1/Oatp1a1	↔(M)	↓(M)	Aleksunes et al. (2012) and Zhu et al. (2013)
Slco1a4/Oatp1a4	↓(M)	↓(M)	Aleksunes et al. (2012), Milona et al. (2010), Shuster et al. (2013), and Zhu et al. (2013)
Slco1b2/Oatp1b2	↓(M)	↓(M)	Aleksunes et al. (2012), Shuster et al. (2013), and Zhu et al. (2013)
Slco2b1/Oatp2b1	↔(M)		Aleksunes et al. (2012)
EFFLUX TRANSPORTERS			
Abca1	↓↔(M)		Aleksunes et al. (2012, 2013) and Shuster et al. (2013)
Abca8a	↓(M)		Shuster et al. (2013)
Abcb1/Mdr1	↓↔(P)		Aleksunes et al. (2013) and Zhang et al. (2008)
Abcb1a/Mdr1a	↓↔(M)		Aleksunes et al. (2013), Milona et al. (2010), Shuster et al. (2013), and Zhang et al. (2008)
Abcb1b/Mdr1b	↔(M)		Zhang et al. (2008)
Abcb4/Mdr2	↓(M)		Aleksunes et al. (2012)
Abcb11/Bsep	↓↔(M,P)	↔(M)	Aleksunes et al. (2012, 2013), Milona et al. (2010), and Zhu et al. (2013)
Abcc1/Mrp1	↔(M)		Aleksunes et al. (2013)
Abcc2/Mrp2	↓↔(M,P)		Aleksunes et al. (2012, 2013)
Abcc3/Mrp3	↓↔(M,P)	↓(M)	Aleksunes et al. (2012, 2013), Milona et al. (2010), Shuster et al. (2013), and Zhu et al. (2013)
Abcc4/Mrp4	↔↑(M,P)	↓(M)	Aleksunes et al. (2012, 2013) and Zhu et al. (2013)
Abcc5/Mrp5	↔(M,P)		Aleksunes et al. (2013)
Abcc6/Mrp6	↓(M,P)		Aleksunes et al. (2012, 2013) and Shuster et al. (2013)
Abcg2/Bcrp	↓↔(M,P)	↓(M)	Aleksunes et al. (2012, 2013) and Zhu et al. (2013)

(Continued)

TABLE 9.4   Transporters in Maternal Rodent Livers[a]—cont'd

Transporter	Mouse	Rat	References
Abcg5	↓ ↔ (M)		Aleksunes et al. (2012, 2013) and Shuster et al. (2013)
Abcg8	↓ ↔ (M)		Aleksunes et al. (2012, 2013) and Shuster et al. (2013)
Atp8b1	↓ (M)		Aleksunes et al. (2012)

[a]*Expression or activity compared with female, nonpregnant liver levels. mRNA expression (M), protein expression (P), and substrate activity are noted. Data were not available for substrate activity. ↑ denotes upregulation, ↓ denotes downregulation, and ↔ denotes no change.*

(apical) membrane, where they extrude substances into the bile. Similar to the SLC transporters, a global down-regulation of efflux transporter expression has been identified in pregnant mice at different time points of gestation spanning days 11—17 (Aleksunes et al., 2012; Shuster et al., 2013; Song et al., 2014). Notably, multidrug resistance—associated protein 3 (Mrp3) mRNA, protein, as well as protein localization to the sinusoidal membrane are all significantly reduced on gestation day 17 (Aleksunes et al., 2012). In addition, gene expression of the multidrug resistance protein 2 (Mdr2), Mrp2, Mrp6, and Abcg5/8 are reduced across multiple gestational days from 11 to 17. Though these data have been explored to a greater extent in mice, decreases in gene expression of Mrp3, Mrp4, and the breast cancer resistance protein (Bcrp) have also been observed in pregnant rats (Zhu et al., 2013). Although many of these transporters, including members of the Mdr and Mrp families, export xenobiotics, they also excrete endogenous substances critical for maintaining pregnancy and fetal growth, such as steroid hormones and cholesterol. A reduction in expression of ABC transporters may be physiologically relevant in pregnancy in order to retain nutrients during a state of high nutritional demand.

NUCLEAR RECEPTORS

During pregnancy, changes in hormone levels and lipid metabolism allow for the proper development of the fetoplacental unit. Elevated levels of female sex steroid hormones, such as progesterone and estradiol, may affect the activity of their cognate hepatic nuclear receptors, which in turn control physiological processes such as metabolism and development (Papacleovoulou et al., 2011; Wen et al., 2013). Nuclear receptors are separated into two groups consisting of endocrine nuclear receptors and orphan nuclear receptors. The endocrine nuclear receptor family, which includes the estrogen, thyroid, glucocorticoid, and progesterone receptors, is activated by hormonal lipids. The orphan nuclear receptor family consists of the farnesoid X receptor (FXR), constitutive androstane receptor (CAR), pregnane X receptor (PXR), liver X receptor (LXR) and peroxisome proliferator—activated receptor (PPAR), which act as lipid sensors. Although endocrine nuclear receptors homodimerize to form active complexes, orphan nuclear receptors generally heterodimerize with the retinoid X receptor (RXR) (reviewed in Xu et al., 2005). Once activated these receptors can induce downstream target genes, including drug metabolizing enzymes, transporters, and additional transcriptional regulatory networks.

Hepatic phases I and II enzymes are transcriptionally cross-regulated by nuclear receptors CAR, FXR, PXR, PPAR, and RXR as well as other transcription factors, including the aryl hydrocarbon receptor and nuclear factor e2−related factor 2 (Papacleovoulou et al., 2011; Waxman, 1999; Wen et al., 2013). In maternal mouse livers, the mRNA expression of Car, Pxr, and Pparα was decreased on gestation days 14 and 17, coinciding with the decline in mRNA expression of Ugts and Gsts (Wen et al., 2013). Similarly, the mRNA and protein expression of Cyp2b10 and Cyp4a14, prototypical targets of Car and Pparα, respectively, were decreased 60−90% when compared with virgin controls. Interestingly, the mRNA of Cyp3a11, a target gene of Pxr was downregulated by 40% on gestational day 17. However, no change in protein expression was observed. Another study looking to explore an observed increase in serum triglyceride and cholesterol levels during the third trimester of pregnancy similarly found a significant decrease in mRNA expression of numerous nuclear receptors in mouse livers on gestation day 19. Specifically, Pparα, β, and γ; Lxrα and β; Fxr; and Rxrα, β, and γ mRNA levels were all profoundly reduced along with several of their target genes such as acyl-CoA oxidase (Ppar), sterol regulatory element−binding protein 1c (Lxr), and Shp (Fxr) (Sweeney et al., 2006). To examine the potential role of hormones in these regulatory changes, the expression of estrogen receptor alpha (Erα) mRNA was quantified on gestational days 14 and 17 and was significantly induced by 200−400% in maternal mouse livers (Wen et al., 2013). The induction of Erα along with elevated levels of sex hormones during pregnancy may act in coordination to regulate the expression and/or activity of other nuclear receptors. It has been shown in primary mouse hepatocytes that Cyp2b10 is induced by estradiol and repressed by progesterone (Kawamoto et al., 2000). As a result, estradiol and progesterone signaling may be responsible for regulating expression of nuclear receptors that in turn modulate levels of various metabolic enzymes during pregnancy.

HORMONAL REGULATION

During pregnancy, altered elimination rates of various drugs suggest that adaptive molecular changes associated with gestation strongly influence phase I and II metabolizing enzymes. Although the underlying mechanisms responsible for altered metabolism remain largely undetermined, physiological changes, including rising hormone concentrations in maternal blood, have been examined as contributing factors. The ability of individual hormones to regulate drug metabolism has been supported by gender-specific differences in the elimination rates of CYP substrates in human females when compared with males (reviewed in Jeong, 2010). Likewise, oral contraceptives elicit a similar effect on CYP enzyme activities to those seen during pregnancy, further supporting the critical involvement of hormones as modifiers of metabolism (McGready et al., 2003).

Estrogen

In pregnant women, levels of estrogens consistently increase until peaking prior to parturition. Circulating 17β-estradiol levels can reach 0.1 μM concentrations at term, ∼100-fold greater than pre-gestational levels (Jeong, 2010). Such high concentrations of a potent hormone may activate and/or repress nuclear receptors, which in turn influence the expression and activity of hepatic drug-metabolizing enzymes.

A number of rodent models have been used to examine the effects of estrogens on the expression profiles of hepatic Cyp enzymes (Table 9.5). A study by Choi et al. (2011) examined the expression and activity levels of phase I enzymes in female rats treated with a subcutaneous injection of 1 mg/kg/day estradiol benzoate or known Cyp inducers. The authors found that after 5 days of treatment, estradiol increased the mRNA expression of Cyp1a2 as well as several isoforms of the Cyp2 family, specifically c6, c7, and c12 (Choi et al., 2011). This finding was consistent with the up-regulation of Cyp2b9 and b10 mRNA expression in primary mouse hepatocytes after estradiol treatment, showing directionally similar changes in orthologs between two rodent species (Nemoto and Sakurai, 1995). Studies also showed that estradiol influences the Cyp3 family, as induction of Cyp3a9 and repression of Cyp3a1 mRNA expression were observed in female nonpregnant rats treated with this hormone (Choi et al., 2011). To explore a potential pathway regulating these enzymes in estradiol-treated rats, the expression of hepatic nuclear receptors, Pxr and Car, was also quantified, and a reduction in expression was observed. In another study conducted to explore any potential species differences between humans and rodents, Choi et al. (2013) treated primary human hepatocytes with estradiol and determined the effects on the expression of various CYP isoforms. Primary human hepatocytes, obtained from five different donors, showed a concentration-dependent induction of CYP2A6, CYP2B6, and CYP3A4 mRNA expression following estradiol treatment that was comparable to CITCO, an inducer of P450 expression via the CAR pathway (Choi et al., 2013). This was consistent with findings from other research groups who also identified the induction of aforementioned CYP isoforms in primary human hepatocytes (Choi et al., 2013; Dickmann and Isoherranen, 2013; Higashi et al., 2007; Koh et al., 2012). In addition, estradiol treatment of primary human hepatocytes resulted in the activation and nuclear translocation of CAR, suggesting translatability of results generated in pregnant rodent models (Koh et al., 2012). Interestingly, with estradiol treatment, there was an increased hydroxylation of diclofenac and p-nitrophenol—indicators of CYP2C9 and CYP2E1 activity, respectively—that did not correlate with changes in mRNA expression (Choi et al., 2013). The variable induction and activity of CYP enzymes suggest the involvement of other hormones, in this regulatory pathway, as well as yet to be determined factors associated with pregnancy.

To assess the influence of estradiol on the expression of phase II metabolizing enzymes (Table 9.6), Chen et al. (2009) treated human HepG2 hepatoma cells transfected to express ERα with exogenous estradiol for 24 hours. There was an up-regulation of UGT1A4 mRNA expression in ERα-overexpressing cells, while no change in mRNA levels was observed in cells transfected with an empty vector, highlighting the importance of specific nuclear receptors in hormonal regulation (Chen et al., 2009). Estradiol treatment also influenced enzymatic activity of UGT1A4, as levels of glucuronidated lamotrigine increased threefold in ERα-transfected HepG2 cells when compared with controls. Though induction of UGT1A4 was seen in response to estradiol, other major UGT isoforms, such as UGT1A1 and UGT2B7, were not affected (Chen et al., 2009; Jeong et al., 2008). Still estradiol has been demonstrated to upregulate different phase II enzymes in addition to the UGT family, such as SULT2A1. Li et al. (2014) showed that estradiol increased the mRNA and protein levels of SULT2A1 in primary human hepatocytes as well as HepG2-ERα-expressing cells

TABLE 9.5 Estrogen Regulation of Phase I Metabolism[a]

Enzyme	Mouse	Rat	Human	References
CYTOCHROME P450s				
Cyp1a2/CYP1A2		↑(M)	↓(M)	Choi et al. (2011) and Jeong (2010)
CYP2A6			↑(M)	Choi et al. (2013), Higashi et al. (2007), and Jeong (2010)
Cyp2b1		↔(M)		Choi et al. (2011)
CYP2B6			↑(M)	Choi et al. (2013), Dickmann and Isoherranen (2013), Jeong (2010), and Koh et al. (2012)
Cyp2b9	↑(M)			Nemoto and Sakurai (1995)
Cyp2b10	↑(M)			Nemoto and Sakurai (1995)
Cyp2c6		↑(M)		Choi et al. (2011)
Cyp2c7		↑(M)		Choi et al. (2011)
CYP2C8			↔(M)	Choi et al. (2013)
CYP2C9			↔(M,P)	Choi et al. (2013)
Cyp2c12		↑(M)		Choi et al. (2011)
CYP2C19			↔(M)	Choi et al. (2013)
Cyp2d2		↔(M)		Choi et al. (2011)
CYP2D6			↔(M)	Choi et al. (2013)
Cyp2e1/CYP2E1		↔(M,P)	↔(M,P)	Choi et al. (2011, 2013)
Cyp3a1		↓(M,P)		Choi et al. (2011)
CYP3A4			↑(M)	Choi et al. (2013) and Jeong (2010)
Cyp3a9		↑(M)		Choi et al. (2011)
Cyp3a41	↑(M)			Sakuma et al. (2002)
Cyp3a44	↑(M)			Sakuma et al. (2002)
Cyp4a10	↓(M)			Zhang and Klaassen (2013)
Cyp4a12a	↑(M)			Zhang and Klaassen (2013)
Cyp4a12b	↑(M)			Zhang and Klaassen (2013)
Cyp4a14	↓(M)			Zhang and Klaassen (2013)
PARAOXONASES				
Pon1	↓(M)			Cheng and Klaassen (2012)

[a]*Expression or activity compared with female nonpregnant liver levels. mRNA expression (M), protein expression (P), and substrate activity are noted. Data were not available for substrate activity. ↑ denotes upregulation, ↓ denotes downregulation, and ↔ denotes no change. Listed studies used estradiol as a form of estrogen.*

TABLE 9.6   Estrogen Regulation of Phase II Metabolism[a]

Enzyme	Mouse	Rat	Human	References
UDP-GLUCURONOSYLTRANSFERASES				
UGT1A1			↔(M)	Jeong et al. (2008)
UGT1A4			↑(M)	Chen et al. (2009)
UGT2B7			↔(M)	Jeong et al. (2008)
SULFOTRANSFERASES				
Sult1a1/SULT1A1	↔(M)		↑(M)	Alnouti and Klaassen (2011) and Li et al. (2014)
Sult1d1	↔(M)			Alnouti and Klaassen (2011)
Sult2a1/a2	↑(M)			Alnouti and Klaassen (2011)
Sult3a1	↑(M)			Alnouti and Klaassen (2011)
Sult1c1	↔(M)			Alnouti and Klaassen (2011)

[a]*Expression or activity compared with female nonpregnant liver levels. mRNA expression (M), protein expression (P), and substrate activity are noted. Data were not available for substrate activity. ↑ denotes upregulation, ↓ denotes downregulation, and ↔ denotes no change. Listed studies used estradiol, estriol, or estrone as forms of estrogen.*

treated with estradiol. The levels of induction were comparable to rifampicin, a known inducer of SULT2A1 expression via PXR, thus exemplifying the degree of regulatory influence of estradiol on phase II enzymes (Li et al., 2014).

One of the few studies exploring the effect of hormones on drug transporter expression (Table 9.7) involved administration of 3 µg/g body weight/day of 17β-estradiol for 5 days to Erα-deficient mice. 17β-estradiol-treated mice exhibited a 2-fold enhancement of hepatic

TABLE 9.7   Estrogen Regulation of Transporters[a]

Enzyme	Mouse	Rat	References
UPTAKE TRANSPORTERS			
Ntcp		↓(M)	Simon et al. (2004)
Slco1a1/Oatp1a1	↔(M)	↓(M,P)	Cheng et al. (2006) and Geier et al. (2003)
Slco1a4/Oatp1a4	↓(M)	↓(M,P)	Cheng et al. (2006) and Geier et al. (2003)
Slco1b2/Oatp1b2		↓(M,P)	Geier et al. (2003)
EFFLUX TRANSPORTERS			
Abca1	↑(M)		Srivastava (2002)
Abcg2/Bcrp	↔(M)		Tanaka et al. (2005)
Mrp2		↑(M)	Simon et al. (2006)

[a]*Expression or activity compared with female nonpregnant liver levels. mRNA expression (M), protein expression (P), and substrate activity are noted. Data were not available for human expression or substrate activity. ↑ denotes upregulation, ↓ denotes downregulation, and ↔ denotes no change. Listed studies used estradiol as a form of estrogen.*

Abca1 mRNA, and the authors proposed a compensatory role of Erβ in this regulation (Srivastava, 2002). Similarly, the mRNA expression of another Abc transporter, Mrp2, was induced in intact male rats in response to estradiol. However, the same treatment had no effect on the Mrp2 mRNA level in intact female rats, suggesting a possible involvement of growth hormone secretory pattern, which differs between sexes (Simon et al., 2006). Exploring the influence of estradiol on the Ntcp transporter, Simon et al. (2004) showed a significant reduction of Ntcp mRNA in male rats injected with 100 μg/kg body weight/day of estradiol daily for 7 days and a dramatic increase in levels of Ntcp mRNA in female rats that underwent an ovariectomy (Simon et al., 2004). Thus, estrogen effectively downregulated the expression of Ntcp. Investigating the effect of estrogen on solute carrier transporters, Geier et al. (2003) observed a significant decrease of basolateral Oatp1a1 (Oatp1), Oatp1a4 (Oatp2), and Oatp1b2 (Oatp4) at the mRNA and protein level in rats treated with ethinylestradiol, a synthetic estrogen, at a dose of 5 mg/kg (Geier et al., 2003). These results correlated with a reduction of Ntcp, Oatp1a4, Mrp2, Mrp3, and Mrp6 expression seen in maternal rodent livers during late pregnancy (Aleksunes et al., 2012; Arrese et al., 2003; Cao et al., 2002; Simon et al., 2006).

Progesterone

Progesterone is a steroid hormone that is involved in the regulation of ovulation and menstruation. As in the case of estrogen, concentrations of progesterone in maternal blood steadily rise during gestation until reaching a peak concentration of 1 μM at term (Jeong, 2010). Due to such a high concentration, progesterone is thought to have the ability to influence hepatic drug metabolizing enzyme expression through nuclear receptors.

To determine the effect of progesterone on the expression profiles of CYP enzymes, Choi et al. (2013) exposed primary human hepatocytes to progesterone for 72 hours. Hormone treatment increased the mRNA expression of CYP2A6, 2B6, 2C8, 3A4, and 3A5 in a concentration-dependent manner. Although there was overlap of CYP mRNA induction between estradiol and progesterone, the patterns of expression were different. That is, while estradiol treatment elicited the greatest enhancement of the CYP isoform 2B6, progesterone showed predominant induction of CYP3A4 mRNA. In addition to their cognate receptors, ER and PR, respectively, estradiol and progesterone were proposed to activate nuclear receptors involved in regulating drug-metabolizing enzymes and transporters. For example, estradiol has been shown to activate CAR and not PXR, whereas progesterone is an activator of PXR and not CAR (Choi et al., 2013). Thus, it is likely that differential effect of hormones in terms of their regulation of phase I enzyme expression is linked, in part, to the types of nuclear receptors activated.

To elucidate whether progesterone has a role in regulating phase II enzymes (Table 9.8), such as UGT1A1 and UGT2B7, Jeong et al. (2008) generated luciferase constructs containing various regions of the human *UGT1A1* promoter cotransfected with ER or PXR into HepG2 cells (Jeong et al., 2008). Progesterone treatment induced the luciferase activity of UGT1A1 by approximately 8-fold in the presence of PXR, whereas estrogen showed no observable induction. A similar experiment conducted with promoter region constructs of the *UGT2B7* gene cotransfected with the aforementioned nuclear receptors exhibited no

TABLE 9.8 Progesterone Regulation of Phase II Metabolism[a]

Enzyme	Human	References
UDP-GLUCURONOSYLTRANSFERASES		
UGT1A1	↑(M)	Jeong et al. (2008)
UGT2B7	↔(M)	Jeong et al. (2008)

[a]*Expression or activity compared with female nonpregnant liver levels. mRNA expression (M), protein expression (P), and substrate activity are noted. Data were not available for rodent expression or substrate activity. ↑ denotes upregulation, ↓ denotes downregulation, and ↔ denotes no change.*

induction of luciferase activity in response to progesterone treatment (Jeong et al., 2008). These results suggest that the inducibility of UGT1A1 by progesterone is driven by a PXR-mediated mechanism.

Placental Lactogen/Prolactin/Growth Hormone

In addition to estrogen and progesterone, peptide hormones of the growth hormone family, such as placental lactogen, growth hormone variant, and prolactin, are increased in the circulation of pregnant women. These peptide hormones have conserved genetic, structural, functional, and binding properties (Lee et al., 2014). Plasma concentrations of prolactin have been shown to increase 10-fold during pregnancy (to levels over 200 ng/mL) when compared with nonpregnant women (Kletzky et al., 1985). Placental lactogen and growth hormone variant are produced by trophoblasts in the placenta and are characterized as pregnancy-specific somatotropins. In terms of biologic function, prolactin is involved in lactation and mammary gland development, whereas placental lactogen and growth hormone variant serve roles in nutrient metabolism (reviewed in Jeong, 2010). These biological functions are activated through hormone binding to either the membrane-bound growth hormone or prolactin receptors, which triggers a number of signaling proteins such as the signal transducer and activator of transcription family.

To determine the effect of these hormones on the expression of major hepatic CYP enzymes (Table 9.9), Lee et al. (2014) treated primary human female hepatocytes with concentrations that reflected maternal serum levels during the third trimester of pregnancy. Treatments with prolactin (150 ng/mL) as well as the growth hormone variant (20 ng/mL) showed no effect on CYP enzyme expression. On the other hand, treatment with placental lactogen (6 μg/mL) caused an increase in CYP2E1 mRNA and protein as well as CYP3A5 mRNA expression. Interestingly, when human hepatocytes were treated with a signaling inhibitor of PI3-kinase, wortmannin, the placental lactogen-induced CYP2E1 mRNA expression was attenuated. It is important to note that the placental lactogen treatment using mouse hepatocytes derived from CYP2E1-humanized mice did not alter Cyp expression, signifying the importance of choosing an appropriate model when studying the effect of pregnancy hormones (Lee et al., 2014).

To examine the potential effect of prolactin on Ugt enzymes, Luquita et al. (2001) analyzed changes of Ugt1 isoforms in rat liver during pregnancy and postpartum. Administration of

TABLE 9.9   Growth Hormone-Related Regulation of Phase I Metabolism[a]

Enzyme	Human	References
PLACENTAL LACTOGEN: CYTOCHROME P450s		
CYP1A2	↔(M)	Lee et al. (2014)
CYP2A6	↔(M)	Lee et al. (2014)
CYP2B6	↔(M)	Lee et al. (2014)
CYP2C9	↔(M)	Lee et al. (2014)
CYP2C19	↔(M)	Lee et al. (2014)
CYP2D6	↔(M)	Lee et al. (2014)
CYP2E1	↑(M,P)	Lee et al. (2014)
CYP3A4	↔(M)	Lee et al. (2014)
CYP3A5	↑(M)	Lee et al. (2014)

[a]*Expression or activity compared with female nonpregnant liver levels. mRNA expression (M), protein expression (P), and substrate activity are noted. Data were not available for rodent expression or substrate activity. ↑ denotes upregulation, ↓ denotes downregulation, and ↔ denotes no change.*

300 μg of ovine prolactin daily for 7 days increased Ugt1a6 mRNA and protein levels as well as *p*-nitrophenol conjugation (Luquita et al., 2001) (Table 9.10). Other Ugt isoforms including 1a1 and 1a5 were unaltered in response to prolactin. Another study examining changes in Ugt expression in response to growth hormone observed a significant decrease in Ugt2b1 and Ugt2b3 mRNA expression in primary rat hepatocytes (Li et al., 1999). These results exemplify the isoform-specific nature of hormone regulation as two members of the growth hormone family had alternate influences on different members of the Ugt family.

Limited studies have also investigated the regulation of transporters by growth hormone-related proteins (Table 9.11). Although growth hormone has been shown to increase mRNA levels of the Mrp2 transporter in primary rat hepatocytes, its protein expression is downregulated during pregnancy, suggesting the role of other hormones in its regulation (Cao et al., 2001; Simon et al., 2006). Primary rat hepatocytes treated with prolactin or growth hormone also showed an increase in mRNA expression levels of Oatp1b2 and Ntcp when compared with controls (Cao et al., 2001; Wood et al., 2005). Ovariectomized rats treated with ovine prolactin had increased Ntcp and bile salt export pump (Bsep) mRNA and protein expression (Cao et al., 2001; Ganguly et al., 1994). Taken together, a global increase of transporter expression in response to members of the growth hormone family is evident in rats. These results suggest that more work needs to be done regarding growth hormones and prolactin in different models.

Cortisol

Cortisol is a steroid hormone released in response to stress and low blood glucose and has been shown to rise anywhere from two- to four-fold in maternal serum over the course of

TABLE 9.10　Growth Hormone-Related Regulation of Phase II Metabolism[a]

Enzyme	Mouse	Human	References
PROLACTIN: UDP-GLUCURONOSYLTRANSFERASES			
UGT1A1		↔(M,P)	Luquita et al. (2001)
UGT1A5		↔(M,P)	Luquita et al. (2001)
UGT1A6		↑(M,P)	Luquita et al. (2001)
PLACENTAL GROWTH HORMONE: UDP-GLUCURONOSYLTRANSFERASES			
UGT1A1		↔(M)	Li et al. (1999)
UGT1A5		↔(M)	Li et al. (1999)
UGT1A6		↔(M)	Li et al. (1999)
UGT2B1		↓(M)	Li et al. (1999)
UGT2B3		↓(M)	Li et al. (1999)
SULFOTRANSFERASES			
Sult1a1	↔(M)		Alnouti and Klaassen (2011)
Sult1d1	↔(M)		Alnouti and Klaassen (2011)
Sult2a1/a2	↑(M)		Alnouti and Klaassen (2011)
Sult3a1	↑(M)		Alnouti and Klaassen (2011)
Sult1c1	↓(M)		Alnouti and Klaassen (2011)

[a]*Expression or activity compared with female nonpregnant liver levels. mRNA expression (M) and protein expression (P) are noted. Data were not available for rat expression or substrate activity. ↑ denotes upregulation, ↓ denotes downregulation, and ↔ denotes no change.*

TABLE 9.11　Growth Hormone-Related Regulation of Transporters[a]

Enzyme	Mouse	Rat	References
UPTAKE TRANSPORTERS			
Ntcp		↑(M,P)	Cao et al. (2001), Ganguly et al. (1994), and Wood et al. (2005)
Slco1a1/Oatp1a1	↔(M)		Cheng et al. (2006)
Slco1b2/Oatp1b2		↑(M)	Cao et al. (2001) and Wood et al. (2005)
EFFLUX TRANSPORTERS			
Bsep		↑(M,P)	Cao et al. (2001)
Mrp2		↑(M)	Cao et al. (2001) and Simon et al. (2006)

[a]*Expression or activity compared with female nonpregnant liver levels. mRNA expression (M) and, protein expression (P) are noted. Data were not available for human expression or substrate activity. ↑ denotes upregulation and ↔ denotes no change.*

gestation (Davis and Sandman, 2010). As a result of its small molecular mass and hydropho-
bicity, cortisol is able to bypass the cell membranes of tissues within the body during pregnancy and bind to distinct receptors to initiate the transcription of target genes (reviewed by
La Marca-Ghaemmaghami et al., 2015). In addition to its actions mediated by the glucocorticoid receptor, corticosteroids have been shown to induce expression levels of nuclear receptors, such as PXR and CAR, which in turn can enhance the expression of CYPs under their
transcriptional regulation (Davis and Sandman, 2010; Pascussi et al., 2000a,b).

Using primary hepatocytes isolated from adrenalectomized or sham-operated mice treated
with a 10 mg/kg/day subcutaneous injection of dexamethasone for 3 days, Sakuma et al.
(2004) showed that corticosteroid-induced Cyp3a11 and Cyp3a41 mRNAs in both models
(Table 9.12). Hypophysectomy completely abolished Cyp3a41 mRNA expression, yet it did
not impact Cyp3a11. Only a combined treatment of dexamethasone and growth hormone
strongly induced the expression of Cyp3a41. Since individual treatment with dexamethasone
had little or no effect on Cyp3a41 mRNA, corticosteroids may be involved in an interdepen-
dent regulation of Cyp3a expression (Sakuma et al., 2004). The findings in this study proved
to be translational as other research groups using primary human hepatocytes observed
greatest CYP1A2, CYP3A4, and CYP3A5 induction after a concurrent administration of dexamethasone and growth hormone (Dhir et al., 2006; Papageorgiou et al., 2013). Treatment with
dexamethasone alone showed an up-regulation of CYP1A2, CYP3A4, and CYP3A5 mRNA
expression; however, it was not as extensive when compared with the coadministration of
dexamethasone and growth hormone (Dhir et al., 2006; Liddle et al., 1998; Papageorgiou
et al., 2013).

To examine the regulatory role of cortisol on Ugt isoforms (Table 9.13), Li et al. (1999) used
primary male rat hepatocytes and found that dexamethasone treatment significantly
increased mRNA expression of Ugt1a1, Ugt1a5, Ugt2b1, and Ugt2b3. The induction of
both phases I and II enzymes by corticosteroids exemplifies its importance in drug metabolism, especially during pregnancy, when levels of cortisol were significantly increased.

TABLE 9.12   Cortisol Regulation of Phase I Metabolism[a]

Enzyme	Mouse	Human	References
CYTOCHROME P450s			
CYP1A2		↑(M,P)	Dhir et al. (2006)
CYP2D6		↔(M,P)	Dhir et al. (2006)
CYP3A4		↑(M,P)	Dhir et al. (2006), Papageorgiou et al. (2013), and Pascussi et al. (2001)
CYP3A5		↑(M)	Papageorgiou et al. (2013)
Cyp3a11	↑(M)		Sakuma et al. (2004)
Cyp3a41	↑(M)		Sakuma et al. (2004)

[a]*Expression or activity compared with female nonpregnant liver levels. mRNA expression (M) and protein expression
(P) are noted. Data were not available for rat expression or substrate activity. ↑ denotes upregulation, ↓ denotes
downregulation, and ↔ denotes no change.*

TABLE 9.13   Cortisol Regulation of Phase II Metabolism[a]

Enzyme	Rat	References
UDP-GLUCURONOSYLTRANSFERASES		
Ugt1a1	↑(M)	Li et al. (1999)
Ugt1a5	↑(M)	Li et al. (1999)
Ugt1a6	↔(M)	Li et al. (1999)
Ugt2b1	↑(M)	Li et al. (1999)
Ugt2b3	↑(M)	Li et al. (1999)

[a]*Expression or activity compared with female nonpregnant liver levels. mRNA expression (M) is noted. Data were not available for mouse or human expression or substrate activity ↑ denotes upregulation and ↔ denotes no change.*

Two studies have shown that dexamethasone induces Mrp2 and Ntcp mRNA as well as protein in primary rat hepatocytes signifying the essential role of pituitary hormones in transporter expression, especially during gestation (Simon et al., 2004; Simon et al., 2006).

EXTRAHEPATIC REGULATION

Although the liver is the primary tissue for drug metabolism and transport, other organs including the kidneys, intestines and placenta contribute to the overall disposition of xenobiotics. Studies in this field have largely focused upon the adaptive regulation of renal transporters involved in secretion and reabsorption with little attention on phase I or II metabolism. The primary cationic uptake transporter Oct2 decreased in the kidneys of pregnant mice between gestation days 10 and 19 (Lee et al., 2013). A global reduction of brush border efflux transporters, including Mate1, Mdr1b, Mrp2, and Mrp4 mRNAs and proteins, was also observed in pregnant mice from gestation days 7—19 (Lee et al., 2013; Shuster et al., 2013; Yacovino et al., 2013). Interestingly, the down-regulation of Mrp4 in kidneys of pregnant mice was attenuated in a mouse model of type I diabetes (Yacovino and Aleksunes, 2012). The exact mechanism(s) underlying the suppression of apical efflux transporters in the kidneys of pregnant mice are not well understood. However, in the context of enhanced glomerular filtration during pregnancy, this may represent an adaptation to reduce solute loss by decreasing tubular secretion.

CASE EXAMPLE: BILE ACID METABOLISM AND TRANSPORT

Alterations in phases I and II enzymes and transport during pregnancy may impact the pharmacokinetics of a number of xenobiotics, particularly in the third trimester when the greatest expression and activity changes have been identified. However, in some cases, the coordinated changes among the three can affect the homeostasis of endogenous

HEPATOCYTE

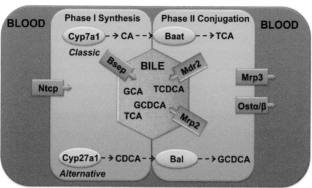

FIGURE 9.1   Major hepatic enzymes and transporters involved in bile acid homeostasis.

compounds. As a case in point, adaptations to bile acid metabolism and transport are considered normal pregnancy-related changes in physiology (Fig. 9.1).

Phase I

CYPs synthesize bile acids in the liver via the classic or alternative pathway. The primary bile acid formed by the classic pathway is cholic acid. Although cholesterol-7α-hydroxylase, or CYP7A1, is the rate-limiting enzyme in this pathway, sterol 12α-hydroxylase, or CYP8B1 is also critical. The primary bile acid formed from the alternative pathway is chenodeoxycholic acid. CYP27A1, 7B1, and 39A1 are important to the alternative pathway. It has been shown in pregnant mice that expression of classic pathway enzymes Cyp7a1 and 8b1 is induced, while alternative pathway enzymes Cyp27a1 and 39a1 are repressed (Aleksunes et al., 2012; Milona et al., 2010). If expression levels in pregnant mice are indicative of activity, these data would suggest the production of more hydrophobic (and often toxic) bile acids via the classic pathway. Cyp7a1, 8b1, 27a1, and 7b1 expression has also been determined throughout gestation in Sprague Dawley rats. Interestingly, the only observable change to mRNA levels was a reduction in Cyp8b1 expression, while expression of other bile acid–synthesizing enzymes remained constant (Zhu et al., 2013).

Phase II

Bile acids are conjugated to taurine or glycine prior to being excreted into bile canaliculi. As is similar with many phase II reactions, this conjugation makes bile acids less toxic and increases their ability to promote the absorption of lipids and lipid soluble vitamins in the intestine. Two critical conjugating enzymes include bile acid CoA ligase (Bal) and bile acid CoA:amino acid N-acetyltransferase (Baat). Similarly to Cyps in the alternative pathway, both Bal and Baat mRNA and protein levels are down-regulated in pregnant mice (Aleksunes et al., 2012). A reduction in conjugation coupled with changes observed in bile acid synthesis may contribute to a net increase in toxicity of the bile acid pool.

Transport

Portal bile acids are taken up into hepatocytes predominantly by the sinusoidal transporter, Ntcp. The canalicular efflux transporters, Bsep and Mrp2 (Keppler et al., 1997; Stieger et al., 2007) are primarily responsible for removing bile acids from the liver. On the other hand, the sinusoidal efflux transporters, organic solute transporter (Ost) α/β and Mrp3, pump small amounts of bile acids into the blood circulation. The literature shows that in mice, both maternal hepatic Ntcp and Bsep mRNA, protein, and localization to their respective membranes are significantly reduced on gestation days 14, 17, and 18. Mrp2 and Mrp3 mRNA expression is similarly down-regulated during the same gestational time points (Aleksunes et al., 2012; Milona et al., 2010). Expression data from pregnant rat livers confirm similar repression of Ntcp and Mrp3 but not Bsep (Zhu et al., 2013).

Although increased levels of estrogen in pregnancy may impact NTCP function, progesterone metabolites have been shown to interfere with NTCP uptake in vitro. Specifically, NTCP activity using taurocholate as a substrate was measured in the presence of allopregnanolone sulfate and epiallopregnanolone sulfate at concentrations observed in women during the third trimester of pregnancy. The investigators found that both progesterone metabolites were competitive inhibitors of Na^+-dependent and Na^+-independent taurocholate uptake in primary human hepatocytes and NTCP-expressing *Xenopus laevis* oocytes (Abu-Hayyeh et al., 2010).

Transcription Factors

In a normal physiological state, bile acid synthesis, conjugation, and recirculation are tightly regulated by multiple transcription factors. Many nuclear receptors suppressed in the maternal mouse liver, including Fxr, Car, Pxr, Lxr, and Pparα, control the expression of important hepatic transporters and enzymes responsible for bile acid recirculation (Aleksunes et al., 2012; Koh et al., 2011; Sweeney et al., 2006; Wen et al., 2013). Conversely, mouse Erα is induced, providing a mechanism for increased estradiol levels during pregnancy to influence cholesterol and lipid pathways (Wen et al., 2013). Although authors saw no changes in expression of Fxr mRNA, an induction of Fxr protein on gestation day 14 in rats was observed. Additionally, Pparα gene expression was induced on gestation day 14, while Erα was repressed on gestation days 10 and 14 (Zhu et al., 2013). Zhu et al. (2013) proposed that in Sprague Dawley rats, unlike mouse models, bile acid homeostasis was sustained during pregnancy through unaltered Fxr regulation. Of the aforementioned nuclear receptors, Fxr and its repression in mice are the most highly studied in relation to maternal bile acid homeostasis.

During mouse pregnancy, elevated bile acids have been attributed to suppressed Fxr function by increased reproductive hormone levels (Abu-Hayyeh et al., 2010, 2013; Aleksunes et al., 2012; Milona et al., 2010). Fxr not only activates the inhibitory transcription factor, Shp, and the intestinal fibroblast growth factor (Fgf15) to regulate bile acid synthesis and transport but can also directly transactivate hepatic bile acid transporters Ntcp, BSEP/Bsep, MDR3, and Ostβ (Ananthanarayanan et al., 2001; Denson et al., 2001; Huang et al., 2003; Lu et al., 2000; Thomas et al., 2010). Fxr-mediated induction of Fgf15 in the intestine is critical in the suppression of bile acid synthesis genes Cyp7a1 and 8b1 in the liver (Inagaki et al., 2005; Yu et al., 2005). In response to bile acid binding in the hepatocyte, Fxr upregulates the transcription of Shp, which works with Fgf15 to suppress the expression of Cyp7a1. Pregnancy is a unique physiological state in which Shp and Ntcp expression are coordinately down-regulated, whereas their relationship is typically inverse, similar to Shp and Cyp7a1 (Aleksunes et al., 2012; Milona et al., 2010). This pattern has also been observed with the bile acid surge at birth in mice (Cui et al., 2012).

Due to the significant role of Bsep in the recirculation of bile acids, mechanisms of repression during mouse pregnancy have been explored in detail, and point to a prominent role of Erα and Fxr. In vivo live imaging of mice with an injected luciferase *Bsep* promoter reporter confirmed decreased Bsep transcription in late pregnancy and inversely correlated with serum estradiol levels. Furthermore, Bsep down-regulation during late gestation was attenuated in Erα-null mice treated with estradiol. The authors propose indirect transcriptional repression of Bsep through the protein—protein interaction of Erα and Fxr, supported by the coimmunoprecipitation of such complexes in vitro and in vivo (Song et al., 2014). In a subsequent study, 17β-estradiol treatment was shown to decrease the Fxr-mediated recruitment of coactivator proliferator-activated receptor gamma coactivator-1, and enhance nuclear receptor corepressor recruitment to the BSEP promoter in Huh7 hepatoma cells (Chen et al., 2015).

Bile acid synthesis is governed by distinct mechanisms; negative feedback from Fxr and Shp, as well as positive feedback from Lxr. Lxr, a positive regulator of Cyp7a1, is inhibited by an interaction with Shp (Brendel et al., 2002), allowing for negative feedback to be dominant in this pathway. Interestingly, the reduction of Shp during pregnancy does not correspond with an induction of Lxr, suggesting it is also repressed by other mechanisms. In addition, CAR/Car and PXR/Pxr have been shown to induce the important bile acid transporters MRP/Mrp2 and Mrp3 in humans and rodents, as well as modify NTCP and BSEP transcription in humans. Pparα has been shown to upregulate mouse Mrp3 and Mdr2 (reviewed in Klaassen and Aleksunes, 2010).

Translational Implications

Differences in expression of genes related to bile acid homeostasis between rodent species raise the question of translational applications of these data. Limited human studies are available to support global down-regulation of conjugation and transport, as well as induction of classic bile acid synthesis enzymes. Conflicting reports have been published regarding serum bile acid levels among nonpregnant and pregnant women. In one of the larger studies ($n = 44-49$ per gestational week), serum bile acid levels in healthy pregnant women were generally consistent throughout gestation and comparable with reference standard nonpregnant values (Egan et al., 2012). Several smaller studies have also quantified individual bile acids in uncomplicated pregnancies as a control group. Castano et al. (2006) observed increased total bile acids, deoxycholic acid, and ursodeoxycholic acid levels in healthy pregnancies ($n = 18$) in comparison to nonpregnant women ($n = 10$). Another study demonstrated that women with uncomplicated pregnancies had highest levels of chenodeoxycholic acid (0.32 μmol/L), followed by cholic acid (0.25 μmol/L) and deoxycholic acid (0.27 μmol/L), though no comparison was made to nonpregnant values (Geenes et al., 2014). Though total bile acids may remain unchanged throughout gestation, media supplemented with serum from healthy pregnant humans caused a downregulation of Shp expression in rat Fao hepatoma cells (Milona et al., 2010). In addition, *FXR* genetic variants, as well as *BSEP* and *MDR3* polymorphisms have been identified as contributors to intrahepatic cholestasis of pregnancy, a bile acid—related disorder specific to gestation (Dixon et al., 2000, 2009; Van Mil et al., 2007). This suggests that any further perturbation of the FXR pathway beyond normal alterations to human pregnant physiology can lead to liver disease.

CONCLUSION AND FUTURE DIRECTIONS

Pregnancy is a period of hormonal flux and has the potential to modify not only physiological parameters but also the expression patterns of various enzymes and transporters directly or indirectly by altering the activity of regulatory nuclear receptors. Recent work has been undertaken to develop physiologically-based pharmacokinetic models of key medications during pregnancy such as indomethacin (Alqahtani and Kaddoumi, 2015), tenofovir (De Sousa Mendes et al., 2015), lithium (Horton et al., 2012) as well as general models for CYP1A2, 2D6 and 3A4 substrates (Gaohua et al., 2012; Ke et al., 2013). Ultimately, a comprehensive understanding of how gestation alters physiology and pharmacokinetics regulation may serve as a guide to optimize drug dosing during pregnancy and ensure therapeutic benefits in mothers with low risk of toxicity to fetuses.

References

Abu-Hayyeh, S., Martinez-Becerra, P., Sheikh Abdul Kadir, S.H., Selden, C., Romero, M.R., Rees, M., Marschall, H.U., Marin, J.J., Williamson, C., 2010. Inhibition of Na^+-taurocholate co-transporting polypeptide-mediated bile acid transport by cholestatic sulfated progesterone metabolites. J. Biol. Chem. 285 (22), 16504—16512.

Abu-Hayyeh, S., Papacleovoulou, G., Lovgren-Sandblom, A., Tahir, M., Oduwole, O., Jamaludin, N.A., Ravat, S., Nikolova, V., Chambers, J., Selden, C., Rees, M., Marschall, H.U., Parker, M.G., Williamson, C., 2013. Intrahepatic cholestasis of pregnancy levels of sulfated progesterone metabolites inhibit farnesoid X receptor resulting in a cholestatic phenotype. Hepatology 57 (2), 716—726.

Aleksunes, L.M., Xu, J., Lin, E., Wen, X., Goedken, M.J., Slitt, A.L., 2013. Pregnancy represses induction of efflux transporters in livers of type I diabetic mice. Pharm. Res. 30 (9), 2209—2220.

Aleksunes, L.M., Yeager, R.L., Wen, X., Cui, J.Y., Klaassen, C.D., 2012. Repression of hepatobiliary transporters and differential regulation of classic and alternative bile acid pathways in mice during pregnancy. Toxicol. Sci. 130 (2), 257—268.

Alnouti, Y., Klaassen, C.D., 2011. Mechanisms of gender-specific regulation of mouse sulfotransferases (Sults). Xenobiotica 41 (3), 187—197.

Alqahtani, S., Kaddoumi, A., 2015. Development of physiologically based pharmacokinetic/pharmacodynamic model for indomethacin disposition in pregnancy. PLoS ONE 10 (10), e0139762.

Ananthanarayanan, M., Balasubramanian, N., Makishima, M., Mangelsdorf, D.J., Suchy, F.J., 2001. Human bile salt export pump promoter is transactivated by the farnesoid X receptor/bile acid receptor. J. Biol. Chem. 276 (31), 28857—28865.

Arrese, M., Trauner, M., Ananthanarayanan, M., Pizarro, M., Solis, N., Accatino, L., Soroka, C., Boyer, J.L., Karpen, S.J., Miquel, J.F., Suchy, F.J., 2003. Down-regulation of the Na^+/taurocholate cotransporting polypeptide during pregnancy in the rat. J. Hepatol. 38 (2), 148—155.

Bader, R.A., Bader, M.E., Rose, D.F., Braunwald, E., 1955. Hemodynamics at rest and during exercise in normal pregnancy as studies by cardiac catheterization. J. Clin. Invest. 34 (10), 1524—1536.

Baldwin, G.R., Moorthi, D.S., Whelton, J.A., MacDonnell, K.F., 1977. New lung functions and pregnancy. Am. J. Obstet. Gynecol. 127 (3), 235—239.

Barron, W.M., Lindheimer, M.D., 1984. Renal sodium and water handling in pregnancy. Obstet. Gynecol. Annu. 13, 35–69.

Beigi, R.H., Han, K., Venkataramanan, R., Hankins, G.D., Clark, S., Hebert, M.F., Easterling, T., Zajicek, A., Ren, Z., Mattison, D.R., Caritis, S.N., Obstetric-Fetal Pharmacology Research Units Network, 2011. Pharmacokinetics of oseltamivir among pregnant and nonpregnant women. Am. J. Obstet. Gynecol. 204 (6 Suppl. 1), S84–S88.

Brendel, C., Schoonjans, K., Botrugno, O.A., Treuter, E., Auwerx, J., 2002. The small heterodimer partner interacts with the liver X receptor alpha and represses its transcriptional activity. Mol. Endocrinol. 16 (9), 2065–2076.

Buckley, D.B., Klaassen, C.D., 2009. Mechanism of gender-divergent UDP-glucuronosyltransferase mRNA expression in mouse liver and kidney. Drug Metab. Dispos. 37 (4), 834–840.

Cao, J., Huang, L., Liu, Y., Hoffman, T., Stieger, B., Meier, P.J., Vore, M., 2001. Differential regulation of hepatic bile salt and organic anion transporters in pregnant and postpartum rats and the role of prolactin. Hepatology 33 (1), 140–147.

Cao, J., Stieger, B., Meier, P.J., Vore, M., 2002. Expression of rat hepatic multidrug resistance-associated proteins and organic anion transporters in pregnancy. Am. J. Physiol. Gastrointest. Liver Physiol. 283 (3), G757–G766.

Castano, G., Lucangioli, S., Sookoian, S., Mesquida, M., Lemberg, A., Di Scala, M., Franchi, P., Carducci, C., Tripodi, V., 2006. Bile acid profiles by capillary electrophoresis in intrahepatic cholestasis of pregnancy. Clin. Sci. (Lond.) 110 (4), 459–465.

Chen, C., Hennig, G.E., McCann, D.J., Manautou, J.E., 2000. Effects of clofibrate and indocyanine green on the hepatobiliary disposition of acetaminophen and its metabolites in male CD-1 mice. Xenobiotica 30 (11), 1019–1032.

Chen, H., Yang, K., Choi, S., Fischer, J.H., Jeong, H., 2009. Up-regulation of UDP-glucuronosyltransferase (UGT) 1A4 by 17beta-estradiol: a potential mechanism of increased lamotrigine elimination in pregnancy. Drug Metab. Dispos. 37 (9), 1841–1847.

Chen, Y., Vasilenko, A., Song, X., Valanejad, L., Verma, R., You, S., Yan, B., Shiffka, S., Hargreaves, L., Nadolny, C., Deng, R., 2015. Estrogen and estrogen receptor-alpha-mediated Transrepression of bile salt export pump. Mol. Endocrinol. 29 (4), 613–626.

Cheng, X., Klaassen, C.D., 2012. Hormonal and chemical regulation of paraoxonases in mice. J. Pharmacol. Exp. Ther. 342 (3), 688–695.

Cheng, X., Maher, J., Lu, H., Klaassen, C.D., 2006. Endocrine regulation of gender-divergent mouse organic anion-transporting polypeptide (Oatp) expression. Mol. Pharmacol. 70 (4), 1291–1297.

Choi, S.Y., Fischer, L., Yang, K., Chung, H., Jeong, H., 2011. Isoform-specific regulation of cytochrome P450 expression and activity by estradiol in female rats. Biochem. Pharmacol. 81 (6), 777–782.

Choi, S.Y., Koh, K.H., Jeong, H., 2013. Isoform-specific regulation of cytochromes P450 expression by estradiol and progesterone. Drug Metab. Dispos. 41 (2), 263–269.

Clark, S.L., Cotton, D.B., Lee, W., Bishop, C., Hill, T., Southwick, J., Pivarnik, J., Spillman, T., DeVore, G.R., Phelan, J., et al., 1989. Central hemodynamic assessment of normal term pregnancy. Am. J. Obstet. Gynecol. 161 (6 Pt 1), 1439–1442.

Cui, J.Y., Aleksunes, L.M., Tanaka, Y., Fu, Z.D., Guo, Y., Guo, G.L., Lu, H., Zhong, X.B., Klaassen, C.D., 2012. Bile acids via FXR initiate the expression of major transporters involved in the enterohepatic circulation of bile acids in newborn mice. Am. J. Physiol. Gastrointest. Liver Physiol. 302 (9), G979–G996.

Davis, E.P., Sandman, C.A., 2010. The timing of prenatal exposure to maternal cortisol and psychosocial stress is associated with human infant cognitive development. Child Dev. 81 (1), 131–148.

Davison, J.M., Dunlop, W., 1980. Renal hemodynamics and tubular function normal human pregnancy. Kidney Int. 18 (2), 152–161.

Daw, J.R., Hanley, G.E., Greyson, D.L., Morgan, S.G., 2011. Prescription drug use during pregnancy in developed countries: a systematic review. Pharmacoepidemiol. Drug Saf. 20 (9), 895–902.

de Haan, G.J., Edelbroek, P., Segers, J., Engelsman, M., Lindhout, D., Devile-Notschaele, M., Augustijn, P., 2004. Gestation-induced changes in lamotrigine pharmacokinetics: a monotherapy study. Neurology 63 (3), 571–573.

De Sousa Mendes, M., Hirt, D., Urien, S., Valade, E., Bouazza, N., Foissac, F., Blanche, S., Treluyer, J.M., Benaboud, S., 2015. Physiologically-based pharmacokinetic modeling of renally excreted antiretroviral drugs in pregnant women. Br. J. Clin. Pharmacol. 80 (5), 1031–1041.

Denson, L.A., Sturm, E., Echevarria, W., Zimmerman, T.L., Makishima, M., Mangelsdorf, D.J., Karpen, S.J., 2001. The orphan nuclear receptor, shp, mediates bile acid-induced inhibition of the rat bile acid transporter, ntcp. Gastroenterology 121 (1), 140–147.

Dhir, R.N., Dworakowski, W., Thangavel, C., Shapiro, B.H., 2006. Sexually dimorphic regulation of hepatic isoforms of human cytochrome p450 by growth hormone. J. Pharmacol. Exp. Ther. 316 (1), 87—94.

Dickmann, L.J., Isoherranen, N., 2013. Quantitative prediction of CYP2B6 induction by estradiol during pregnancy: potential explanation for increased methadone clearance during pregnancy. Drug Metab. Dispos. 41 (2), 270—274.

Dixon, P.H., Weerasekera, N., Linton, K.J., Donaldson, O., Chambers, J., Egginton, E., Weaver, J., Nelson-Piercy, C., de Swiet, M., Warnes, G., Elias, E., Higgins, C.F., Johnston, D.G., McCarthy, M.I., Williamson, C., 2000. Hetero-zygous MDR3 missense mutation associated with intrahepatic cholestasis of pregnancy: evidence for a defect in protein trafficking. Hum. Mol. Genet. 9 (8), 1209—1217.

Dixon, P.H., van Mil, S.W., Chambers, J., Strautnieks, S., Thompson, R.J., Lammert, F., Kubitz, R., Keitel, V., Glantz, A., Mattsson, L.A., Marschall, H.U., Molokhia, M., Moore, G.E., Linton, K.J., Williamson, C., 2009. Contri-bution of variant alleles of ABCB11 to susceptibility to intrahepatic cholestasis of pregnancy. Gut 58 (4), 537—544.

Dunlop, W., 1981. Serial changes in renal haemodynamics during normal human pregnancy. Br. J. Obstet. Gynaecol. 88 (1), 1—9.

Egan, N., Bartels, A., Khashan, A.S., Broadhurst, D.I., Joyce, C., O'Mullane, J., O'Donoghue, K., 2012. Reference stan-dard for serum bile acids in pregnancy. BJOG 119 (4), 493—498.

Ejiri, N., Katayama, K., Doi, K., 2005a. Induction of cytochrome P450 isozymes by phenobarbital in pregnant rat and fetal livers and placenta. Exp. Mol. Pathol. 78 (2), 150—155.

Ejiri, N., Katayama, K., Kiyosawa, N., Baba, Y., Doi, K., 2005b. Microarray analysis on phase II drug metabolizing enzymes expression in pregnant rats after treatment with pregnenolone-16alpha-carbonitrile or phenobarbital. Exp. Mol. Pathol. 79 (3), 272—277.

Elkus, R., Popovich Jr., J., 1992. Respiratory physiology in pregnancy. Clin. Chest Med. 13 (4), 555—565.

Fortin, M.C., Aleksunes, L.M., Richardson, J.R., 2013. Alteration of the expression of pesticide-metabolizing enzymes in pregnant mice: potential role in the increased vulnerability of the developing brain. Drug Metab. Dispos. 41 (2), 326—331.

Fotopoulou, C., Kretz, R., Bauer, S., Schefold, J.C., Schmitz, B., Dudenhausen, J.W., Henrich, W., 2009. Prospectively assessed changes in lamotrigine-concentration in women with epilepsy during pregnancy, lactation and the neonatal period. Epilepsy Res. 85 (1), 60—64.

Ganguly, T.C., Liu, J., Hyde, J.F., Hagenbuch, B., Meier, P.J., Vore, M., 1994. Prolactin increases hepatic Na^+/taur-ocholate co-transport activity and messenger RNA post partum. Biochem. J. 303 (Pt 1), 33—36.

Gaohua, L., Abduljalil, K., Jamei, M., Johnson, T.N., Rostami-Hodjegan, A., 2012. A pregnancy physiologically based pharmacokinetic (p-PBPK) model for disposition of drugs metabolized by CYP1A2, CYP2D6 and CYP3A4. Br. J. Clin. Pharmacol. 74 (5), 873—885.

Geenes, V., Lovgren-Sandblom, A., Benthin, L., Lawrance, D., Chambers, J., Gurung, V., Thornton, J., Chappell, L., Khan, E., Dixon, P., Marschall, H.U., Williamson, C., 2014. The reversed feto-maternal bile acid gradient in intra-hepatic cholestasis of pregnancy is corrected by ursodeoxycholic acid. PLoS ONE 9 (1), e83828.

Geier, A., Dietrich, C.G., Gerloff, T., Haendly, J., Kullak-Ublick, G.A., Stieger, B., Meier, P.J., Matern, S., Gartung, C., 2003. Regulation of basolateral organic anion transporters in ethinylestradiol-induced cholestasis in the rat. Bio-chim. Biophys. Acta 1609 (1), 87—94.

He, X.J., Ejiri, N., Nakayama, H., Doi, K., 2005. Effects of pregnancy on CYPs protein expression in rat liver. Exp. Mol. Pathol. 78 (1), 64—70.

He, X.J., Yamauchi, H., Suzuki, K., Ueno, M., Nakayama, H., Doi, K., 2007. Gene expression profiles of drug-metabolizing enzymes (DMEs) in rat liver during pregnancy and lactation. Exp. Mol. Pathol. 83 (3), 428—434.

Hebert, M.F., Easterling, T.R., Kirby, B., Carr, D.B., Buchanan, M.L., Rutherford, T., Thummel, K.E., Fishbein, D.P., Unadkat, J.D., 2008. Effects of pregnancy on CYP3A and P-glycoprotein activities as measured by disposition of midazolam and digoxin: a University of Washington specialized center of research study. Clin. Pharmacol. Ther. 84 (2), 248—253.

Heikkinen, T., Ekblad, U., Palo, P., Laine, K., 2003. Pharmacokinetics of fluoxetine and norfluoxetine in pregnancy and lactation. Clin. Pharmacol. Ther. 73 (4), 330—337.

Higashi, E., Fukami, T., Itoh, M., Kyo, S., Inoue, M., Yokoi, T., Nakajima, M., 2007. Human CYP2A6 is induced by estrogen via estrogen receptor. Drug Metab. Dispos. 35 (10), 1935—1941.

Hogstedt, S., Lindberg, B., Rane, A., 1983. Increased oral clearance of metoprolol in pregnancy. Eur. J. Clin. Pharma-col. 24 (2), 217—220.

Horton, S., Tuerk, A., Cook, D., Cook, J., Dhurjati, P., 2012. Maximum recommended dosage of lithium for pregnant women based on a PBPK model for lithium absorption. Adv. Bioinform. 2012, 352729.

Huang, L., Zhao, A., Lew, J.L., Zhang, T., Hrywna, Y., Thompson, J.R., de Pedro, N., Royo, I., Blevins, R.A., Pelaez, F., Wright, S.D., Cui, J., 2003. Farnesoid X receptor activates transcription of the phospholipid pump MDR3. J. Biol. Chem. 278 (51), 51085–51090.

Hytten, F.E., Paintin, D.B., 1963. Increase in plasma volume during normal pregnancy. J. Obstet. Gynaecol. Br. Emp. 70, 402–407.

Inagaki, T., Choi, M., Moschetta, A., Peng, L., Cummins, C.L., McDonald, J.G., Luo, G., Jones, S.A., Goodwin, B., Richardson, J.A., Gerard, R.D., Repa, J.J., Mangelsdorf, D.J., Kliewer, S.A., 2005. Fibroblast growth factor 15 functions as an enterohepatic signal to regulate bile acid homeostasis. Cell Metab. 2 (4), 217–225.

Jeong, H., 2010. Altered drug metabolism during pregnancy: hormonal regulation of drug-metabolizing enzymes. Expert Opin. Drug Metab. Toxicol. 6 (6), 689–699.

Jeong, H., Choi, S., Song, J.W., Chen, H., Fischer, J.H., 2008. Regulation of UDP-glucuronosyltransferase (UGT) 1A1 by progesterone and its impact on labetalol elimination. Xenobiotica 38 (1), 62–75.

Kawamoto, T., Kakizaki, S., Yoshinari, K., Negishi, M., 2000. Estrogen activation of the nuclear orphan receptor CAR (constitutive active receptor) in induction of the mouse Cyp2b10 gene. Mol. Endocrinol. 14 (11), 1897–1905.

Ke, A.B., Nallani, S.C., Zhao, P., Rostami-Hodjegan, A., Isoherranen, N., Unadkat, J.D., 2013. A physiologically based pharmacokinetic model to predict disposition of CYP2D6 and CYP1A2 metabolized drugs in pregnant women. Drug Metab. Dispos. 41 (4), 801–813.

Ke, A.B., Nallani, S.C., Zhao, P., Rostami-Hodjegan, A., Unadkat, J.D., 2014. Expansion of a PBPK model to predict disposition in pregnant women of drugs cleared via multiple CYP enzymes, including CYP2B6, CYP2C9 and CYP2C19. Br. J. Clin. Pharmacol. 77 (3), 554–570.

Keppler, D., Konig, J., Buchler, M., 1997. The canalicular multidrug resistance protein, cMRP/MRP2, a novel conjugate export pump expressed in the apical membrane of hepatocytes. Adv. Enzym. Regul. 37, 321–333.

Klaassen, C.D., Aleksunes, L.M., 2010. Xenobiotic, bile acid, and cholesterol transporters: function and regulation. Pharmacol. Rev. 62 (1), 1–96.

Kletzky, O.A., Rossman, F., Bertolli, S.I., Platt, L.D., Mishell Jr., D.R., 1985. Dynamics of human chorionic gonadotropin, prolactin, and growth hormone in serum and amniotic fluid throughout normal human pregnancy. Am. J. Obstet. Gynecol. 151 (7), 878–884.

Koerner, M., Yerby, M., Friel, P., McCormick, K., 1989. Valproic acid disposition and protein binding in pregnancy. Ther. Drug Monit. 11 (3), 228–230.

Koh, K.H., Jurkovic, S., Yang, K., Choi, S.Y., Jung, J.W., Kim, K.P., Zhang, W., Jeong, H., 2012. Estradiol induces cytochrome P450 2B6 expression at high concentrations: implication in estrogen-mediated gene regulation in pregnancy. Biochem. Pharmacol. 84 (1), 93–103.

Koh, K.H., Pan, X., Shen, H.W., Arnold, S.L., Yu, A.M., Gonzalez, F.J., Isoherranen, N., Jeong, H., 2014a. Altered expression of small heterodimer partner governs cytochrome P450 (CYP) 2D6 induction during pregnancy in CYP2D6-humanized mice. J. Biol. Chem. 289 (6), 3105–3113.

Koh, K.H., Pan, X., Zhang, W., McLachlan, A., Urrutia, R., Jeong, H., 2014b. Kruppel-like factor 9 promotes hepatic cytochrome P450 2D6 expression during pregnancy in CYP2D6-humanized mice. Mol. Pharmacol. 86 (6), 727–735.

Koh, K.H., Xie, H., Yu, A.M., Jeong, H., 2011. Altered cytochrome P450 expression in mice during pregnancy. Drug Metab. Dispos. 39 (2), 165–169.

La Marca-Ghaemmaghami, P., et al., 2015. Stress during pregnancy: experienced stress, stress hormones, and protective factors. European Psychologist 20 (2), 102–119.

Lassiter, T.L., Padilla, S., Mortensen, S.R., Chanda, S.M., Moser, V.C., Barone Jr., S., 1998. Gestational exposure to chlorpyrifos: apparent protection of the fetus? Toxicol. Appl. Pharmacol. 152 (1), 56–65.

Lee, N., Hebert, M.F., Prasad, B., Easterling, T.R., Kelly, E.J., Unadkat, J.D., Wang, J., 2013. Effect of gestational age on mRNA and protein expression of polyspecific organic cation transporters during pregnancy. Drug Metab. Dispos. 41 (12), 2225–2232.

Lee, J.K., Chung, H.J., Fischer, L., Fischer, J., Gonzalez, F.J., Jeong, H., 2014. Human placental lactogen induces CYP2E1 expression via PI 3-kinase pathway in female human hepatocytes. Drug Metab. Dispos. 42 (4), 492–499.

Levy, D.M., Williams, O.A., Magides, A.D., Reilly, C.S., 1994. Gastric emptying is delayed at 8–12 weeks' gestation. Br. J. Anaesth. 73 (2), 237–238.

Li, W., Ning, M., Koh, K.H., Kim, H., Jeong, H., 2014. 17beta-Estradiol induces sulfotransferase 2A1 expression through estrogen receptor alpha. Drug Metab. Dispos 42 (4), 796–802.

Li, Y.Q., Prentice, D.A., Howard, M.L., Mashford, M.L., Desmond, P.V., 1999. The effect of hormones on the expression of five isoforms of UDP-glucuronosyltransferase in primary cultures of rat hepatocytes. Pharm. Res. 16 (2), 191–197.

Liddle, C., Goodwin, B.J., George, J., Tapner, M., Farrell, G.C., 1998. Separate and interactive regulation of cytochrome P450 3A4 by triiodothyronine, dexamethasone, and growth hormone in cultured hepatocytes. J. Clin. Endocrinol. Metab. 83 (7), 2411–2416.

Lu, T.T., Makishima, M., Repa, J.J., Schoonjans, K., Kerr, T.A., Auwerx, J., Mangelsdorf, D.J., 2000. Molecular basis for feedback regulation of bile acid synthesis by nuclear receptors. Mol. Cell 6 (3), 507–515.

Luquita, M.G., Catania, V.A., Pozzi, E.J., Veggi, L.M., Hoffman, T., Pellegrino, J.M., Ikushiro, S., Emi, Y., Iyanagi, T., Vore, M., Mottino, A.D., 2001. Molecular basis of perinatal changes in UDP-glucuronosyltransferase activity in maternal rat liver. J. Pharmacol. Exp. Ther. 298 (1), 49–56.

Matsumoto, J., Yokota, H., Yuasa, A., 2002. Developmental increases in rat hepatic microsomal UDP-glucuronosyltransferase activities toward xenoestrogens and decreases during pregnancy. Environ. Health Perspect. 110 (2), 193–196.

McGready, R., Stepniewska, K., Seaton, E., Cho, T., Cho, D., Ginsberg, A., Edstein, M.D., Ashley, E., Looareesuwan, S., White, N.J., Nosten, F., 2003. Pregnancy and use of oral contraceptives reduces the biotransformation of proguanil to cycloguanil. Eur. J. Clin. Pharmacol. 59 (7), 553–557.

Milona, A., Owen, B.M., Cobbold, J.F., Willemsen, E.C., Cox, I.J., Boudjelal, M., Cairns, W., Schoonjans, K., Taylor-Robinson, S.D., Klomp, L.W., Parker, M.G., White, R., van Mil, S.W., Williamson, C., 2010. Raised hepatic bile acid concentrations during pregnancy in mice are associated with reduced farnesoid X receptor function. Hepatology 52 (4), 1341–1349.

Nakai, A., Miyake, H., Oya, A., Asakura, H., Koshino, T., Araki, T., 2002. Reproducibility of pulsed Doppler measurements of the maternal renal circulation in normal pregnancies and those with pregnancy-induced hypertension. Ultrasound Obstet. Gynecol. 19 (6), 598–604.

Nemoto, N., Sakurai, J., 1995. Glucocorticoid and sex hormones as activating or modulating factors for expression of Cyp2b-9 and Cyp2b-10 in the mouse liver and hepatocytes. Arch. Biochem. Biophys. 319 (1), 286–292.

Ning, M., Koh, K.H., Pan, X., Jeong, H., 2015. Hepatocyte nuclear factor (HNF) 4alpha transactivation of cytochrome P450 (Cyp) 2d40 promoter is enhanced during pregnancy in mice. Biochem. Pharmacol. 94 (1), 46–52.

Ohman, I., Beck, O., Vitols, S., Tomson, T., 2008. Plasma concentrations of lamotrigine and its 2-N-glucuronide metabolite during pregnancy in women with epilepsy. Epilepsia 49 (6), 1075–1080.

Pan, X., Jeong, H., 2015. Estrogen-induced cholestasis leads to repressed CYP2D6 expression in CYP2D6-humanized mice. Mol. Pharmacol. 88 (1), 106–112.

Papacleovoulou, G., Abu-Hayyeh, S., Williamson, C., 2011. Nuclear receptor-driven alterations in bile acid and lipid metabolic pathways during gestation. Biochim. Biophys. Acta 1812 (8), 879–887.

Papageorgiou, I., Grepper, S., Unadkat, J.D., 2013. Induction of hepatic CYP3A enzymes by pregnancy-related hormones: studies in human hepatocytes and hepatic cell lines. Drug Metab. Dispos. 41 (2), 281–290.

Parry, E., Shields, R., Turnbull, A.C., 1970. Transit time in the small intestine in pregnancy. J. Obstet. Gynaecol. Br. Commonw. 77 (10), 900–901.

Pascussi, J.M., Drocourt, L., Fabre, J.M., Maurel, P., Vilarem, M.J., 2000a. Dexamethasone induces pregnane X receptor and retinoid X receptor-alpha expression in human hepatocytes: synergistic increase of CYP3A4 induction by pregnane X receptor activators. Mol. Pharmacol. 58 (2), 361–372.

Pascussi, J.M., Drocourt, L., Gerbal-Chaloin, S., Fabre, J.M., Maurel, P., Vilarem, M.J., 2001. Dual effect of dexamethasone on CYP3A4 gene expression in human hepatocytes. Sequential role of glucocorticoid receptor and pregnane X receptor. Eur. J. Biochem. 268 (24), 6346–6358.

Pascussi, J.M., Gerbal-Chaloin, S., Fabre, J.M., Maurel, P., Vilarem, M.J., 2000b. Dexamethasone enhances constitutive androstane receptor expression in human hepatocytes: consequences on cytochrome P450 gene regulation. Mol. Pharmacol. 58 (6), 1441–1450.

Peck, T.M., Arias, F., 1979. Hematologic changes associated with pregnancy. Clin. Obstet. Gynecol. 22 (4), 785–798.

Pennell, P.B., Newport, D.J., Stowe, Z.N., Helmers, S.L., Montgomery, J.Q., Henry, T.R., 2004. The impact of pregnancy and childbirth on the metabolism of lamotrigine. Neurology 62 (2), 292–295.

Pernoll, M.L., Metcalfe, J., Schlenker, T.L., Welch, J.E., Matsumoto, J.A., 1975. Oxygen consumption at rest and during exercise in pregnancy. Respir. Physiol. 25 (3), 285–293.

Perucca, E., Crema, A., 1982. Plasma protein binding of drugs in pregnancy. Clin. Pharmacokinet. 7 (4), 336–352.

Pillai, V.C., Han, K., Beigi, R.H., Hankins, G.D., Clark, S., Hebert, M.F., Easterling, T.R., Zajicek, A., Ren, Z., Caritis, S.N., Venkataramanan, R., 2015. Population pharmacokinetics of oseltamivir in non-pregnant and pregnant women. Br. J. Clin. Pharmacol. 80 (5), 1042–1050.

Pritchard, J.A., 1965. Changes in the blood volume during pregnancy and delivery. Anesthesiology 26, 393–399.

Quinney, S.K., Mohamed, A.N., Hebert, M.F., Haas, D.M., Clark, S., Umans, J.G., Caritis, S.N., Li, L., 2012. A semi-mechanistic metabolism model of CYP3A substrates in pregnancy: predicting changes in midazolam and nifedipine pharmacokinetics. CPT Pharmacometrics Syst. Pharmacol. 1, e2.

Reimers, A., Helde, G., Brathen, G., Brodtkorb, E., 2011. Lamotrigine and its N2-glucuronide during pregnancy: the significance of renal clearance and estradiol. Epilepsy Res. 94 (3), 198–205.

Reisinger, T.L., Newman, M., Loring, D.W., Pennell, P.B., Meador, K.J., 2013. Antiepileptic drug clearance and seizure frequency during pregnancy in women with epilepsy. Epilepsy Behav. 29 (1), 13–18.

Riva, R., Albani, F., Contin, M., Baruzzi, A., Altomare, M., Merlini, G.P., Perucca, E., 1984. Mechanism of altered drug binding to serum proteins in pregnant women: studies with valproic acid. Ther. Drug Monit. 6 (1), 25–30.

Robson, S.C., Mutch, E., Boys, R.J., Woodhouse, K.W., 1990. Apparent liver blood flow during pregnancy: a serial study using indocyanine green clearance. Br. J. Obstet. Gynaecol. 97 (8), 720–724.

Rubler, S., Damani, P.M., Pinto, E.R., 1977. Cardiac size and performance during pregnancy estimated with echocardiography. Am. J. Cardiol. 40 (4), 534–540.

Sabers, A., 2012. Algorithm for lamotrigine dose adjustment before, during, and after pregnancy. Acta Neurol. Scand. 126 (1), e1–4.

Sakuma, T., Endo, Y., Mashino, M., Kuroiwa, M., Ohara, A., Jarukamjorn, K., Nemoto, N., 2002. Regulation of the expression of two female-predominant CYP3A mRNAs (CYP3A41 and CYP3A44) in mouse liver by sex and growth hormones. Arch. Biochem. Biophys. 404 (2), 234–242.

Sakuma, T., Kitajima, K., Nishiyama, M., Endo, Y., Miyauchi, K., Jarukamjorn, K., Nemoto, N., 2004. Collaborated regulation of female-specific murine Cyp3a41 gene expression by growth and glucocorticoid hormones. Biochem. Biophys. Res. Commun. 314 (2), 495–500.

Shi, D., Yang, J., Yang, D., LeCluyse, E.L., Black, C., You, L., Akhlaghi, F., Yan, B., 2006. Anti-influenza prodrug oseltamivir is activated by carboxylesterase human carboxylesterase 1, and the activation is inhibited by antiplatelet agent clopidogrel. J. Pharmacol. Exp. Ther. 319 (3), 1477–1484.

Shuster, D.L., Bammler, T.K., Beyer, R.P., Macdonald, J.W., Tsai, J.M., Farin, F.M., Hebert, M.F., Thummel, K.E., Mao, Q., 2013. Gestational age-dependent changes in gene expression of metabolic enzymes and transporters in pregnant mice. Drug Metab. Dispos. 41 (2), 332–342.

Simon, F.R., Fortune, J., Iwahashi, M., Qadri, I., Sutherland, E., 2004. Multihormonal regulation of hepatic sinusoidal Ntcp gene expression. Am. J. Physiol. Gastrointest. Liver Physiol. 287 (4), G782–G794.

Simon, F.R., Iwahashi, M., Hu, L.J., Qadri, I., Arias, I.M., Ortiz, D., Dahl, R., Sutherland, E., 2006. Hormonal regulation of hepatic multidrug resistance-associated protein 2 (Abcc2) primarily involves the pattern of growth hormone secretion. Am. J. Physiol. Gastrointest. Liver Physiol. 290 (4), G595–G608.

Sit, D., Perel, J.M., Luther, J.F., Wisniewski, S.R., Helsel, J.C., Wisner, K.L., 2010. Disposition of chiral and racemic fluoxetine and norfluoxetine across childbearing. J. Clin. Psychopharmacol. 30 (4), 381–386.

Sit, D.K., Perel, J.M., Helsel, J.C., Wisner, K.L., 2008. Changes in antidepressant metabolism and dosing across pregnancy and early postpartum. J. Clin. Psychiatry 69 (4), 652–658.

Song, X., Vasilenko, A., Chen, Y., Valanejad, L., Verma, R., Yan, B., Deng, R., 2014. Transcriptional dynamics of bile salt export pump during pregnancy: mechanisms and implications in intrahepatic cholestasis of pregnancy. Hepatology 60 (6), 1993–2007.

Srivastava, R.A., 2002. Estrogen-induced regulation of the ATP-binding cassette transporter A1 (ABCA1) in mice: a possible mechanism of atheroprotection by estrogen. Mol. Cell Biochem. 240 (1–2), 67–73.

Stieger, B., Meier, Y., Meier, P.J., 2007. The bile salt export pump. Pflugers Arch. 453 (5), 611–620.

Sweeney, T.R., Moser, A.H., Shigenaga, J.K., Grunfeld, C., Feingold, K.R., 2006. Decreased nuclear hormone receptor expression in the livers of mice in late pregnancy. Am. J. Physiol. Endocrinol. Metab. 290 (6), E1313–E1320.

Tanaka, Y., Slitt, A.L., Leazer, T.M., Maher, J.M., Klaassen, C.D., 2005. Tissue distribution and hormonal regulation of the breast cancer resistance protein (Bcrp/Abcg2) in rats and mice. Biochem. Biophys. Res. Commun. 326 (1), 181–187.

Thomas, A.M., Hart, S.N., Kong, B., Fang, J., Zhong, X.B., Guo, G.L., 2010. Genome-wide tissue-specific farnesoid X receptor binding in mouse liver and intestine. Hepatology 51 (4), 1410–1419.

Topletz, A.R., Le, H.N., Lee, N., Chapman, J.D., Kelly, E.J., Wang, J., Isoherranen, N., 2013. Hepatic Cyp2d and Cyp26a1 mRNAs and activities are increased during mouse pregnancy. Drug Metab. Dispos. 41 (2), 312–319.

Tracy, T.S., Venkataramanan, R., Glover, D.D., Caritis, S.N., 2005. Temporal changes in drug metabolism (CYP1A2, CYP2D6 and CYP3A Activity) during pregnancy. Am. J. Obstet. Gynecol. 192 (2), 633–639.

Tran, T.A., Leppik, I.E., Blesi, K., Sathanandan, S.T., Remmel, R., 2002. Lamotrigine clearance during pregnancy. Neurology 59 (2), 251–255.

Van Mil, S.W., Milona, A., Dixon, P.H., Mullenbach, R., Geenes, V.L., Chambers, J., Shevchuk, V., Moore, G.E., Lammert, F., Glantz, A.G., Mattsson, L.A., Whittaker, J., Parker, M.G., White, R., Williamson, C., 2007. Functional variants of the central bile acid sensor FXR identified in intrahepatic cholestasis of pregnancy. Gastroenterology 133 (2), 507–516.

Ververs, F.F., Voorbij, H.A., Zwarts, P., Belitser, S.V., Egberts, T.C., Visser, G.H., Schobben, A.F., 2009. Effect of cytochrome P450 2D6 genotype on maternal paroxetine plasma concentrations during pregnancy. Clin. Pharmacokinet. 48 (10), 677–683.

Wadelius, M., Darj, E., Frenne, G., Rane, A., 1997. Induction of CYP2D6 in pregnancy. Clin. Pharmacol. Ther. 62 (4), 400–407.

Walker, A.A., Dickmann, L., Isoherranen, N., 2011. Pregnancy decreases rat CYP1A2 activity and expression. Drug Metab. Dispos. 39 (1), 4–7.

Waxman, D.J., 1999. P450 gene induction by structurally diverse xenochemicals: central role of nuclear receptors CAR, PXR, and PPAR. Arch. Biochem. Biophys. 369 (1), 11–23.

Wen, X., Donepudi, A.C., Thomas, P.E., Slitt, A.L., King, R.S., Aleksunes, L.M., 2013. Regulation of hepatic phase II metabolism in pregnant mice. J. Pharmacol. Exp. Ther. 344 (1), 244–252.

Wood, M., Ananthanarayanan, M., Jones, B., Wooton-Kee, R., Hoffman, T., Suchy, F.J., Vore, M., 2005. Hormonal regulation of hepatic organic anion transporting polypeptides. Mol. Pharmacol. 68 (1), 218–225.

Woodruff, T.J., Zota, A.R., Schwartz, J.M., 2011. Environmental chemicals in pregnant women in the United States: NHANES 2003-2004. Environ. Health Perspect. 119 (6), 878–885.

Xu, C., Li, C.Y., Kong, A.N., 2005. Induction of phase I, II and III drug metabolism/transport by xenobiotics. Arch. Pharm. Res. 28 (3), 249–268.

Yacovino, L.L., Aleksunes, L.M., 2012. Renal efflux transporter expression in pregnant mice with Type I diabetes. Toxicol. Lett. 211 (3), 304–311.

Yacovino, L.L., Gibson, C.J., Aleksunes, L.M., 2013. Down-regulation of brush border efflux transporter expression in the kidneys of pregnant mice. Drug Metab. Dispos. 41 (2), 320–325.

Yu, C., Wang, F., Jin, C., Huang, X., McKeehan, W.L., 2005. Independent repression of bile acid synthesis and activation of c-Jun N-terminal kinase (JNK) by activated hepatocyte fibroblast growth factor receptor 4 (FGFR4) and bile acids. J. Biol. Chem. 280 (18), 17707–17714.

Zhang, H., Wu, X., Wang, H., Mikheev, A.M., Mao, Q., Unadkat, J.D., 2008. Effect of pregnancy on cytochrome P450 3a and P-glycoprotein expression and activity in the mouse: mechanisms, tissue specificity, and time course. Mol. Pharmacol. 74 (3), 714–723.

Zhang, Y., Klaassen, C.D., 2013. Hormonal regulation of Cyp4a isoforms in mouse liver and kidney. Xenobiotica 43 (12), 1055–1063.

Zhu, Q.N., Xie, H.M., Zhang, D., Liu, J., Lu, Y.F., 2013. Hepatic bile acids and bile acid-related gene expression in pregnant and lactating rats. PeerJ 1, e143.

Estrogen-Metabolizing Enzymes in Systemic and Local Liver Injuries: A Case Study of Disease–Drug Interaction

X. Chai[1,2], S. Zeng[2], W. Xie[1]

[1]University of Pittsburgh, Pittsburgh, PA, United States;
[2]Zhejiang University, Hangzhou, China

O U T L I N E

Estrogen Sulfotransferase and Steroid
Sulfatase in Estrogen Homeostasis: An
Introduction   241

Estrogen Sulfotransferase and Its
Regulation in Sepsis Response   243

Estrogen Sulfotransferase and Its
Regulation in Liver Ischemia and
Reperfusion Response   245

Steroid Sulfatase and Its Regulation in
Estrogen Homeostasis and Inflammation
in Chronic Liver Disease   248

Conclusions and Perspectives   251

Acknowledgment   251

References   252

ESTROGEN SULFOTRANSFERASE AND STEROID SULFATASE IN ESTROGEN HOMEOSTASIS: AN INTRODUCTION

Estrogen is not only a key hormone in reproduction, but its functions have also been implicated in numerous pathophysiological conditions, ranging from breast cancer, cognitive function, bone homeostasis, and energy homeostasis to name a few (Hewitt et al., 2005; Simpson et al., 2005). As an essential hormone, the synthesis and metabolism of estrogen must be tightly regulated.

Estrogen sulfation and desulfation represent an important and unique mechanism to control estrogen homeostasis by a reversible metabolic process of conjugation and deconjugation, rather than the destruction of estrogens (Hobkirk, 1993) (Fig. 10.1). Estrogens can be sulfated and deactivated by several sulfotransferases such as the estrogen sulfotransferase (EST or SULT1E1), SULT1A1, and SULT2A1 (Falany, 1997). It is believed that EST is the primary EST at the physiological concentrations due to its high affinity at nanomolar concentrations of estrogens (Zhang et al., 1998; Kakuta et al., 1998). Unlike estrogens, estrogen sulfates cannot bind to the estrogen receptor (ER) and thus are hormonally inactive (Song, 2001; Song et al., 1995). However, estrogen sulfates have higher concentrations and prolonged half-life in the circulation, acting as a reservoir for regenerating active estrogens through the steroid sulfatase (STS)-mediated desulfation reaction (Reed et al., 2005).

EST belongs to the sulfotransferases (SULTs) family of phase II conjugating enzymes that play an essential role in the metabolism and homeostasis of endobiotics and xenobiotics. EST is a cytosolic sulfotransferase best known for its activity in sulfonating and deactivating estrogens, an antiinflammatory hormone. Consistent with the role of EST in estrogen deactivation, EST ablation in male mice resulted in structural and functional lesions in the male reproductive system (Qian et al., 2001). Female $EST^{-/-}$ mice exhibited spontaneous fetal loss due to placental thrombosis caused by insufficient estrogen deactivation and increased ER activation (Tong et al., 2005). The basal expression of hepatic EST is low, but its expression is highly inducible in response to ligands for nuclear receptors, such as the liver X receptor (Gong et al., 2007), glucocorticoid receptor (Gong et al., 2008), and constitutive androstane receptor (Alnouti and Klaassen, 2008; Sueyoshi et al., 2011).

STS is believed to be the only enzyme responsible for the conversion of hormonally inactive estrogen sulfates to the active estrogens. Consistent with the role of STS in hormonal homeostasis, STS gene deletion or mutation is known to be associated with reproductive manifestations, such as cryptorchidism in males and failed labor progression in females due to disrupted steroid hormone homeostasis (Traupe and Happle, 1983). Increased expression of STS has been detected in malignant breast tissues and predicts a poor prognosis (Miyoshi et al., 2003), suggesting an important function of STS in enhancing local estrogen

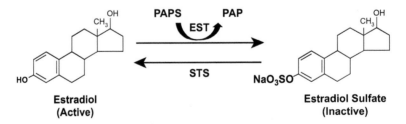

Estradiol
(Active)

Estradiol Sulfate
(Inactive)

FIGURE 10.1   **Estrogen sulfotransferase (EST) and steroid sulfatase (STS) in estrogen homeostasis.** Estrogen sulfation and desulfation represent an important and unique mechanism to control estrogen homeostasis by a reversible metabolic process of conjugation and deconjugation. EST deactivates estrogens by sulfo-conjugation using 3′-phosphoadenosine 5′-phosphosulfate (PAPS) as the sulfate donor. STS converts the hormonally inactive estrogen sulfates to the active estrogens.

signaling and promoting the development of hormone-dependent breast cancer. Indeed, chemical inhibitors of STS have been developed and explored as antibreast cancer agents (Purohit and Foster, 2012; Shah et al., 2016).

Despite the appreciated biological significance of STS, little is known about the transcriptional regulation of this enzyme. Cytokines have been suggested to regulate the expression and activity of STS, but the conclusions have been a subject of debate. Interleukin-1 decreased the expression and activity of STS in endometrial stromal cells (Matsuoka et al., 2002). However, interleukin-6 and tumor necrosis factor α (TNFα) were reported to increase STS activity in breast cancer cells, probably through posttranslational mechanisms (Newman et al., 2000). There is a likelihood that the effects of cytokines on the expression of STS depend on the cellular context.

ESTROGEN SULFOTRANSFERASE AND ITS REGULATION IN SEPSIS RESPONSE

Sepsis is defined as the host's deleterious and nonresolving systemic inflammatory response to microbial infections. Sepsis is one of the leading causes of death in the intensive care unit. The lipopolysacharide (LPS) treatment and cecal ligation and puncture (CLP) are two commonly used mouse models of sepsis. LPS, or endotoxin, is one of the major pattern recognition molecules. LPS is a model compound to trigger an inflammatory response (Ulevitch and Tobias, 1995). LPS is known to elicit its inflammatory actions through the Toll-like receptor 4 (TLR4), a member of the pattern recognition receptor family that mediates innate and adaptive immune response (Poltorak et al., 1998). Activation of TLR4 will lead to the activation of nuclear factor κB (NF-κB), a transcriptional factor that regulates a battery of inflammatory genes (Deng et al., 2013). CLP is another widely used rodent model of sepsis that also triggers marked inflammatory response (Remick et al., 2000; Deitch, 2005; Buras et al., 2005). The CLP model involves feces-derived polymicrobial infection. It has been reported that TLR4 contributes to bacterial clearance and the host inflammatory response in the setting of Gram-negative bacterial infection (Cai et al., 2009; Tsai et al., 2011).

The antiinflammatory activities of estrogens have long been recognized but not without controversies, including in the context of endotoxemia. Evidences that support the benefit of the antiinflammatory activities of estrogens include: (1) in postmenopausal women, estrogen replacement demonstrates prophylactic effects in the prevention of recurrent urinary tract infections (Cardozo et al., 2001; Eriksen, 1999; Perrotta et al., 2008) and (2) hormonal replacement therapy after menopause is also protective of disease activity in women with inflammatory bowel disease (Kane and Reddy, 2008). However, estrogens or ER agonists have also been reported to increase serum TNF levels and mortality in endotoxemic mice (Zuckerman et al., 1995; Ikejima et al., 1998; Trentzsch et al., 2003; Rettew et al., 2009). Knowing that EST is a key enzyme in the metabolic deactivation of estrogens through the EST-mediated sulfation, it is unclear whether and how the hepatic expression and regulation of EST affect the host's response to sepsis.

We recently reported that EST ablation sensitizes mice to sepsis (Chai et al., 2015). It is known that the expression of many drug-metabolizing enzymes, including several SULT isoforms, is suppressed by inflammation (Morgan, 1997; Aitken et al., 2006; Bell and

Strobel, 2012). Therefore, we were initially surprised that the CLP and LPS models of sepsis induced the expression of EST (Chai et al., 2015). We also showed that the CLP- and LPS-responsive induction of EST was sufficient to compromise the activity of estrogen. In the LPS model, treatment of mice with LPS reduced the circulating level of estradiol, increased the urinary output of estrogen sulfate, and attenuated the estrogen responsive uterine epithelial proliferation and gene expression in EST-dependent manner. The induction of EST was shown to be liver specific, because the expression of EST in the white adipose tissue was not affected. Surprisingly, EST ablation sensitizes mice to sepsis-induced death, and this phenotype was recapitulated in wild-type (WT) mice pretreated with Triclosan (5-chloro-2(2,4-dichlorophenoxy)-phenol), a pharmacological inhibitor of EST (Wang et al., 2004; James et al., 2010). Mechanistically, we showed that EST ablation attenuates sepsis-induced inflammatory responses due to compromised estrogen deactivation, leading to increased sepsis lethality. In contrast, transgenic overexpression of EST promotes estrogen deactivation and sensitizes mice to CLP-induced inflammatory response. We went on to show that the induction of EST by sepsis is NF-κB dependent, and the mouse EST gene is an NF-κB target gene, as supported by our promoter analysis. An NF-κB binding site was identified in the mouse EST gene promoter. We also showed that treatment with pyrrolidine dithiocarbamate (PDTC), a pharmacological inhibitor of NF-κB (Lawrence et al., 2001), attenuated CLP- and LPS-responsive induction of EST. These results together demonstrated that EST is a transcriptional target of NF-κB. The roles of EST and its regulation by inflammation are summarized in Fig. 10.2. In the same study, we showed that the CLP- and LPS-responsive induction of EST was TLR4 dependent, because this induction was decreased in two independent strains of TLR4 mutant mice (Poltorak et al., 1998; Nace et al., 2013). We also showed that pharmacological depletion of Kupffer cells by treating mice with gadolinium chloride (Harstad and Klaassen, 2002) attenuated but did not abolish the CLP- and LPS-responsive induction of EST, suggesting that Kupffer cells are required for the optimal induction of EST by sepsis.

This study revealed an unexpected role of EST in sepsis response. Sepsis induced hepatic EST gene expression and compromised estrogenic activity in the liver. Reciprocally, the expression and regulation of EST affected the host's sensitivity to sepsis. EST ablation and overexpression attenuated and enhanced the sepsis-responsive inflammatory response, respectively. The heightened CLP-induced death in EST$^{-/-}$ mice, although paradoxical, was consistent with previous reports that ER agonists increase mortality in endotoxemic

FIGURE 10.2 **Summarized effect of estrogen sulfotransferase (EST) and its regulation on sepsis response.** Sepsis induces the hepatic EST gene expression in a nuclear factor κB (NF-κB)-dependent manner and consequently compromises estrogenic activity in the liver. The inactivation of estrogen, an antiinflammatory hormone, may be necessary for the host to launch an efficient inflammatory response, which is a key survival response.

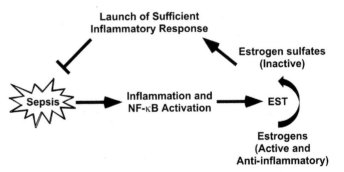

mice (Zuckerman et al., 1995; Ikejima et al., 1998; Trentzsch et al., 2003; Rettew et al., 2009). Our results were also consistent with a clinical report that higher estrogen levels were associated with a greater risk of mortality in critically injured adults (Dossett et al., 2008).

In addition to their clinical significance, our results are also of relevance in environmental health and drug development. Specifically, the CLP sensitizing effect of EST ablation was recapitulated in WT mice treated with the EST inhibitor Triclosan. Triclosan is widely used in consumer products as an antibacterial agent, although its antibacterial benefit has recently been questioned. Triclosan is increasingly found in the environment, such as in sewage sludge and wastewater (Prosser et al., 2014; Gautam et al., 2014). Indeed, Triclosan is readily detectable in human plasma and urine (Dann and Hontela, 2011; Calafat et al., 2008). Triclosan inhibits EST from transferring a sulfuryl moiety from the sulfate donor 3'-phosphoadenosine 5'-phosphosulfate onto estrogen by binding to the estrogen-binding site on EST, causing the formation of Triclosan-sulfate conjugate instead of the estrogen-sulfate conjugate (Wang et al., 2004; James et al., 2010). Our results urge caution in avoiding unwanted side effects when the EST-inhibiting pharmaceutical or neutraceutical agents are used in patients with sepsis.

The sepsis induction of EST and the establishment of EST as an NF-κB target gene were intriguing, considering that many of the drug-metabolizing enzymes are suppressed by inflammation and NF-κB (Morgan, 1997). To our knowledge, EST is one of a very small number of drug-metabolizing enzymes whose expression was reported to be induced by inflammation. The inflammatory responsive induction of EST may represent a double-edged sword. Although the consequent increase in estrogen deprivation has a potential to exacerbate inflammation as suggested by the results from our EST transgenic mice, the inflammation sensitizing effect of EST has a potential benefit in helping with the host's ability to launch an efficient inflammatory response, a key survival response that releases proinflammatory cytokines and chemokines with a subsequent recruitment of inflammatory cells (Leventhal and Schroppel, 2012) (Fig. 10.2). The reciprocal regulation of inflammation and EST represents a yet to be explored mechanism of endocrine regulation of inflammation, which may be explored to improve the clinical management of sepsis.

ESTROGEN SULFOTRANSFERASE AND ITS REGULATION IN LIVER ISCHEMIA AND REPERFUSION RESPONSE

Liver ischemia and reperfusion (I/R) injury occurs in various clinical settings when the blood flow to the liver is blocked or the liver is in a low-flow state. Examples of these clinical situations include liver resection, solid organ transplantation, cardiac and vascular surgery, massive trauma, hemorrhage shock, and cardiogenic shock (Saidi and Kenari, 2014). The I/R injury can cause a series of clinical manifestations, ranging from asymptomatic elevation of liver enzymes to acute liver failure or even death (Serracino-Inglott et al., 2001).

The pathogenesis of hepatic I/R injury is a dynamic process including the deprivation of blood and oxygen supply, followed by their restoration. The pathological events associated with I/R include a direct hypoxic damage as the result of ischemia, as well as a delayed and more severe oxidative damage that eventually leads to the activation of inflammatory pathways (Zhai et al., 2011). During the hypoxic phase, sublethal cellular damage leads to the release of reactive oxygen species, damaging the associated molecular pattern of macrophages and hepatocytes. Reperfusion augments the injury by triggering the sterile inflammatory responses, causing irreversible liver damage (Klune and Tsung, 2010). Meanwhile, a series of protective pathways are also activated and as such, the extent of organ damage is largely determined by the balance between the detrimental and protective systems. There are two transcriptional factors, the hypoxia-inducible factor-1 (HIF-1) and nuclear factor erythroid 2–related factor 2 (Nrf2), which play important roles in protecting the liver from I/R injury. Stabilization and accumulation of HIF-1 or Nrf2 can lead to the activation of an array of genes to adapt the cells to hypoxic or oxidative damages, and thus affect numerous cellular functions, such as cell apoptosis, proliferation, survival, metabolism, and angiogenesis (Zhai et al., 2011; Dery et al., 2005).

Both clinical and animal studies have shown a sexual dimorphic response of the liver to I/R. Many studies suggested that female livers are more tolerant than male livers under stress conditions, suggesting estrogen as a responsible and protective factor for this sexual dimorphism (Harada et al., 1985; Jarrar et al., 2000; Lee et al., 2000; Jain et al., 2000). The proposed mechanisms for the protective effect of estrogens on liver I/R include inhibition of apoptosis (Lin et al., 2012), an increased serum level of nitric oxide and decreased serum level of TNFα (Eckhoff et al., 2002), regulation of heat-shock protein expression (Shen et al., 2007), and selective modulation of MAPK kinase activities (Vilatoba et al., 2005). However, it came to our attention that most of these experiments were performed by challenging male mice or ovariectomized female animals with pharmacological doses of estrogens, whereas the dynamics of the endogenous estrogens and their metabolism during I/R remains unknown. Considering the potential side effects associated with the pharmacological estrogen therapies (Staren and Omer, 2004), it is necessary to develop novel therapeutic strategies to attenuate hepatic I/R injury through the regulation of endogenous estrogen metabolism.

We recently reported that the hepatic expression and activity of EST were markedly induced in a mouse model of I/R, which was associated with a higher level of estrone sulfate and decreased expression of estrogen responsive genes in the liver in an EST-dependent manner (Guo et al., 2015). Mechanistically, oxidative stress-induced activation of Nrf2, instead of the hypoxia-inducible activation of HIF-1, was responsible for the EST induction, because the I/R responsive induction of EST was abolished in the Nrf2$^{-/-}$ mice. Moreover, a pharmacological activation of Nrf2 was sufficient to induce the expression of EST in primary hepatocytes. We went on to show that Nrf2 regulates EST through the binding of Nrf2 to two antioxidant response elements (AREs) in the promoter region of the mouse EST gene, establishing EST as a direct transcriptional target of Nrf2. At the pathophysiological level and in the female mice, EST ablation attenuated the I/R injury as a result of decreased estrogen deprivation, whereas this benefit was abolished upon ovariectomy. These results suggested that the upregulation of EST in the liver may have played a pathogenic role in I/R injury, because EST ablation in female mice attenuated I/R responsive liver injury in an estrogen-dependent manner. Interestingly, the effect of EST ablation was highly sex specific, because the EST$^{-/-}$ male mice exhibited heightened I/R injury. Reciprocally, both estrogens and EST regulate the expression and activity of Nrf2. Estrogen deprivation by ovariectomy abolished the I/R responsive Nrf2 accumulation in female mice, whereas the compromised estrogen deprivation in EST$^{-/-}$ mice was associated with an increased Nrf2 accumulation. Our results suggested a novel I/R responsive feedback mechanism to limit the activity of Nrf2, in which

Nrf2 induces the expression of EST, which subsequently increases estrogen deactivation and limits the estrogen responsive activation of Nrf2 (Fig. 10.3).

An interesting finding from this study is the sex-specific effect of EST ablation on I/R. In contrast to its protective effect in female mice, EST ablation sensitized male mice to I/R injury. Previous reports suggested that estrogens protected male mice from I/R injury (Eckhoff et al., 2002; Vilatoba et al., 2005). However, most of the reported protections were observed in male animals that were treated with pharmacological doses of estrogens. Our results suggested differential effects between the administration of pharmacological doses of estrogens and alteration in endogenous estrogen metabolism. The increased sensitivity to I/R in male $EST^{-/-}$ mice was abolished upon castration, suggesting that the sensitization was androgen dependent. Indeed, androgens have been reported to play a role in liver I/R injury (Soljancic et al., 2013). The detailed mechanism for the sex-specific effect of EST ablation on I/R injury remains to be better defined. Interestingly and consistent with the EST ablation, the loss of Nrf2 effect was also gender specific, because the male $Nrf2^{-/-}$ mice showed heightened sensitivity to I/R liver injury as shown by us and others (Chai et al., 2015; Guo et al., 2015; Kudoh et al., 2014; Ke et al., 2013), whereas the female $Nrf2^{-/-}$ mice showed attenuated sensitivity to I/R liver injury (Guo et al., 2015).

Together, our results suggested that the induction of hepatic EST, which was mediated by the oxidative stress-induced Nrf2 activation, may have played a pathogenic role in the I/R liver injury. As such, both EST ablation and Nrf2 ablation conferred a protection in female mice. Pharmacological inhibition of EST, at least in females, might represent a novel therapeutic approach to manage hepatic I/R injury. It is encouraging that major progress has been made in the identification and characterization of chemical EST inhibitors (James et al., 2010).

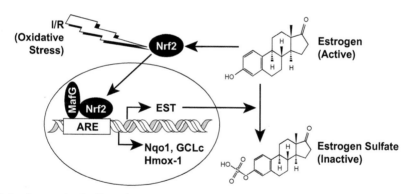

FIGURE 10.3 **Summarized effect of estrogen sulfotransferase (EST) and its regulation on liver ischemia and reperfusion (I/R) response.** Liver I/R induces the hepatic EST gene expression in an oxidative stress and Nrf2-dependent manner and consequently compromises estrogenic activity in the liver. The induction of EST in female mice appears to be pathogenic, because EST ablation protected mice from I/R injury. However, the effect of EST ablation is gender specific, as the male EST null mice exhibited heightened sensitivity to I/R injury. The detailed mechanism for the sex-specific effect of EST ablation on I/R injury remains to be defined. *ARE*, antioxidant response element; *Nrf2*, nuclear factor erythroid 2–related factor 2. *From Guo, Y., Hu, B., Huang, H., Tsung, A., Gaikwad, N.W., Xu, M., Jiang, M., Ren, S., Fan, J., Billiar, T.R., Huang, M., Xie, W., 2015. Estrogen sulfotransferase is an oxidative stress-responsive gene that gender-specifically affects liver ischemia/reperfusion injury. J. Biol. Chem. 290, 14754–14764, © The American Society for Biochemistry and Molecular Biology.*

STEROID SULFATASE AND ITS REGULATION IN ESTROGEN HOMEOSTASIS AND INFLAMMATION IN CHRONIC LIVER DISEASE

Abnormal estrogen metabolism in liver disease has been long recognized in the clinic. Concomitants of liver diseases are clinical signs and symptoms like palmar erythema, spider nevus, gynecomastia, and infertility due to disturbed homeostasis of steroid hormones, especially the estrogens (Li et al., 1999). Studies have reported increased estrogen levels and signs of endocrine disturbance in patients with chronic liver diseases (Adlercreutz, 1970). The hormone levels are positively correlated to the severity of the liver disease (Gavaler, 1995), whereas treating patients toward improved liver function resulted in regression of endocrine disturbance (Long and Simmons, 1951). The liver is the primary site of estrogen metabolism through phase I oxidation reactions, which are mainly catalyzed by CYP1A2 and CYP3A4 (Zhu and Conney, 1998), and phase II conjugation reactions mediated by EST (Falany, 1997). It is thought that damage to the liver impairs its capacity to metabolize and inactivate estrogens, resulting in increased estrogen levels in the circulation (Glass et al., 1940). However, there have been reports that changes in steroid hormone levels may occur before the liver functions are compromised (Becker, 1993), suggesting additional mechanisms by which liver disease causes estrogen excess. Specifically, having known that STS plays a key role in converting the inactive but abundant estrogens to active estrogens, it is unclear whether the expression of STS is regulated in chronic liver disease and if so, whether the regulation of STS also contributes to the estrogen excess. Although estrogens are known to be the antiinflammatory hormones, it is unclear whether the estrogen excess can affect the clinical outcome of the underlying liver diseases.

The development of many chronic inflammatory liver diseases is more common in men than in women. The prognosis of hepatocellular carcinoma is also worse for male than for female patients (El-Serag et al., 2001). These gender differences may be accounted for by sex hormones. Although it is not a classic target organ of sex steroid hormones, the liver has been shown to express functional ER and respond to estrogen stimulation (Porter et al., 1983). Since estrogens are known for their antiinflammatory activities (Straub, 2007), they may provide a benefit in inhibiting the progression of chronic inflammatory liver diseases.

In a recent report, we showed that the hepatic expression of STS was induced in patients with chronic inflammatory liver diseases, which was accompanied by increased circulating estrogen levels (Jiang et al., 2016). The frequent induction of STS in chronic inflammatory liver diseases was first suggested in our bioinformatics analysis of the Gene Expression Omnibus (www.ncbi.nlm.nih.gov/geo) database (GSE32504), in which we found the expression of STS was induced in subjects with elevated levels of C-reactive protein, an inflammation marker that also predicts disease progression and clinical outcome in patients with liver disease (Cervoni et al., 2012). Immunohistochemistry staining of STS on liver sections from control, cirrhosis, or chronic hepatitis subjects showed that the incidence of chronic hepatitis and cirrhosis was positively associated with the expression of STS. Subsequently, we found the human STS gene, but not the mouse Sts gene, was induced by inflammatory stimuli in primary human hepatocytes or human hepatic cell lines. The inflammatory stimuli we tested include LPS, TNF-α (Ding and Yin, 2004), and phorbol-12-myristate-13-acetate (Holden et al., 2008), all known to activate NF-κB. We went on to show that the human STS is a novel NF-κB target gene. Three NF-κB binding sites were identified in the human STS gene promoter, and two of them were found to be functionally relevant. At the functional level, the inflammatory induction of STS facilitated the conversion of inactive estrogen sulfates to active estrogens, and consequently attenuated the inflammatory response. In contrast, genetic small interfering RNA (siRNA) knockdown or pharmacological inhibition of STS by STX64 (Purohit et al., 2000), or a direct blockade of estrogen signaling by the ER antagonist Fulvestrant (also called ICI 182,780) sensitized liver cells to the transcriptional activation of NF-κB and inflammatory response. Our results suggest a negative feedback loop in chronic inflammatory liver diseases, in which the inflammatory activation of NF-κB induces STS gene expression. The induced STS facilitates the conversion of inactive estrogen sulfates to active estrogens, which in return attenuates the NF-κB-mediated inflammation via the estrogen/ER signaling, thereby completing the negative feedback loop (Fig. 10.4). Our results also provided a potential explanation of why changes in steroid hormone levels in patients can occur before the liver functions are compromised (Becker, 1993).

One of our most interesting and surprising findings is the inflammatory induction of STS and the establishment of STS as an NF-κB target gene. This finding is intriguing because most drug-metabolizing enzymes as well as transporters are suppressed by inflammation and NF-κB (Klein et al., 2015). It is interesting to note that the induction of STS was human-specific because LPS treatment had little effect on the expression of Sts in the mouse liver. The species specificity of the regulation may be due to the marked divergence between the human and mouse STS genes. The genomic DNA of the mouse Sts gene spans approximately 9-kb, which is substantially smaller than its 146-kb human counterpart (Salido et al., 1996; Yen et al., 1988). Despite the much-appreciated biological significance of STS, the transcriptional regulation of this gene has been poorly understood. It has been reported that the human STS gene promoter resembled neither a tightly regulated gene that often contains a TATA box to position the RNA polymerase, nor a housekeeping gene that is usually GC rich and contains binding sites for the Sp1 transcriptional factor. The human STS promoter is GC poor and lacks the TATA box and Sp1 binding sites (Li et al., 1996). In the current study, we established the human STS gene as a transcriptional target of NF-κB. NF-κB transactivates STS gene expression through its binding sites in the STS gene promoter.

The biological and clinical relevance of the inflammatory regulation of STS is intriguing. Our results clearly show that the inflammatory induction of STS enhances estrogen activity, which subsequently attenuates the NF-κB activation and inflammatory response, possibly through the inhibition of IKK activation. The NF-κB and STS mediated negative feedback loop to limit the NF-κB activity may however represent a double-edged sword. Although the consequent increase in estrogen activity can limit inflammation as suggested by our results, the induction of STS does have the potential to prevent the host's ability to launch an efficient and pro-survival inflammatory response. The same notion for the double-edged sword effect of estrogens was suggested in our recent work showing that ablation of the estrogen deactivating gene EST actually sensitized mice to sepsis-induced lethality (Chai et al., 2015). It is possible that the significance of this negative feedback loop in liver diseases is disease stage-specific, because the NF-κB-mediated inflammation in hepatocytes plays a dual role in the progression of liver

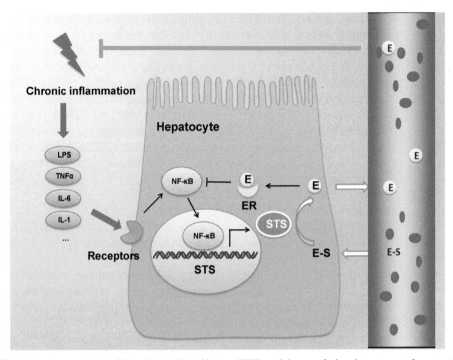

FIGURE 10.4 **Summarized effect of steroid sulfatase (STS) and its regulation in estrogen homeostasis and inflammation in chronic liver disease.** A proposed STS-mediated negative feedback loop in chronic inflammatory liver disease that limits the activity of nuclear factor κB (NF-κB) and attenuates inflammation. During chronic inflammation, inflammatory mediators such as lipopolysaccharide (LPS) and tumor necrosis factor α (TNFα) act on hepatocytes to elicit NF-κB activation. NF-κB then induces the expression of STS, which converts inactive estrogen sulfates to active estrogens and increases the estrogen level in the liver and circulation. The estrogens/ER signaling in return suppresses the NF-κB response and inhibits inflammation. *From Jiang, M., Klein, M., Zanger, U.M., Mohammad, M.K., Cave, M.C., Gaikwad, N.W., Dias, N.J., Selcer, K.W., Guo, Y., He, J., Zhang, X., Shen, Q., Qin, W., Li, J., Li, S., Xie, W., 2016. Inflammatory regulation of steroid sulfatase: a novel mechanism to control estrogen homeostasis and inflammation in chronic liver disease. J. Hepatol. 64, 44–52. © European Association for the Study of the Liver.*

diseases. In the early stages of liver diseases, activation of NF-κB helps to fight infection and prevent hepatocyte death by inducing the antiapoptotic genes. In the late stages, however, NF-κB also promotes the survival of hepatocytes harboring oncogenic mutations, which increase the risk of hepatocellular carcinoma. Future studies are necessary to pinpoint the stage when NF-κB activation becomes oncogenic, so that more precise treatment can be launched. On the other hand, the antiinflammatory effect of estrogen may not be limited to the suppression of NF-κB. Activation of the estrogen signaling has been reported to inhibit the development of fatty liver, which is an important cause of hepatic inflammation (Monteiro et al., 2014). Although estrogens may have beneficial effect in inhibiting inflammation, potential adverse effects, such as tumor promotion, risk of cardiovascular disease and feminization of males, limit the utility of systemic estrogen therapies. It will be ideal that selective ER modulators can be developed to protect against liver injury without causing adverse effects to extrahepatic tissues. More studies are needed to validate STS activation or other estrogen-related therapies in the management of chronic liver diseases.

Among the limitations is that although the chemical inhibitors we used in this study, such as the STS inhibitor STX64, NF-κB inhibitor PDTC, and ER antagonist Fulvestrant/ICI 182,780, are well-established inhibitors to manipulate protein activities, we cannot exclude the possibility that these chemicals may interfere with the off-target regulatory pathways (Atanasov et al., 2003). It is encouraging to note that in the case of STS and NF-κB, the results from the use of pharmacological inhibitors were consistent with those obtained from the genetic siRNA knockdowns. In conclusion, our results provide a novel endocrine basis for the estrogen excess in chronic liver diseases, pointing to a critical and comprehensive role of the hepatic microenvironment in the regulation of estrogen homeostasis. We propose that the inflammatory regulation of STS represents a novel mechanism to control estrogen homeostasis and inflammation, including in the context of chronic liver diseases.

CONCLUSIONS AND PERSPECTIVES

In this chapter, we present several cases of our own work in which the expression of estrogen-metabolizing enzymes EST and STS is subjected to the regulation by systemic or local liver injuries, including sepsis, liver I/R, and chronic liver disease. These are prototypical examples of the so-called disease—drug interaction, in which diseases affect the metabolism of the liver. In the meantime, the expression or lack of expression of EST can affect an animal's sensitivity to sepsis and I/R. In the case of STS, inhibition of STS can sensitize the inflammatory response of hepatic cells. It is conceivable that the disease—drug interactions can be extended to: (1) other types of diseases, (2) the metabolism of drugs or endogenous chemicals (endobiotics) other than estrogens, (3) drug-metabolizing enzymes other than EST and STS, and (4) metabolism in the extrahepatic tissues.

Drug metabolism and disposition are critical in maintaining the chemical and functional homeostasis of xenobiotics/drugs and endobiotics. The liver plays an essential role in drug metabolism and disposition not only because of its large size, but also due to its abundant expression of enzymes and transporters. Accumulated evidence suggests that many hepatic and systemic diseases can affect drug metabolism and disposition by regulating the expression and/or activity of enzymes and transporters in the liver. Reciprocally, the expression and activity of DMEs can affect animals' sensitivity to local and systemic liver injuries. Understanding the disease effect on drug metabolism is clinically important due to the concern of disease—drug interactions. Future studies are necessary to understand the mechanism by which liver injury regulates drug metabolism to better manage the disease—drug interactions. Human studies are also urgently needed to determine whether the animal results can be recapitulated in human patients.

Acknowledgment

The original research described in this chapter was supported in part by the National Institutes of Health (NIH) grants ES023438 and DK099232 (to W.X.). W.X. is supported in part by the Joseph Koslow Endowed Professorship from the University of Pittsburgh School of Pharmacy.

References

Adlercreutz, H., 1970. Oestrogen metabolism in liver disease. J. Endocrinol. 46, 129–163.

Aitken, A.E., Richardson, T.A., Morgan, E.T., 2006. Regulation of drug-metabolizing enzymes and transporters in inflammation. Annu. Rev. Pharmacol. Toxicol. 46, 123–149.

Alnouti, Y., Klaassen, C.D., 2008. Regulation of sulfotransferase enzymes by prototypical microsomal enzyme inducers in mice. J. Pharmacol. Exp. Ther. 324, 612–621.

Atanasov, A.G., Tam, S., Rocken, J.M., Baker, M.E., Odermatt, A., 2003. Inhibition of 11 beta-hydroxysteroid dehydrogenase type 2 by dithiocarbamates. Biochem. Biophys. Res. Commun. 308, 257–262.

Becker, U., 1993. The influence of ethanol and liver disease on sex hormones and hepatic oestrogen receptors in women. Dan. Med. Bull. 40, 447–459.

Bell, J.C., Strobel, H.W., 2012. Regulation of cytochrome P450 4F11 by nuclear transcription factor-κB. Drug Metab. Dispos. 40, 205–211.

Buras, J.A., Holzmann, B., Sitkovsky, M., 2005. Animal models of sepsis: setting the stage. Nat. Rev. Drug Discov. 4, 854–865.

Cai, S., Batra, S., Shen, L., Wakamatsu, N., Jeyaseelan, S., 2009. Both TRIF- and MyD88-dependent signaling contribute to host defense against pulmonary *Klebsiella* infection. J. Immunol. 183, 6629–6638.

Calafat, A.M., Ye, X., Wong, L.Y., Reidy, J.A., Needham, L.L., 2008. Urinary concentrations of triclosan in the U.S. population: 2003–2004. Environ. Health Perspect. 116, 303–307.

Cardozo, L., Lose, G., McClish, D., Versi, E., de Koning Gans, H., 2001. A systematic review of estrogens for recurrent urinary tract infections: third report of the hormones and urogenital therapy (HUT) committee. Int. Urogynecol. J. Pelvic Floor Dysfunct. 12, 15–20.

Cervoni, J.P., Thevenot, T., Weil, D., Muel, E., Barbot, O., Sheppard, F., Monnet, E., Di Martino, V., 2012. C-reactive protein predicts short-term mortality in patients with cirrhosis. J. Hepatol. 56, 1299–1304.

Chai, X., Guo, Y., Jiang, M., Hu, B., Li, Z., Fan, J., Deng, M., Billiar, T.R., Kucera, H.R., Gaikwad, N.W., Xu, M., Lu, P., Yan, J., Fu, H., Liu, Y., Yu, L., Huang, M., Zeng, S., Xie, W., 2015. Oestrogen sulfotransferase ablation sensitizes mice to sepsis. Nat. Commun. 6, 7979.

Dann, A.B., Hontela, A., 2011. Triclosan: environmental exposure, toxicity and mechanisms of action. J. Appl. Toxicol. 31, 285–311.

Deitch, E.A., 2005. Rodent models of intra-abdominal infection. Shock 24 (Suppl. 1), 19–23.

Deng, M., Scott, M.J., Loughran, P., Gibson, G., Sodhi, C., Watkins, S., Hackam, D., Billiar, T.R., 2013. Lipopolysaccharide clearance, bacterial clearance, and systemic inflammatory responses are regulated by cell type-specific functions of TLR4 during sepsis. J. Immunol. 190, 5152–5160.

Dery, M.A., Michaud, M.D., Richard, D.E., 2005. Hypoxia-inducible factor 1: regulation by hypoxic and non-hypoxic activators. Int. J. Biochem. Cell Biol. 37, 535–540.

Ding, W.X., Yin, X.M., 2004. Dissection of the multiple mechanisms of TNF-alpha-induced apoptosis in liver injury. J. Cell Mol. Med. 8, 445–454.

Dossett, L.A., Swenson, B.R., Heffernan, D., Bonatti, H., Metzger, R., Sawyer, R.G., May, A.K., 2008. High levels of endogenous estrogens are associated with death in the critically injured adult. J. Trauma 64, 580–585.

Eckhoff, D.E., Bilbao, G., Frenette, L., Thompson, J.A., Contreras, J.L., 2002. 17-Beta-estradiol protects the liver against warm ischemia/reperfusion injury and is associated with increased serum nitric oxide and decreased tumor necrosis factor-alpha. Surgery 132, 302–309.

El-Serag, H.B., Mason, A.C., Key, C., 2001. Trends in survival of patients with hepatocellular carcinoma between 1977 and 1996 in the United States. Hepatology 33, 62–65.

Eriksen, B., 1999. A randomized, open, parallel-group study on the preventive effect of an estradiol-releasing vaginal ring (Estring) on recurrent urinary tract infections in postmenopausal women. Am. J. Obstet. Gynecol. 180, 1072–1079.

Falany, C.N., 1997. Enzymology of human cytosolic sulfotransferases. FASEB J. 11, 206–216.

Gautam, P., Carsella, J.S., Kinney, C.A., 2014. Presence and transport of the antimicrobials triclocarban and triclosan in a wastewater-dominated stream and freshwater environment. Water Res. 48, 247–256.

Gavaler, J.S., 1995. Alcohol effects on hormone levels in normal postmenopausal women and in postmenopausal women with alcohol-induced cirrhosis. Recent Dev. Alcohol. 12, 199–208.

Glass, S.J., Edmondson, H.A., Soll, S.N., 1940. Sex hormone changes associated with liver disease. Endocrinology 27, 749–752.

Gong, H., Guo, P., Zhai, Y., Zhou, J., Uppal, H., Jarzynka, M.J., Song, W.C., Cheng, S.Y., Xie, W., 2007. Estrogen deprivation and inhibition of breast cancer growth in vivo through activation of the orphan nuclear receptor liver X receptor. Mol. Endocrinol. 21, 1781–1790.

Gong, H., Jarzynka, M.J., Cole, T.J., Lee, J.H., Wada, T., Zhang, B., Gao, J., Song, W.C., DeFranco, D.B., Cheng, S.Y., Xie, W., 2008. Glucocorticoids antagonize estrogens by glucocorticoid receptor-mediated activation of estrogen sulfotransferase. Cancer Res. 68, 7386–7393.

Guo, Y., Hu, B., Huang, H., Tsung, A., Gaikwad, N.W., Xu, M., Jiang, M., Ren, S., Fan, J., Billiar, T.R., Huang, M., Xie, W., 2015. Estrogen sulfotransferase is an oxidative stress-responsive gene that gender-specifically affects liver ischemia/reperfusion injury. J. Biol. Chem. 290, 14754–14764.

Harada, H., Pavlick, K.P., Hines, I.N., Hoffman, J.M., Bharwani, S., Gray, L., Wolf, R.E., Grisham, M.B., 1985. Selected contribution: effects of gender on reduced-size liver ischemia and reperfusion injury. J. Appl. Physiol. 2001 (91), 2816–2822.

Harstad, E.B., Klaassen, C.D., 2002. Gadolinium chloride pretreatment prevents cadmium chloride-induced liver damage in both wild-type and MT-null mice. Toxicol. Appl. Pharmacol. 180, 178–185.

Hewitt, S.C., Harrell, J.C., Korach, K.S., 2005. Lessons in estrogen biology from knockout and transgenic animals. Annu. Rev. Physiol. 67, 285–308.

Hobkirk, R., 1993. Steroid sulfation Current concepts. Trends Endocrinol. Metab. 4, 69–74.

Holden, N.S., Squires, P.E., Kaur, M., Bland, R., Jones, C.E., Newton, R., 2008. Phorbol ester-stimulated NF-kappaB-dependent transcription: roles for isoforms of novel protein kinase C. Cell. Signal. 20, 1338–1348.

Ikejima, K., Enomoto, N., Iimuro, Y., Ikejima, A., Fang, D., Xu, J., Forman, D.T., Brenner, D.A., Thurman, R.G., 1998. Estrogen increases sensitivity of hepatic Kupffer cells to endotoxin. Am. J. Physiol. 274, G669–G676.

Jain, A., Reyes, J., Kashyap, R., Dodson, S.F., Demetris, A.J., Ruppert, K., Abu-Elmagd, K., Marsh, W., Madariaga, J., Mazariegos, G., Geller, D., Bonham, C.A., Gayowski, T., Cacciarelli, T., Fontes, P., Starzl, T.E., Fung, J.J., 2000. Long-term survival after liver transplantation in 4,000 consecutive patients at a single center. Ann. Surg. 232, 490–500.

James, M.O., Li, W., Summerlot, D.P., Rowland-Faux, L., Wood, C.E., 2010. Triclosan is a potent inhibitor of estradiol and estrone sulfonation in sheep placenta. Environ. Int. 36, 942–949.

Jarrar, D., Wang, P., Cioffi, W.G., Bland, K.I., Chaudry, I.H., 2000. The female reproductive cycle is an important variable in the response to trauma-hemorrhage. Am. J. Physiol. Heart Circ. Physiol. 279 (3), H1015–H1021.

Jiang, M., Klein, M., Zanger, U.M., Mohammad, M.K., Cave, M.C., Gaikwad, N.W., Dias, N.J., Selcer, K.W., Guo, Y., He, J., Zhang, X., Shen, Q., Qin, W., Li, J., Li, S., Xie, W., 2016. Inflammatory regulation of steroid sulfatase: a novel mechanism to control estrogen homeostasis and inflammation in chronic liver disease. J. Hepatol. 64, 44–52.

Kakuta, Y., Pedersen, L.C., Chae, K., Song, W.C., Leblanc, D., London, R., Carter, C.W., Negishi, M., 1998. Mouse steroid sulfotransferases: substrate specificity and preliminary X-ray crystallographic analysis. Biochem. Pharmacol. 55, 313–317.

Kane, S.V., Reddy, D., 2008. Hormonal replacement therapy after menopause is protective of disease activity in women with inflammatory bowel disease. Am. J. Gastroenterol. 103, 1193–1196.

Ke, B., Shen, X.D., Zhang, Y., Ji, H., Gao, F., Yue, S., Kamo, N., Zhai, Y., Yamamoto, M., Busuttil, R.W., Kupiec-Weglinski, J.W., 2013. KEAP1-NRF2 complex in ischemia-induced hepatocellular damage of mouse liver transplants. J. Hepatol. 59, 1200–1207.

Klein, M., Thomas, M., Hofmann, U., Seehofer, D., Damm, G., Zanger, U.M., 2015. A systematic comparison of the impact of inflammatory signaling on absorption, distribution, metabolism, and excretion gene expression and activity in primary human hepatocytes and HepaRG cells. Drug Metab. Dispos. 43, 273–283.

Klune, J.R., Tsung, A., 2010. Molecular biology of liver ischemia/reperfusion injury: established mechanisms and recent advancements. Surg. Clin. North Am. 90, 665–677.

Kudoh, K., Uchinami, H., Yoshioka, M., Seki, E., Yamamoto, Y., 2014. Nrf2 activation protects the liver from ischemia/reperfusion injury in mice. Ann. Surg. 260, 118–127.

Lawrence, T., Gilroy, D.W., Colville-Nash, P.R., Willoughby, D.A., 2001. Possible new role for NF-kappaB in the resolution of inflammation. Nat. Med. 7, 1291–1297.

Lee, C.C., Chau, G.Y., Lui, W.Y., Tsay, S.H., King, K.L., Loong, C.C., Hshia, C.Y., Wu, C.W., 2000. Better post-resectional survival in female cirrhotic patients with hepatocellular carcinoma. Hepatogastroenterology 47, 446–449.

Leventhal, J.S., Schroppel, B., 2012. Toll-like receptors in transplantation: sensing and reacting to injury. Kidney Int. 81, 826–832.

Li, X.M., Alperin, E.S., Salido, E., Gong, Y., Yen, P., Shapiro, L.J., 1996. Characterization of the promoter region of human steroid sulfatase: a gene which escapes X inactivation. Somat. Cell Mol. Genet. 22, 105–117.

Li, C.P., Lee, F.Y., Hwang, S.J., Chang, F.Y., Lin, H.C., Lu, R.H., Hou, M.C., Chu, C.J., Chan, C.C., Luo, J.C., Lee, S.D., 1999. Spider angiomas in patients with liver cirrhosis: role of alcoholism and impaired liver function. Scand. J. Gastroenterol. 34, 520–523.

Lin, F.S., Shen, S.Q., Chen, Z.B., Yan, R.C., 2012. 17beta-estradiol attenuates reduced-size hepatic ischemia/reperfusion injury by inhibition apoptosis via mitochondrial pathway in rats. Shock 37, 183–190.

Long, R.S., Simmons, E.E., 1951. The liver and estrogen metabolism; report of cases. AMA Arch. Intern. Med. 88, 762–769.

Matsuoka, R., Yanaihara, A., Saito, H., Furusawa, Y., Toma, Y., Shimizu, Y., Yanaihara, T., Okai, T., 2002. Regulation of estrogen activity in human endometrium: effect of IL-1beta on steroid sulfatase activity in human endometrial stromal cells. Steroids 67, 655–659.

Miyoshi, Y., Ando, A., Hasegawa, S., Ishitobi, M., Taguchi, T., Tamaki, Y., Noguchi, S., 2003. High expression of steroid sulfatase mRNA predicts poor prognosis in patients with estrogen receptor-positive breast cancer. Clin. Cancer Res. 9, 2288–2293.

Monteiro, R., Teixeira, D., Calhau, C., 2014. Estrogen signaling in metabolic inflammation. Mediators Inflamm. 2014, 615917.

Morgan, E.T., 1997. Regulation of cytochromes P450 during inflammation and infection. Drug Metab. Rev. 29, 1129–1188.

Nace, G.W., Huang, H., Klune, J.R., Eid, R.E., Rosborough, B.R., Korff, S., Li, S., Shapiro, R.A., Stolz, D.B., Sodhi, C.P., Hackam, D.J., Geller, D.A., Billiar, T.R., Tsung, A., 2013. Cellular-specific role of toll-like receptor 4 in hepatic ischemia-reperfusion injury in mice. Hepatology 58, 374–387.

Newman, S.P., Purohit, A., Ghilchik, M.W., Potter, B.V., Reed, M.J., 2000. Regulation of steroid sulphatase expression and activity in breast cancer. J. Steroid. Biochem. Mol. Biol. 75, 259–264.

Perrotta, C., Aznar, M., Mejia, R., Albert, X., Ng, C.W., 2008. Oestrogens for preventing recurrent urinary tract infection in postmenopausal women. Cochrane Database Syst. Rev. 2, CD005131.

Poltorak, A., He, X., Smirnova, I., Liu, M.-Y., Huffel, C.V., Du, X., Birdwell, D., Alejos, E., Silva, M., Galanos, C., Freudenberg, M., Ricciardi-Castagnoli, P., Layton, B., Beutler, B., 1998. Defective LPS signaling in C3H/HeJ and C57BL/10ScCr mice: mutations in Tlr4 gene. Science 282, 2085–2088.

Porter, L.E., Elm, M.S., Van Thiel, D.H., Dugas, M.C., Eagon, P.K., 1983. Characterization and quantitation of human hepatic estrogen receptor. Gastroenterology 84, 704–712.

Prosser, R.S., Lissemore, L., Topp, E., Sibley, P.K., 2014. Bioaccumulation of triclosan and triclocarban in plants grown in soils amended with municipal dewatered biosolids. Environ. Toxicol. Chem. 33, 975–984.

Purohit, A., Foster, P.A., 2012. Steroid sulfatase inhibitors for estrogen- and androgen-dependent cancers. J. Endocrinol. 212, 99–110.

Purohit, A., Woo, L.W., Potter, B.V., Reed, M.J., 2000. In vivo inhibition of estrone sulfatase activity and growth of nitrosomethylurea-induced mammary tumors by 667 COUMATE. Cancer Res. 60, 3394–3396.

Qian, Y.M., Sun, X.J., Tong, M.H., Li, X.P., Richa, J., Song, W.C., 2001. Targeted disruption of the mouse estrogen sulfotransferase gene reveals a role of estrogen metabolism in intracrine and paracrine estrogen regulation. Endocrinology 142, 5342–5350.

Reed, M.J., Purohit, A., Woo, L.W., Newman, S.P., Potter, B.V., 2005. Steroid sulfatase: molecular biology, regulation, and inhibition. Endocr. Rev. 26, 171–202.

Remick, D.G., Newcomb, D.E., Bolgos, G.L., Call, D.R., 2000. Comparison of the mortality and inflammatory response of two models of sepsis: lipopolysaccharide vs. cecal ligation and puncture. Shock 13, 110–116.

Rettew, J.A., Huet, Y.M., Marriott, I., 2009. Estrogens augment cell surface TLR4 expression on murine macrophages and regulate sepsis susceptibility in vivo. Endocrinology 150, 3877–3884.

Saidi, R.F., Kenari, S.K., 2014. Liver ischemia/reperfusion injury: an overview. J. Invest. Surg. 27, 366–379.

Salido, E.C., Li, X.M., Yen, P.H., Martin, N., Mohandas, T.K., Shapiro, L.J., 1996. Cloning and expression of the mouse pseudoautosomal steroid sulphatase gene (Sts). Nat. Genet. 13, 83–86.

Serracino-Inglott, F., Habib, N.A., Mathie, R.T., 2001. Hepatic ischemia-reperfusion injury. Am. J. Surg. 181, 160–166.

Shah, R., Singh, J., Singh, D., Jaggi, A.S., Singh, N., 2016. Sulfatase inhibitors for recidivist breast cancer treatment: a chemical review. Eur. J. Med. Chem. 114, 170–190.

Shen, S.Q., Zhang, Y., Xiong, C.L., 2007. The protective effects of 17beta-estradiol on hepatic ischemia-reperfusion injury in rat model, associated with regulation of heat-shock protein expression. J. Surg. Res. 140, 67–76.

Simpson, E.R., Misso, M., Hewitt, K.N., Hill, R.A., Boon, W.C., Jones, M.E., Kovacic, A., Zhou, J., Clyne, C.D., 2005. Estrogen—the good, the bad, and the unexpected. Endocr. Rev. 26, 322–330.

Soljancic, A., Ruiz, A.L., Chandrashekar, K., Maranon, R., Liu, R., Reckelhoff, J.F., Juncos, L.A., 2013. Protective role of testosterone in ischemia-reperfusion-induced acute kidney injury. Am. J. Physiol. Regul. Integr. Comp. Physiol. 304, R951–R958.

Song, W.C., Moore, R., McLachlan, J.A., Negishi, M., 1995. Molecular characterization of a testis-specific estrogen sulfotransferase and aberrant liver expression in obese and diabetogenic C57BL/KsJ-db/db mice. Endocrinology 136, 2477–2484.

Song, W.C., 2001. Biochemistry and reproductive endocrinology of estrogen sulfotransferase. Ann. N. Y. Acad. Sci. 948, 43–50.

Staren, E.D., Omer, S., 2004. Hormone replacement therapy in postmenopausal women. Am. J. Surg. 188, 136–149.

Straub, R.H., 2007. The complex role of estrogens in inflammation. Endocr. Rev. 28, 521–574.

Sueyoshi, T., Green, W.D., Vinal, K., Woodrum, T.S., Moore, R., Negishi, M., 2011. Garlic extract diallyl sulfide (DAS) activates nuclear receptor CAR to induce the Sult1e1 gene in mouse liver. PLoS ONE 6, e21229.

Tong, M.H., Jiang, H., Liu, P., Lawson, J.A., Brass, L.F., Song, W.-C., 2005. Spontaneous fetal loss caused by placental thrombosis in estrogen sulfotransferase-deficient mice. Nat. Med. 11, 153–159.

Traupe, H., Happle, R., 1983. Clinical spectrum of steroid sulfatase deficiency: X-linked recessive ichthyosis, birth complications and cryptorchidism. Eur. J. Pediatr. 140, 19–21.

Trentzsch, H., Stewart, D., De Maio, A., 2003. Genetic background conditions the effect of sex steroids on the inflammatory response during endotoxic shock. Crit. Care Med. 31, 232–236.

Tsai, T.H., Chen, S.F., Huang, T.Y., Tzeng, C.F., Chiang, A.S., Kou, Y.R., Lee, T.S., Shyue, S.K., 2011. Impaired Cd14 and Cd36 expression, bacterial clearance, and Toll-like receptor 4-Myd88 signaling in caveolin-1-deleted macrophages and mice. Shock 35, 92–99.

Ulevitch, R.J., Tobias, P.S., 1995. Receptor-dependent mechanisms of cell stimulation by bacterial endotoxin. Annu. Rev. Immunol. 13, 437–457.

Vilatoba, M., Eckstein, C., Bilbao, G., Frennete, L., Eckhoff, D.E., Contreras, J.L., 2005. 17beta-estradiol differentially activates mitogen-activated protein-kinases and improves survival following reperfusion injury of reduced-size liver in mice. Transplant. Proc. 37, 399–403.

Wang, L.Q., Falany, C.N., James, M.O., 2004. Triclosan as a substrate and inhibitor of 3'-phosphoadenosine 5'-phosphosulfate-sulfotransferase and UDP-glucuronosyl transferase in human liver fractions. Drug Metab. Dispos. 32, 1162–1169.

Yen, P.H., Marsh, B., Allen, E., Tsai, S.P., Ellison, J., Connolly, L., Neiswanger, K., Shapiro, L.J., 1988. The human X-linked steroid sulfatase gene and a Y-encoded pseudogene: evidence for an inversion of the Y chromosome during primate evolution. Cell 55, 1123–1135.

Zhai, Y., Busuttil, R.W., Kupiec-Weglinski, J.W., 2011. Liver ischemia and reperfusion injury: new insights into mechanisms of innate-adaptive immune-mediated tissue inflammation. Am. J. Transplant. 11, 1563–1569.

Zhang, H., Varlamova, O., Vargas, F.M., Falany, C.N., Leyh, T.S., 1998. Sulfuryl transfer: the catalytic mechanism of human estrogen sulfotransferase. J. Biol. Chem. 273, 10888–10892.

Zhu, B.T., Conney, A.H., 1998. Functional role of estrogen metabolism in target cells: review and perspectives. Carcinogenesis 19, 1–27.

Zuckerman, S.H., Bryan-Poole, N., Evans, G.F., Short, L., Glasebrook, A.L., 1995. In vivo modulation of murine serum tumour necrosis factor and interleukin-6 levels during endotoxemia by oestrogen agonists and antagonists. Immunology 86, 18–24.

Xenobiotic Receptors in the Crosstalk Between Drug Metabolism and Energy Metabolism

P. Lu, W. Xie

University of Pittsburgh, Pittsburgh, PA, United States

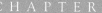

O U T L I N E

Introduction	258	
Xenobiotic Receptors as Master Regulators of Drug Metabolism	258	
Discovery of Aryl Hydrocarbon Receptor	258	
Discovery of Pregnane X Receptor and Constitutive Androstane Receptor	259	
Drug Metabolism can be Affected by Energy Metabolism	260	
Effect of Nonalcoholic Fatty Liver Disease and Nonalcoholic Steatohepatitis on Drug Metabolism	260	
Effect of Diabetes and Insulin Resistance on Drug Metabolism	261	
Effect of Circadian Clock and Feeding —Fasting Switch on Drug Metabolism	263	
Energy Metabolism can be Affected by Drug Metabolism and Xenobiotic Receptors	264	

Aryl Hydrocarbon Receptor in Energy Metabolism   264

Pregnane X Receptor and Constitutive Androstane Receptor in Energy Metabolism   266

Pregnane X Receptor and Constitutive Androstane Receptor in Lipid Metabolism   266

Pregnane X Receptor and Constitutive Androstane Receptor in Glucose Metabolism and Insulin Resistance   268

Pregnane X Receptor and Constitutive Androstane Receptor in Lipoprotein Homeostasis   269

Conclusion and Perspectives   270

References   271

INTRODUCTION

The aryl hydrocarbon receptor (AhR), pregnane X receptor (PXR), and the constitutive androstane receptor (CAR) are three liver-enriched xenobiotic receptors. These xenobiotic receptors transcriptionally regulate the expression of drug-metabolizing enzymes (DMEs) and transporters, which are essential components of xenobiotic response in protecting the hosts from the accumulation of harmful chemicals. More recent research has uncovered interesting endobiotic functions of these xenobiotic receptors, including their regulation of the energy metabolism and energy homeostasis. Meanwhile, disruptions of energy homeostasis, such as type 2 diabetes and obesity, have an impact on drug metabolism. This chapter will focus on the recent progress on the integral role of AhR, PXR, and CAR in the crosstalk between drug metabolism and energy homeostasis.

XENOBIOTIC RECEPTORS AS MASTER REGULATORS OF DRUG METABOLISM

Exposures to xenobiotics such as drug and environmental chemicals have profound influence on human health. DMEs and transporters play key roles in the metabolism, detoxification, and elimination of chemical insults and drugs introduced into the human body. The metabolism and clearance of xenobiotics are accomplished by the concerted action of phase I cytochrome P450 (CYP) enzymes, phase II conjugating enzymes, and "phase III" drug transporters (Anzenbacher and Anzenbacherova, 2001). The P450 enzymes catalyze the monooxygenase reactions of lipophilic compounds facilitated by the reducing power of the NADPH P450 oxidoreductase (Guengerich, 2001; Nebert and Gonzalez, 1987). Phase II conjugating enzymes are several families of transferases, such as the sulfotransferases (SULTs), glutathione S-transferases (GSTs), and UDP-glucuronosyltransferases (UGTs), which conjugate polar functional groups onto xenobiotics (McCarver and Hines, 2002). Phase III transporters include members of ABC transporter proteins and the solute carrier family that facilitate the xenobiotic/drug excretion (Ayrton and Morgan, 2008). Although in most cases, biotransformations of xenobiotics lead to pharmacologically inactive metabolites, they may also activate so-called prodrugs to pharmacologically active products or even to toxic metabolites (Handschin and Meyer, 2003).

Discovery of Aryl Hydrocarbon Receptor

Most DMEs are inducible upon exposures to xenobiotics (Waxman and Azaroff, 1992; Hankinson, 1995). However, the molecular basis underlying this drug-induced metabolism remained largely unknown for a long time. The discovery of xenobiotic receptors stemmed from the concept that xenobiotic induction of DMEs was mediated by a receptor through a transcriptional machinery, which is the so-called "induction-receptor" hypothesis. The plausibility of this hypothesis took a great leap forward with the discovery of the dioxin receptor or the AhR in 1976 (Poland et al., 1976). AhR is a ligand-activated transcription factor that belongs to the basic helix—loop—helix (bHLH)/Per-Arnt-Sim (PAS) family (Hoffman et al.,

1991). Upon binding to its agonists, such as 2,3,7,8-tetrachlorodibenzo-p-dioxin (TCDD) or 3-methylcholanthrene (3-MC), AhR dissociates from its cytoplasmic complex and translocates into the nucleus, forms a heterodimer with its partner AhR nuclear translocator (Arnt), binds to the dioxin response elements (DREs) located in the promoter of its target genes, and activates their transcription. Examples of AhR target genes include phase I CYP1As and CYP1B1, phase II UGT1As, and TCDD-inducible poly (ADP-ribose) polymerase (TiPARP) (Hankinson, 1995; Diani-Moore et al., 2010). The evidence that AhR null mice showed impairment in the normal development of the liver, immune system, heart, and vascular tissues suggested the existence of endogenous AhR ligands as well as the physiological functions of AhR beyond mediating xenobiotic metabolism (Denison and Nagy, 2003; Fernandez-Salguero et al., 1995; Lahvis et al., 2000; Schmidt et al., 1996). In recent years, several endogenous AhR ligands have been found, including the tetrapyroles, arachidonic acid metabolites, tryptophan catabolite, and modified low-density lipoprotein (LDL) (Denison and Nagy, 2003; Opitz et al., 2011; McMillan and Bradfield, 2007).

Discovery of Pregnane X Receptor and Constitutive Androstane Receptor

Compared with AhR whose discovery preceded the era of receptor cloning and resulted from efforts to understand the mechanism of TCDD-induced xenobiotic metabolism, the xenobiotic nuclear receptors PXR (NR1I2) and CAR (NR1I3) were discovered as "orphan receptors" without knowing their ligands and functions (Okey, 2007). PXR and CAR share several important characteristics of xenobiotic receptors. They are expressed predominantly in the liver and small intestine where their target genes are located and are capable of binding to a wide variety of structurally diverse chemicals including endogenous and synthetic steroids, pharmaceutical agents, and xenobiotic chemicals. Similar to AhR, PXR and CAR are nucleocytoplasmic shuttling proteins, and both subcellular compartmentalization and intracellular trafficking are crucial in their transcriptional functions. Upon ligand binding, PXR and CAR form heterodimers with the retinoid X receptor (RXR) and trigger the transcription of their target genes. PXR and CAR not only showed an overlap in their ligands, but also shared many target genes including phase I and phase II DMEs and drug transporters (Xie et al., 2004; Wada et al., 2009). As xenobiotic receptors, a key difference between PXR/CAR and AhR is that the PXR/CAR target enzymes, such as the CYP3A and CYP2C enzymes, are most relevant to the metabolism and disposition of clinical drugs.

In addition to their implications in drug metabolism and drug—drug interactions, PXR and CAR have also been proposed to have numerous endobiotic functions by regulating genes involved in the metabolism of endobiotics, including bilirubin, bile acids, and steroid hormones (Timsit and Negishi, 2007). Of note, there are marked species differences in the ligand-dependent activation of PXR and CAR, which is attributed to the sequence divergence in their ligand-binding domains. For instance, pregnenolone 16α-carbonitrile (PCN), a synthetic antiglucocorticoid, is a potent agonist for the mouse and rat PXR but has little effect on the human and rabbit PXR. In contrast, rifampicin, a macrolide antibiotic, activates the human and rabbit PXR, but has little effect on the rat and mouse PXR (Jones et al., 2000). Similarly, 1,4-bis[2-(3,5-dichloropyridyloxy)]benzene (TCPOBOP), a potent mouse CAR ligand, cannot activate either the rat or human CAR, whereas androstanol represses mouse but not the human CAR (Moore et al., 2000). The creations of PXR and CAR null mice (Xie et al., 2000; Wei et al., 2000; Staudinger et al., 2001) as well as the PXR and CAR humanized mice (Xie et al., 2000; Zhang et al., 2002) have made it possible to address the species specificity of xenobiotic responses in vivo.

DRUG METABOLISM CAN BE AFFECTED BY ENERGY METABOLISM

Drug metabolism can vary considerably due to various pathophysiological factors, including liver diseases and diabetes mellitus, due to the disease effect on the expression and/or activity of DMEs and transporters. Given the dramatically increased number of patients suffering from metabolic syndrome such as steatosis, obesity, and diabetes, it is of great value to understand the impact of energy disturbance on the pharmacokinetics and efficacy of drug therapy. Xenobiotic receptors including AhR, PXR, and CAR may function as the links between drug metabolism and energy metabolism.

Effect of Nonalcoholic Fatty Liver Disease and Nonalcoholic Steatohepatitis on Drug Metabolism

The metabolic syndrome is now becoming a leading public health issue that includes steatosis, nonalcoholic steatohepatitis (NASH), obesity, and type II diabetes. The liver is the major site of fatty acid synthesis and triglyceride storage. Hepatic steatosis, also referred to as simple fatty liver or nonalcoholic fatty liver disease (NAFLD), is generally defined as the presence of cytoplasmic triglyceride droplets in more than 5% of the hepatocytes (Cohen et al., 2011). NAFLD is commonly associated with metabolic syndromes including obesity and type 2 diabetes and can lead to NASH, which is an advanced stage of steatosis with hallmarks of inflammation and progressive fibrosis (Tilg and Moschen, 2010).

Steatosis may arise from an imbalance between triglyceride acquisition and removal due to increased fatty acid synthesis and uptake, decreased fatty acid β-oxidation, and reduced triglyceride secretion. The fatty acids used for hepatic triglyceride formation are originated from de novo synthesis, diet, or lipolysis of the adipose tissue. Carbohydrate feeding promotes de novo lipogenesis by inducing the key enzymes involved in this pathway such as the fatty acid synthase (Venkatesh et al., 2014), stearoyl CoA desaturase 1 (SCD-1), and acetyl coenzyme A carboxylase 1 (ACC-1), all of which are under the transcriptional control of the master lipogenic transcriptional factor sterol response element—binding protein-1c (SREBP-1c). Lipoprotein lipase (LPL) and adipocyte triglyceride hydrolase (ATGL) catalyze the hydrolysis of the triglyceride in the chylomicrons and adipocytes, respectively; thereby releasing free fatty acids into the circulation. The liver takes up free fatty acids via the fatty acid transport protein or fatty acid translocase (FAT/CD36) when there is an excess of circulating fatty acids. Once in the liver, fatty acids can be oxidized to produce energy and ketone bodies, reesterified to triglyceride, or exported as very-low-density lipoproteins (VLDL). Carnitine palmitoyltransferase 1 (CPT1) and mitochondrial 3-hydroxy-3-methylglutarate-CoA synthase (HMGCS) are key enzymes in β-oxidation and ketogenesis, respectively. Apolipoprotein B100 (ApoB100) is the key component that controls the overall rate of VLDL production and secretion (Nguyen et al., 2008). NASH occurs in a subset of patients with steatosis and is characterized by the presence of liver inflammation and fibrogenesis. Hepatic steatosis does not always result in liver injuries and requires a second "hit" to progress to NASH (James and Day, 1998). It is currently hypothesized that insulin resistance and oxidative stress, in combination with the inflammatory cytokine dysregulation, eventually trigger hepatocyte death, resulting in further inflammatory signaling and activation of the hepatic stellate cells in a fibrotic repair response (Jou et al., 2008).

Patients with NAFLD and NASH were reported to have impaired drug metabolism and increased risk of drug toxicity compared with normal subjects (Barshop et al., 2011; Fiatarone et al., 1991; Blouin and Warren, 1999; Cheymol, 2000; Tarantino et al., 2007, 2009). Indeed, downregulation of CYP enzyme has been found in animal models of steatosis and NASH (Leclercq et al., 1998; Su et al., 1999; Gomez-Lechon et al., 2009) and in in vitro models of fat-overloaded hepatocytes (Donato et al., 2007). Moreover, the reduction in hepatic CYP enzymes is correlated to the degree of liver fat content (Leclercq et al., 1998). The expression of phase II conjugating enzymes, such as the SULT enzymes, can also be regulated by NAFLD and NASH. For example, patients with the progression to NASH were reported to have decreased SULT1A2 and SULT1A1 expressions (Younossi et al., 2005; Stepanova et al., 2010). An induction in SULT2A1/2 expression was observed in ob/ob male mice (Cheng et al., 2008), whereas a reduction in SULT2A1 protein level and activity was found in high-fat diet (HFD)-fed mice (Koide et al., 2011). Our recent studies showed induced hepatic expression of SULT2B1b and steroid sulfatase in an obese mouse model as well as during the fed to fasting transition (Shi et al., 2014). Additionally, hepatic UGT expression was observed to decrease in animal models of steatosis (Koide et al., 2011; Osabe et al., 2008; Kirpich et al., 2011).

The regulation of DMEs by hepatic steatosis is largely dependent on the xenobiotic receptors. Li et al. (2007) provided evidence in rat primary hepatocytes that polyunsaturated fatty acids downregulate phenobarbital-induced CYP2B1 expression through attenuation of CAR translocation from the cytosol into the nucleus, which resulted in diminished binding of the CAR/RXR heterodimer onto the nuclear receptor–binding site 1 (NR-1) of the CYP 2B1 gene promoter. A hallmark of fatty liver disease is the increased hepatic expression of the SREBP-1, which is a key lipogenic transcription factor. It has been reported that SREBP-1 repressed drug-induced hepatic CYP expression via functioning as a non-DNA-binding inhibitor of PXR and CAR and blocking their interaction with nuclear receptor cofactors (Roth et al., 2008a). The regulation of lipid disturbance on drug metabolism can also be mediated by the crosstalk between the xenobiotic receptor CAR and the lipogenic nuclear receptor liver X receptor (LXR) (Gao and Xie, 2010). LXR can *trans*-suppress the activity of CAR through competition for the nuclear receptor coactivators (Zhai et al., 2010).

Effect of Diabetes and Insulin Resistance on Drug Metabolism

Fatty liver is a well-known predisposing factor for type 2 diabetes and insulin resistance. Fat accumulation in the liver generates increased free fatty acids and proinflammatory lipid metabolites that can impair insulin signaling and result in insulin resistance (Shoelson et al., 2006). The influence of diabetes mellitus on drug metabolism has been known for some time. Investigation in human patients with type 1 diabetes showed faster drug elimination that can be reversed by insulin treatment, suggesting an interplay between the insulin action and drug metabolism (Zysset and Wietholtz, 1988; Goldstein et al., 1990). This observation was consistent with the report in the streptozotocin-induced type 1 diabetic mouse model, in which the mice showed an increased expression of CYP2B that can be corrected by insulin treatment (Sakuma et al., 2001). The induction of CYP2B seemed to be mediated by CAR-dependent induction of peroxisome proliferator—activated receptor γ coactivator 1α (PGC1α) and AMP-activated protein kinase (AMPK) (Dong et al., 2009a). The effect of type 2 diabetes on CYP gene expression is somewhat controversial and model specific. Yoshinari et al. (2006) reported downregulation of CYP2B1/2 and CAR expression in the Zucker rats, but upregulation of CYP2B10 and CAR expression in the leptin receptor deficient db/db mice. This CYP2B10 induction in db/db mice is probably mediated by the induction of hepatocyte nuclear factor 4α (HNF4α) and RXR, the heterodimer partner of CAR (Yoshinari et al., 2006). Moreover, the effects of diabetes on drug metabolism can be sex dependent at least in animal models (Skett and Joels, 1985). A study from our group reported a sex-specific effect of estrogen sulfotransferase (EST) in mouse models of type 2 diabetes (Gao et al., 2012). EST is the conjugating enzyme responsible for the sulfonation and inactivation of estrogens, and hepatic EST expression is induced in the ob/ob diabetic mouse model (Gao et al., 2012). Specifically, EST ablation improved metabolic function in ob/ob, dexamethasone-, and HFD-induced female mouse models of type 2 diabetes, which appeared to have resulted from increased estrogenic activity in the liver. But interestingly, loss of EST in ob/ob males exacerbated the diabetic phenotype, which was due to the decreased islet β-cell mass and failure of glucose-stimulated insulin secretion as a result of inflammation in the white adipose tissue (Gao et al., 2012). These results suggest that inhibition of EST, at least in females, may represent a novel approach to manage type 2 diabetes. Besides, acute and chronic diabetes mellitus may also have a differential effect on drug metabolism in rats (Skett and Joels, 1985).

Cell culture studies also supported the effect of diabetes on drug metabolism. Consistent with the observations in type 1 diabetes, insulin removal in rat primary hepatocytes enhanced dexamethasone- and β-naphthoflavone-induced expressions of CYP3A and CYP1A (Sidhu and Omiecinski, 1999). In contrast, De Waziers et al. (1995) showed suppressed expression of CYP2B and CYP2E by insulin in rat hepatoma cells. The interplay between insulin and drug metabolism could be explained by forkhead box O1 protein (FOXO1), which is a member of the insulin-sensitive transcription factor family that functions as a coactivator of CAR- and PXR-mediated transcription (Kodama et al., 2004). It was suggested that in conditions of insulin deprivation, such as type 1 diabetes, FOXO1 translocates into the nucleus, becomes activated, and increases the transcriptional activity of CAR and PXR. AhR seemed to be also implicated in low-glucose responsive regulation of CYP enzymes. It was reported that low-glucose conditions induced the expression of CYP1A/B enzymes in human hepatoma cells, which was associated with increased nuclear translocation of AhR, a positive regulator of CYP1A/B (Terashima et al., 2011). The effects of diabetes on drug metabolism are summarized in Fig. 11.1.

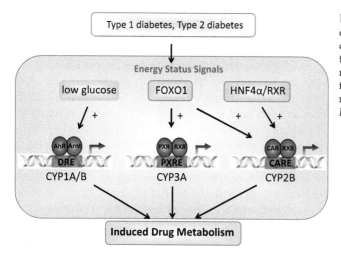

FIGURE 11.1 Summary of the effect of diabetes on drug metabolism. *AhR*, aryl hydrocarbon receptor; *Arnt*, AhR nuclear translocator; *CAR*, constitutive androstane receptor; *CYP*, cytochrome P450; *FOXO1*, forkhead box O1 protein; *HNF4α*, hepatocyte nuclear factor 4α; *PXR*, pregnane X receptor; *RXR*, retinoid X receptor.

Effect of Circadian Clock and Feeding–Fasting Switch on Drug Metabolism

Diurnal rhythm and feeding–fasting switch can also affect drug metabolism. The mammalian circadian timing system comprises a complex network with a master pacemaker located in the suprachiasmatic nucleus (SCN) of the hypothalamus (Partch et al., 2014). The phase of SCN pacemakers is entrained by both daily light–dark cycles and feeding-fasting rhythms. Molecular regulation of diurnal rhythm on a daily basis requires the activity of the PAS domain transcription factor family, circadian locomotor output cycles kaput (CLOCK) and its partner brain and muscle ARNT-like protein 1 (BMAL1). CLOCK and BMAL1 heterodimerize and drive the transcription of the PAS domain-containing Period (Per) genes (Jung et al., 2003). Structural similarity between the clock elements and the PAS domain protein AhR suggests that circadian rhythm has an impact on AhR activity. Several studies in animal models showed that AhR and Arnt expression in the liver fluctuate in accordance with the diurnal rhythm (Richardson et al., 1998; Huang et al., 2002). Circadian changes in its downstream target gene CYP1A1 indicate that activation of the AhR signaling pathway is rhythmic under physiological conditions (Mukai et al., 2008). It was suggested that light-stimulated generation of endogenous AhR ligand tryptophan photoproducts triggers AhR activation and contributes to the alteration of AhR signaling by circadian rhythm (Mukai and Tischkau, 2007). The diurnal changes in hepatic CYP1A1 expression in response to TCDD were abolished by targeted disruption of Per1 and Per2, suggesting a potential interaction between AhR signaling and the circadian clock (Qu et al., 2010). Another group also reported that mutation of CLOCK decreased AhR expression and repressed benzo[α]pyrene-induced CYP1A1 expression (Tanimura et al., 2011). Moreover, enhancer box (E-box) element, the binding site of CLOCK/BMAL1, was found in the AhR gene promoter, suggesting a direct regulation of AhR transcription by the CLOCK/BMAL1 heterodimer (Garrison and Denison, 2000); whether AhR activity is influenced by fasting–feeding switch needs to be demonstrated.

Regulation of DMEs by fasting has been reported in both animal models and humans (Qu et al., 1998; Longo et al., 2000; Murray, 2006; Lammers et al., 2015), which may in part occur through the altered activity of CAR and PXR during fasting (Buler et al., 2011). Fasting markedly increases the expression of CAR and its target genes such as CYP2B10, UGT1A1, SULT2A1, and OATP2 (Ding et al., 2006). Interestingly, cyclic adenosine monophosphate (cAMP), which is increased by fasting, produced a similar pattern of gene regulation (Ding et al., 2006). CAR nuclear translocation can be induced by AMPK activation, which is in part triggered by increased availability of cAMP (Shindo et al., 2007; Blattler et al., 2007), suggesting a key role of CAR activation during fasting response. HNF4α and peroxisome proliferator-activated receptor alpha (PPARα) were reported to be the major mediators for fasting-responsive induction of CAR, because this induction was nearly abolished in either HNF4α or PPARα knockout mice (Wieneke et al., 2007; Ding et al., 2006). HNF4α and PPARα response elements were found in the CAR gene promoter, suggesting CAR as a direct transcriptional target of HNF4α and PPARα. The induction of CAR by HNF4α may be furthered by PGC1α, an HNF4α coactivator that is also induced by fasting (Wieneke et al., 2007; Ding et al., 2006). PGC1α also coactivates CAR on the CYP2B10 promoter and possibly others, which may contribute to the amplification of CAR downstream genes. Fasting-activated PGC-1α and sirtuin 1 (SIRT1) may also mediate the induction of PXR expression by fasting (Buler et al., 2011). The expression of CAR and its target genes also exhibit circadian fluctuation (Zhang et al., 2009; Yang et al., 2006), suggesting that the circadian clock also has an impact on the expression of CAR.

ENERGY METABOLISM CAN BE AFFECTED BY DRUG METABOLISM AND XENOBIOTIC RECEPTORS

While AhR, PXR, and CAR were initially characterized as xenobiotic receptors, subsequent observations have pointed to their equally important endobiotic functions, including their effects on energy metabolism.

Aryl Hydrocarbon Receptor in Energy Metabolism

It has long been suggested that the systemic TCDD toxicity involves an overall perturbation of energy homeostasis (Potter et al., 1986). Earlier work-associated exposures to AhR agonists with dyslipidemia by reporting that TCDD and related halogenated aromatic hydrocarbons (HAHs) produced marked fatty liver in several species (Albro et al., 1978; Kohli et al., 1979; Jones and Greig, 1975). In agreement with these animal results, dioxin exposure in human populations has also been reported to be associated with an increased incidence of fatty liver (Lee et al., 2006). The accumulation of hepatic triglycerides was accompanied by an induction in liver weight and liver to body weight ratios (Hinton et al., 1978). Increased de novo fatty acid synthesis (Gorski et al., 1988), decreased fatty acid oxidation (Lakshman et al., 1991), and increased half-life of liver lipid moieties (Hinton et al., 1978) have been suggested to account for the hepatic steatosis in AhR agonist–treated rats. However, some other studies showed decreased hepatic fatty acid synthesis in both animal models and primary human hepatocytes upon TCDD treatment, which was associated with reduced expressions of key lipogenic genes, including Fasn, SCD-1, and Acaca (Tanos et al., 2012; Lakshman et al., 1988; Fletcher et al., 2005). Cautions need to apply when interpreting these phenotypes because TCDD itself is toxic to the cells and animals. Recently, we showed that mice overexpressing a constitutively activated AhR (CA-AhR) in the liver developed a spontaneous steatosis without causing a general hepatotoxicity. The steatosis in CA-AhR transgenic mice was manifested by increased fatty acid uptake and decreased VLDL-triglyceride secretion. CD36, the fatty acid translocase, was identified as a novel AhR target gene that mediated the steatotic effect (Lee et al., 2010). In another independent study, mice fed with the AhR ligand 3-MC, an AhR agonist less toxic than TCDD, showed hepatosteatotic phenotype through a similar mechanism (Kawano et al., 2010).

Using the same CA-AhR transgenic mice, we showed that activation of AhR can also sensitize mice to NASH, an advanced stage of NAFLD with the hallmarks of inflammation and progressive fibrosis (Tilg and Moschen, 2010). The CA-AhR transgenic mice showed heightened sensitivity to methionine- and choline-deficient (Chen et al., 1998) diet-induced NASH through decreasing the activity of superoxide dismutase 2 (SOD2) and increasing mitochondrial reactive oxygen species production in the liver. Mechanistically, the mitochondrial sirtuin deacetylase Sirt3, which can enhance the scavenging of superoxide through the activation of mitochondrial SOD2, was inhibited by AhR. The AhR-responsive inhibition of Sirt3, a NAD^+-dependent deacetylase, was likely due to the depletion of cellular concentration of NAD^+ because of the activation of TiPARP by AhR (He et al., 2013a). Sensitization of mice to the MCD diet—induced NASH was also demonstrated in wild-type (WT) mice treated with TCDD. Interestingly, the antioxidative role of AhR has also been reported. For example, the nuclear factor erythroid 2—related factor 2 (Nrf2), a master regulator of antioxidative responses, was directly induced by AhR activation, which in turn protected against the oxidative stress (Lu et al., 2011). Other reported AhR inducible cytoprotective genes include the NAD(P)H:quinone oxidoreductase 1 (Nqo1), GSTs, and UGTs (Nebert et al., 2000). These results suggested that AhR might have a rather complex role in the liver's handling of oxidative stress.

Dyslipidemia is a well-known predisposing factor for the development of type 2 diabetes. With the potential effects of AhR on dyslipidemia, it is reasonable to hypothesize that AhR can affect the pathogenesis of diabetes as well. Indeed, both animal models and human studies suggested an association between TCDD exposure and increased incidence of diabetes (Remillard and Bunce, 2002; Henriksen et al., 1997; Matsumura, 1995), but the underlying mechanism was poorly defined. TCDD-induced reduction in glucose uptake has been reported in adipose tissue, liver, and pancreas (Enan et al., 1992a,b; Kern et al., 2002), primarily through the decreased expression of glucose transporter 4 (GLUT4) (Liu and Matsumura, 1995). Another suggested mechanism was the inhibition of hepatic phosphoenolpyruvate carboxykinase (PEPCK) and glucose 6-phosphatase (G6Pase), which resulted in an impairment of gluconeogenesis (Weber et al., 1991). In a human study, nondiabetic veterans with high-blood TCDD levels were found more likely to develop insulin resistance (Cranmer et al., 2000). TCDD-treated animals showed β-cell dysfunction, including reduced insulin production and secretion (Enan et al., 1992b; Ebner et al., 1988). Based on the fact that loss of PPARγ is diabetogenic, and the PPARγ agonists thiazolidinediones sensitize tissues to the insulin actions, it was also suggested that the diabetogenic effects of TCDD might be through antagonizing the PPARγ functions (Remillard and Bunce, 2002). Again, the toxic nature of TCDD may compromise the interpretation of these results. Our recent report suggested the AHR-fibroblast growth factor 21 (FGF21) endocrine signaling pathway may help to explain

AHR as an environmental modifier that integrates signals from chemical exposure in the regulation of lipid and energy metabolism (Lu et al., 2015). By using the CA-hAHR transgenic mice, we showed that despite fatty liver, activation of human AHR in the liver prevented mice from HFD-induced obesity and type 2 diabetes. The endocrine hormone FGF21 was identified as a direct AHR transcriptional target and the mediator for the metabolic benefit of AHR in disassociating fatty liver from insulin resistance (Lu et al., 2015).

The AhR heterodimerization partner Arnt, also known as hypoxia-inducible factor 1β (HIF1β), is a ubiquitously expressed nuclear protein that also belongs to the bHLH/PAS family of transcription factors (Reisz-Porszasz et al., 1994). Recent findings showed that the expression of Arnt was reduced in both liver and β cells of obese individuals with type 2 diabetes (Gunton et al., 2005; Wang et al., 2009), suggesting an important role of Arnt in the development of metabolic disease. Further studies demonstrated that the deficiency of Arnt activity in β cells and liver contributed to impaired insulin secretion and dysregulation of glucose homeostasis, respectively (Gunton et al., 2005; Wang et al., 2009).

Insulin resistance is associated with elevated plasma levels of VLDL and LDL (Haidari et al., 2002; Federico et al., 2006). Subsequent atherosclerotic lesion is a serious cause for the cardiovascular complications that occur in the patients with type 2 diabetes. A significant positive correlation between high serum TCDD and plasma cholesterol and triglyceride levels was observed in subjects exposed to chloracne, and among US Vietnam war veterans who were exposed to high levels of TCDD (IARC, 1997; Geusau et al., 2001; Martin, 1984). A follow-up study on a cohort of former TCDD workers showed that exposure to TCDD caused atherosclerotic plaques and ischemic heart disease (Pelclova et al., 2002). Animal studies confirmed that TCDD induced a marked dyslipidemia characterized by the induction of total cholesterol, VLDL, LDL, and triglyceride levels (Brewster et al., 1988; Minami et al., 2008; Swift et al., 1981). Mechanistically and of particular relevance to triglyceride metabolism, the adipose activity of LPL, which hydrolyses triglyceride and promotes its cellular uptake, was reduced in both animals and adipocyte cultures after TCDD treatment (Kern et al., 2002; Brewster and Matsumura, 1984). As for the cause of hypercholesterolemia, TCDD caused a downregulation of LDLR on the plasma membrane of hepatocytes, leading to a decreased cholesterol internalization and elevated levels of plasma cholesterol (Bombick et al., 1984). However, it remains to be determined whether the effect of TCDD on the expression of adipose LPL and liver LDLR is AhR dependent. The effects of AhR on energy metabolism are summarized in Fig. 11.2.

Pregnane X Receptor and Constitutive Androstane Receptor in Energy Metabolism

Pregnane X Receptor and Constitutive Androstane Receptor in Lipid Metabolism

In recent years, the previously known xenobiotic receptors PXR and CAR have emerged for their pivotal endobiotic functions, including the regulation of lipid homeostasis (Zhou et al., 2006, 2009; Gao and Xie, 2012). A number of studies suggested PXR has a steatogenic effect. Transgenic mice overexpressing a constitutively activated PXR in the liver developed hepatomegaly and marked hepatic steatosis resulting from an accumulation of triglycerides. In independent pharmacological models, treatment of human PXR (hPXR) "humanized" mice with the hPXR agonist rifampicin elicited a similar steatotic phenotype (Zhou et al.,

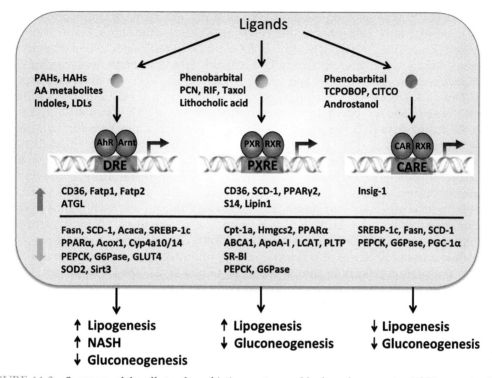

FIGURE 11.2 Summary of the effects of xenobiotic receptors aryl hydrocarbon receptor (AhR), pregnane X receptor (PXR), and constitutive androstane receptor (CAR) on energy metabolism. *ABCA1*, ATP-binding cassette transporter A1; *AGTL*, adipocyte triglyceride hydrolase; *Arnt*, AhR nuclear translocator; *CARE*, CAR response element; *CITCO*, 6-(4-chlorophenyl)-imidazo[2,1-b]thiazole-5-carbaldehyde; *DRE*, dioxin response element; *GLUT4*, glucose transporter 4; *HAHs*, halogenated aromatic hydrocarbons; *LDL*, low-density lipoprotein; *PAHs*, polycyclic aromatic hydrocarbons; *PCN*, pregnenolone 16alpha-carbonitrile; *PEPCK*, phosphoenolpyruvate carboxykinase; *PLTP*, phospholipid transfer protein; *PPAR*, peroxisome proliferator-activated receptor; *PXRE*, PXR response element; *RIF*, rifampicin; *RXR*, retinoid X receptor; *SCD-1*, stearoyl CoA desaturase 1; *SOD2*, superoxide dismutase 2; *SR-BI*, scavenge receptor B-I; *TCPOBOP*, 1,4-bis[2-(3,5-dichloropyridyloxy)]benzene.

2006; Cheng et al., 2012). The steatotic effect of PXR was also supported by the finding that hepatic steatosis was suppressed in mice lacking PXR after partial hepatectomy (Dai et al., 2008). The prosteatotic effect of PXR was also demonstrated in human hepatocytes and hepatoma cell lines by either pharmacological or genetic activation of PXR (Moya et al., 2010). It was previously reported that treatment of mice with the PXR agonist PCN conferred resistance to lithocholic acid (LCA)-induced hepatotoxicity (Xie et al., 2001). Recently, it was suggested that in addition to the PXR-mediated induction of DMEs, PCN-mediated stimulation of lipogenesis might have also contributed to the protection against LCA-induced liver injury (Miyata et al., 2010). Consistent with the notion that steatosis is the first step in the development of NAFLD, a case–control association study investigating 290 individuals revealed that PXR genetic variants might contribute to disease severity in NAFLD by influencing the individual susceptibility to progress to more severe stages of the disease (Sookoian et al., 2010). A recent study using primary hepatocytes showed that PXR acetylation status alone can regulate lipogenesis independent of ligand activation (Biswas et al., 2011).

Mechanistically, the steatotic effect of PXR is likely the result of a combined effect of increased hepatic fatty acid uptake, increased lipogenesis, and suppression of fatty acid β-oxidation (Zhou et al., 2006). Activation of PXR increased fatty acid uptake through the induction of hepatic CD36, and several other accessory lipogenic enzymes, including SCD-1, long chain free fatty acid elongase, and PPARγ2 (Zhou et al., 2006). Promoter analysis established CD36 as a direct transcriptional target of PXR. Moreover, PPARγ2, a positive regulator of CD36, was also shown to be a direct transcriptional target of PXR (Zhou et al., 2008). These results suggested that PXR regulated CD36 gene expression directly or through crosstalk with PPARγ (Wada et al., 2009; Lee et al., 2008). Independent reports suggested that activation of PXR induced de novo lipogenesis through the direct induction of the thyroid hormone-responsive spot 14 protein (S14), which is known to transduce hormone-related and nutrient-related signals to genes that are involved in lipogenesis (Moreau et al., 2009). Our recent results suggested that lipin-1, the expression of which is known to increase triglyceride synthesis, was a potential PXR target, providing yet another possible explanation for the lipogenic effect of PXR in the liver (He et al., 2013b). In addition to increased lipogenesis, the steatotic effect of PXR was also associated with suppression of several genes involved in fatty acid β-oxidation such as PPARα and thiolase (Zhou et al., 2006). CPT1a and HMGCS2, respective rate-limiting enzymes of β-oxidation and ketogenesis, were inhibited after treatment of mice with PCN, and this effect was achieved by direct binding of activated PXR to Forkhead box A2 (FoxA2), thereby preventing FoxA2 binding to its target genes including CPT1a and HMGCS2 (Nakamura et al., 2007).

In contrast to the overall lipogenic effect of PXR, activation of CAR suppresses lipogenesis. Treatment with the CAR agonist TCPOBOP alleviated hepatic steatosis and inhibited the expression of lipogenic genes including SREBP-1c, ACC-1, FAS, and SCD-1 in both diet-induced and genetic obese mouse models (Dong et al., 2009b; Gao et al., 2009). For the mechanism of the inhibitory effect of CAR on lipogenesis (Roth et al., 2008b), it was reported that activation of CAR induced the expression of Insig-1, a protein with antilipogenic properties, and resulted in a reduction in the level of active SREBP-1. Promoter analysis suggested Insig-1 as a direct CAR target gene. An independent study from our group suggested that activation of CAR can *trans*-suppress the lipogenic nuclear receptor LXR by inhibiting the recruitment of LXRα to the SREBP-1c gene promoter (Zhai et al., 2010).

Pregnane X Receptor and Constitutive Androstane Receptor in Glucose Metabolism and Insulin Resistance

In addition to impacting on lipid metabolism, PXR and CAR also play a role in glucose homeostasis and insulin resistance. The effect of PXR on glucose metabolism and insulin resistance has been controversial. We recently reported that PXR ablation alleviated HFD-induced insulin resistance. In an independent model, introducing the PXR$^{-/-}$ allele into the ob/ob background also relieved the diabetic phenotype. The ob/ob mice deficient of PXR showed an inhibition of gluconeogenesis and an increased rate of glucose disposal during euglycemic clamp. In contrast, transgenic activation of PXR worsened the diabetic phenotype (He et al., 2013b). The detrimental effect of PXR activation on glucose metabolism was supported by an independent report that administration of PXR agonists PCN and rifampin impaired postprandial glucose tolerance during the oral glucose tolerance test in rats and healthy human subjects, which might be due to a downregulation of hepatic GLUT2, the major hepatic glucose transporter facilitating the glucose influx at high plasma glucose (Rysa et al., 2013). It was noted that treatment of WT mice with PCN has been reported to inhibit G6Pase and PEPCK gene expression (Kodama et al., 2004, 2007), but those observations were made in mice fed with chow diet after an acute PXR ligand treatment. The discrepancies may have resulted from different nutritional and/or metabolic status, a notion that is also supported by our observation that the suppression of G6Pase and PEPCK gene expression seen in chow-fed VP-PXR transgenic mice (Zhou et al., 2006) was absent in ob/ob mice that carry the same transgene (He et al., 2013b).

Treatment with the CAR agonist TCPOBOP inhibited gluconeogenesis and alleviated insulin resistance in both the HFD and ob/ob mouse models in a CAR-dependent manner (Dong et al., 2009b; Gao et al., 2009). In contrast, the CAR null mice showed spontaneous defect in insulin sensitivity (Dong et al., 2009b; Gao et al., 2009). The antidiabetic effect of CAR in mice was consistent with the clinical observation that diabetic patients who received phenobarbital showed decreased plasma glucose and improved insulin sensitivity (Lahtela et al., 1985). The expression of the gluconeogenic enzyme genes PEPCK and G6Pase was suppressed in CAR-activated mice. Several mechanisms have been proposed to explain the inhibitory effect of CAR on gluconeogenesis. Early studies reported that liganded CAR represses the binding of FoxO1 to the insulin responsive sequence element on the promoters of gluconeogenic enzyme genes (Kodama et al., 2004; Yarushkin et al., 2013). CAR can also compete with HNF4α for the direct repeat spaced by one nucleotide (DR1)-binding motif and dissociate the coactivator PGC1α from HNF4α, thereby suppressing gluconeogenesis (Yarushkin et al., 2013; Miao et al., 2006). In addition, CAR competitively binds to HNF4α coactivators SRC2/GRIP1 and PGC1α, and thus attenuates the expression of gluconeogenic genes (Miao et al., 2006). Moreover, HNF4α-mediated gluconeogenic transactivation is also regulated by the nuclear translocation of HNF4α, in which acetylation of HNF4α plays an essential role. Our previous study reported that the cholesterol sulfotransferase (SULT2B1b) inhibits gluconeogenesis through deacetylation of HNF4α (Shi et al., 2014). SULT2B1b is a CAR responsive gene, representing another mechanism by which CAR inhibits gluconeogenesis. A recent study from our group showed that CAR suppressed hepatic gluconeogenic gene expression through posttranslational regulation of the subcellular localization and degradation of PGC1α (Gao et al., 2015). Specifically, activated CAR translocated into the nucleus and served as an adaptor protein to recruit PGC1α to the Cullin1 E3 ligase complex for proteasomal degradation, in which the promyelocytic leukemia protein-nuclear bodies function as a critical scaffold (Gao et al., 2015). Both drug metabolism and gluconeogenesis are energy-demanding processes. It is our opinion that the negative regulation of PGC1α by CAR may represent a cellular adaptive mechanism to accommodate energy-restricted conditions.

Pregnane X Receptor and Constitutive Androstane Receptor in Lipoprotein Homeostasis

PXR and CAR also play a role in regulating lipoprotein homeostasis. Treatment of patients with HIV infection or epileptic patients with HIV protease inhibitors or antiepileptic drugs, both of which are potent PXR agonists, increased total and LDL cholesterol levels (Riddler et al., 2003; Carr et al., 1998; Dussault et al., 2001; Shafran et al., 2005; Eiris et al., 1995; Aynaci et al., 2001). Several dietary components such as Cafestol and sulforaphane, which could alter plasma lipid levels, were found to be PXR agonists or antagonists (Ricketts et al., 2007; Zhou et al., 2007). In animal models, activation of PXR led to increased levels of the atherogenic lipoproteins VLDL and LDL (Zhou et al., 2009; de Haan et al., 2009). A genome-wide association study showed that genetic variants in PXR could affect plasma LDL levels in humans (Lu et al., 2010). It was proposed that alterations of several genes involved in high-density lipoprotein (HDL) metabolism accounted for the atherogenic effect of PXR. These include the decreased expression of ATP-binding cassette transporter A1 and ApoA-I that are required for HDL assembly, reduced expression of lecithin-cholesterol acyltransferase and phospholipid transfer protein (PLTP) that are important for HDL maturation, and decreased expression of scavenge receptor B-I that is important for lipoprotein clearance (de Haan et al., 2009; Sporstol et al., 2005). However, in several other studies, activation of PXR has been shown to exert a beneficial effect by increasing the HDL levels, which was associated with increased ApoA-I levels (Bachmann et al., 2004; Masson et al., 2005). In addition, the effect of lovastatin on lowering cholesterol in human liver cells was found to be dependent on PXR activation (Plee-Gautier et al., 2012). The mechanism for these discrepancies remains to be understood.

The effects of CAR activation on plasma lipoprotein levels in rodents and humans are inconclusive or ambiguous. TCPOBOP, a CAR agonist, decreased plasma HDL and ApoA-I levels in WT and human ApoA-I transgenic mice (Masson et al., 2008); whereas the CAR null mice exhibited higher HDL levels under cholestatic conditions after bile duct ligation (Stedman et al., 2005). Phenobarbital, another CAR agonist, was shown to increase plasma cholesterol and lipoprotein levels (Aynaci et al., 2001). In contrast, treatment with phenytoin, a nonspecific CAR agonist, increased the HDL levels in humans (Goerdt et al., 1995; Miller et al., 1995). Activation of CAR was able to stimulate the elimination of cholesterol derived from HDL via its conversion into bile acids during diet-induced hypercholesterolemia, which improves the cholesterol homeostasis (Sberna et al., 2011). The effects of PXR and CAR on energy metabolism are summarized in Fig. 11.2.

CONCLUSION AND PERSPECTIVES

Cytochrome P450s and other DMEs are involved in the metabolism of many prescription drugs. Differences in drug response are common among patients, and the causes are multifactorial including genetic, environmental, and disease determinants. The crosstalk between energy metabolism and drug metabolism provides an excellent example of how alterations in energy metabolism, such as those seen in obesity and type 2 diabetes, affect drug metabolism. Meanwhile, "xenobiotic receptors" such as AhR, PXR, and CAR can have an isoform-specific effect on the homeostasis of lipids and glucose and insulin resistivity. The crosstalk between energy metabolism and drug metabolism does make biological sense, because drug metabolism is also an energy-demanding process. It is conceivable that this crosstalk may represent a cellular adaptive mechanism to accommodate energy-restricted conditions.

At the translational level, our understanding on the interplay between drug metabolism and energy metabolism as well as the roles of xenobiotic receptors in this crosstalk may offer a molecular basis for predicting alterations in drug response and providing a rationale for dose adjustment in patients with type 2 diabetes and obesity. Through the crosstalk with transcription factors involved in lipogenesis and gluconeogenesis, activation of AhR, PXR, and CAR also have a significant impact on energy homeostasis. It is therefore tempting to speculate that pharmacological modulation of these xenobiotic receptors may be beneficial in managing metabolic diseases.

References

Albro, P.W., Corbett, J.T., Harris, M., Lawson, L.D., 1978. Effects of 2,3,7,8-tetrachlorodibenzo-p-dioxin on lipid profiles in tissue of the Fischer rat. Chem. Biol. Interact. 23, 315–330.

Anzenbacher, P., Anzenbacherova, E., 2001. Cytochromes P450 and metabolism of xenobiotics. Cell Mol. Life Sci. 58, 737–747.

Aynaci, F.M., Orhan, F., Orem, A., Yildirmis, S., Gedik, Y., 2001. Effect of Antiepileptic drugs on plasma lipoprotein (a) and other lipid levels in childhood. J. Child Neurol. 16, 367–369.

Ayrton, A., Morgan, P., 2008. Role of transport proteins in drug discovery and development: a pharmaceutical perspective. Xenobiotica 38, 676–708.

Bachmann, K., Patel, H., Batayneh, Z., Slama, J., White, D., Posey, J., Ekins, S., Gold, D., Sambucetti, L., 2004. PXR and the regulation of apoA1 and HDL-cholesterol in rodents. Pharmacol. Res. 50, 237–246.

Barshop, N.J., Capparelli, E.V., Sirlin, C.B., Schwimmer, J.B., Lavine, J.E., 2011. Acetaminophen pharmacokinetics in children with nonalcoholic fatty liver disease. J. Pediatr. Gastroenterol. Nutr. 52, 198–202.

Biswas, A., Pasquel, D., Tyagi, R.K., Mani, S., 2011. Acetylation of pregnane X receptor protein determines selective function independent of ligand activation. Biochem. Biophys. Res. Commun. 406, 371–376.

Blattler, S.M., Rencurel, F., Kaufmann, M.R., Meyer, U.A., 2007. In the regulation of cytochrome P450 genes, phenobarbital targets LKB1 for necessary activation of AMP-activated protein kinase. Proc. Natl. Acad. Sci. USA. 104, 1045–1050.

Blouin, R.A., Warren, G.W., 1999. Pharmacokinetic considerations in obesity. J. Pharm. Sci. 88, 1–7.

Bombick, D.W., Matsumura, F., Madhukar, B.V., 1984. TCDD (2,3,7,8-tetrachlorodibenzo-p-dioxin) causes reduction in the low density lipoprotein (LDL) receptor activities in the hepatic plasma membrane of the guinea pig and rat. Biochem. Biophys. Res. Commun. 118, 548–554.

Brewster, D.W., Matsumura, F.T.C.D.D., 1984. (2,3,7,8-tetrachlorodibenzo-p-dioxin) reduces lipoprotein lipase activity in the adipose tissue of the guinea pig. Biochem. Biophys. Res. Commun. 122, 810–817.

Brewster, D.W., Bombick, D.W., Matsumura, F., 1988. Rabbit serum hypertriglyceridemia after administration of 2,3,7,8-tetrachlorodibenzo-p-dioxin (TCDD). J. Toxicol. Environ. Health 25, 495–507.

Buler, M., Aatsinki, S.M., Skoumal, R., Hakkola, J., 2011. Energy sensing factors PGC-1α and SIRT1 modulate PXR expression and function. Biochem. Pharmacol. 82, 2008–2015.

Carr, A., Samaras, K., Burton, S., Law, M., Freund, J., Chisholm, D.J., Cooper, D.A., 1998. A syndrome of peripheral lipodystrophy, hyperlipidaemia and insulin resistance in patients receiving HIV protease inhibitors. AIDS 12, F51–F58.

Cohen, J.C., Horton, J.D., Hobbs, H.H., 2011. Human fatty liver disease: old questions and new insights. Science 332, 1519–1523.

Chen, I., McDougal, A., Wang, F., Safe, S., 1998. Aryl hydrocarbon receptor-mediated antiestrogenic and antitumorigenic activity of diindolylmethane. Carcinogenesis 19, 1631–1639.

Cheng, Q., Aleksunes, L.M., Manautou, J.E., Cherrington, N.J., Scheffer, G.L., Yamasaki, H., Slitt, A.L., 2008. Drug-metabolizing enzyme and transporter expression in a mouse model of diabetes and obesity. Mol. Pharm. 5, 77–91.

Cheng, J., Krausz, K.W., Tanaka, N., Gonzalez, F.J., 2012. Chronic exposure to rifaximin causes hepatic steatosis in pregnane X receptor-humanized mice. Toxicol. Sci. 129, 456–468.

Cheymol, G., 2000. Effects of obesity on pharmacokinetics implications for drug therapy. Clin. Pharmacokinet. 39, 215–231.

Cranmer, M., Louie, S., Kennedy, R.H., Kern, P.A., Fonseca, V.A., 2000. Exposure to 2,3,7,8-tetrachlorodibenzo-p-dioxin (TCDD) is associated with hyperinsulinemia and insulin resistance. Toxicol. Sci. 56, 431–436.

Dai, G., He, L., Bu, P., Wan, Y.J., 2008. Pregnane X receptor is essential for normal progression of liver regeneration. Hepatology 47, 1277–1287.

De Waziers, I., Garlatti, M., Bouguet, J., Beaune, P.H., Barouki, R., 1995. Insulin down-regulates cytochrome P450 2B and 2E expression at the post-transcriptional level in the rat hepatoma cell line. Mol. Pharmacol. 47, 474–479.

Denison, M.S., Nagy, S.R., 2003. Activation of the aryl hydrocarbon receptor by structurally diverse exogenous and endogenous chemicals. Annu. Rev. Pharmacol. Toxicol. 43, 309–334.

Diani-Moore, S., Ram, P., Li, X., Mondal, P., Youn, D.Y., Sauve, A.A., Rifkind, A.B., 2010. Identification of the aryl hydrocarbon receptor target gene TiPARP as a mediator of suppression of hepatic gluconeogenesis by 2,3,7,8-tetrachlorodibenzo-p-dioxin and of nicotinamide as a corrective agent for this effect. J. Biol. Chem. 285, 38801–38810.

Ding, X., Lichti, K., Kim, I., Gonzalez, F.J., Staudinger, J.L., 2006. Regulation of constitutive androstane receptor and its target genes by fasting, cAMP, hepatocyte nuclear factor α, and the coactivator peroxisome proliferator-activated receptor γ coactivator-1α. J. Biol. Chem. 281, 26540–26551.

Donato, M.T., Jimenez, N., Serralta, A., Mir, J., Castell, J.V., Gomez-Lechon, M.J., 2007. Effects of steatosis on drug-metabolizing capability of primary human hepatocytes. Toxicol. In Vitro 21, 271–276.

Dong, B., Qatanani, M., Moore, D.D., 2009a. Constitutive androstane receptor mediates the induction of drug metabolism in mouse models of type 1 diabetes. Hepatology 50, 622–629.

Dong, B., Saha, P.K., Huang, W., Chen, W., Abu-Elheiga, L.A., Wakil, S.J., Stevens, R.D., Ilkayeva, O., Newgard, C.B., Chan, L., Moore, D.D., 2009b. Activation of nuclear receptor CAR ameliorates diabetes and fatty liver disease. Proc. Natl. Acad. Sci. USA. 106, 18831–18836.

Dussault, I., Lin, M., Hollister, K., Wang, E.H., Synold, T.W., Forman, B.M., 2001. Peptide mimetic HIV protease inhibitors are ligands for the orphan receptor SXR. J. Biol. Chem. 276, 33309–33312.

Ebner, K., Brewster, D.W., Matsumura, F., 1988. Effects of 2,3,7,8-tetrachlorodibenzo-p-dioxin on serum insulin and glucose levels in the rabbit. J. Environ. Sci. Health B 23, 427–438.

Eiris, J.M., Lojo, S., Del Rio, M.C., Novo, I., Bravo, M., Pavon, P., Castro-Gago, M., 1995. Effects of long-term treatment with antiepileptic drugs on serum lipid levels in children with epilepsy. Neurology 45, 1155–1157.

Enan, E., Liu, P.C., Matsumura, F., 1992a. 2,3,7,8-Tetrachlorodibenzo-p-dioxin causes reduction of glucose transporting activities in the plasma membranes of adipose tissue and pancreas from the guinea pig. J. Biol. Chem. 267, 19785–19791.

Enan, E., Liu, P.C., Matsumura, F.T.C.D.D., 1992b. (2,3,7,8-tetrachlorodibenzo-P-dioxin) causes reduction in glucose uptake through glucose transporters on the plasma membrane of the guinea pig adipocyte. J. Environ. Sci. Health B 27, 495–510.

Federico, L.M., Naples, M., Taylor, D., Adeli, K., 2006. Intestinal insulin resistance and aberrant production of apolipoprotein B48 lipoproteins in an animal model of insulin resistance and metabolic dyslipidemia: evidence for activation of protein tyrosine phosphatase-1B, extracellular signal-related kinase, and sterol regulatory element-binding protein-1c in the fructose-fed hamster intestine. Diabetes 55, 1316–1326.

Fernandez-Salguero, P., Pineau, T., Hilbert, D.M., McPhail, T., Lee, S.S., Kimura, S., Nebert, D.W., Rudikoff, S., Ward, J.M., Gonzalez, F.J., 1995. Immune system impairment and hepatic fibrosis in mice lacking the dioxin-binding Ah receptor. Science 268, 722–726.

Fiatarone, J.R., Coverdale, S.A., Batey, R.G., Farrell, G.C., 1991. Non-alcoholic steatohepatitis: impaired antipyrine metabolism and hypertriglyceridaemia may be clues to its pathogenesis. J. Gastroenterol. Hepatol. 6, 585–590.

Fletcher, N., Wahlstrom, D., Lundberg, R., Nilsson, C.B., Nilsson, K.C., Stockling, K., Hellmold, H., Hakansson, H., 2005. 2,3,7,8-Tetrachlorodibenzo-p-dioxin (TCDD) alters the mRNA expression of critical genes associated with cholesterol metabolism, bile acid biosynthesis, and bile transport in rat liver: a microarray study. Toxicol. Appl. Pharmacol. 207, 1–24.

Gao, J., Xie, W., 2010. Pregnane X receptor and constitutive androstane receptor at the crossroads of drug metabolism and energy metabolism. Drug Metab. Dispos. 38, 2091–2095.

Gao, J., Xie, W., 2012. Targeting xenobiotic receptors PXR and CAR for metabolic diseases. Trends Pharmacol. Sci. 33, 552–558.

Gao, J., He, J., Zhai, Y., Wada, T., Xie, W., 2009. The constitutive androstane receptor is an anti-obesity nuclear receptor that improves insulin sensitivity. J. Biol. Chem. 284, 25984–25992.

Gao, J., He, J., Shi, X., Stefanovic-Racic, M., Xu, M., O'Doherty, R.M., Garcia-Ocana, A., Xie, W., 2012. Sex-specific effect of estrogen sulfotransferase on mouse models of type 2 diabetes. Diabetes 61, 1543–1551.

Gao, J., Yan, J., Xu, M., Ren, S., Xie, W., 2015. CAR suppresses hepatic gluconeogenesis by facilitating the ubiquitination and degradation of PGC1α. Mol. Endocrinol. http://dx.doi.org/10.1210/me.2015-1145.

Garrison, P.M., Denison, M.S., 2000. Analysis of the murine AhR gene promoter. J. Biochem. Mol. Toxicol. 14, 1–10.

Geusau, A., Abraham, K., Geissler, K., Sator, M.O., Stingl, G., Tschachler, E., 2001. Severe 2,3,7,8-tetrachlorodibenzo-p-dioxin (TCDD) intoxication: clinical and laboratory effects. Environ. Health Perspect. 109, 865—869.

Goerdt, C., Keith, M., Rubins, H.B., 1995. Effects of phenytoin on plasma high-density lipoprotein cholesterol levels in men with low levels of high-density lipoprotein cholesterol. J. Clin. Pharmacol. 35, 767—775.

Goldstein, S., Simpson, A., Saenger, P., 1990. Hepatic drug metabolism is increased in poorly controlled insulin-dependent diabetes mellitus. Acta Endocrinol. 123, 550—556.

Gomez-Lechon, M.J., Jover, R., Donato, M.T., 2009. Cytochrome p450 and steatosis. Curr. Drug Metab. 10, 692—699.

Gorski, J.R., Weber, L.W., Rozman, K., 1988. Tissue-specific alterations of de novo fatty acid synthesis in 2,3,7,8-tetrachlorodibenzo-p-dioxin (TCDD)-treated rats. Arch. Toxicol. 62, 146—151.

Guengerich, F.P., 2001. Common and uncommon cytochrome P450 reactions related to metabolism and chemical toxicity. Chem. Res. Toxicol. 14, 611—650.

Gunton, J.E., Kulkarni, R.N., Yim, S., Okada, T., Hawthorne, W.J., Tseng, Y.H., Roberson, R.S., Ricordi, C., O'Connell, P.J., Gonzalez, F.J., Kahn, C.R., 2005. Loss of ARNT/HIF1β mediates altered gene expression and pancreatic-islet dysfunction in human type 2 diabetes. Cell 122, 337—349.

de Haan, W., de Vries-van der Weij, J., Mol, I.M., Hoekstra, M., Romijn, J.A., Jukema, J.W., Havekes, L.M., Princen, H.M., Rensen, P.C., 2009. PXR agonism decreases plasma HDL levels in ApoE3-Leiden.CETP mice. Biochim. Biophys. Acta 1791, 191—197.

Haidari, M., Leung, N., Mahbub, F., Uffelman, K.D., Kohen-Avramoglu, R., Lewis, G.F., Adeli, K., 2002. Fasting and postprandial overproduction of intestinally derived lipoproteins in an animal model of insulin resistance. Evidence that chronic fructose feeding in the hamster is accompanied by enhanced intestinal de novo lipogenesis and ApoB48-containing lipoprotein overproduction. J. Biol. Chem. 277, 31646—31655.

Handschin, C., Meyer, U.A., 2003. Induction of drug metabolism: the role of nuclear receptors. Pharmacol. Rev. 55, 649—673.

Hankinson, O., 1995. The aryl hydrocarbon receptor complex. Annu. Rev. Pharmacol. Toxicol. 35, 307—340.

He, J., Hu, B., Shi, X., Weidert, E.R., Lu, P., Xu, M., Huang, M., Kelley, E.E., Xie, W., 2013a. Activation of the aryl hydrocarbon receptor sensitizes mice to nonalcoholic steatohepatitis by deactivating mitochondrial sirtuin deacetylase Sirt3. Mol. Cell Biol. 33, 2047—2055.

He, J., Gao, J., Xu, M., Ren, S., Stefanovic-Racic, M., O'Doherty, R.M., Xie, W., 2013b. PXR ablation alleviates diet-induced and genetic obesity and insulin resistance in mice. Diabetes 62, 1876—1887.

Henriksen, G.L., Ketchum, N.S., Michalek, J.E., Swaby, J.A., 1997. Serum dioxin and diabetes mellitus in veterans of Operation Ranch Hand. Epidemiology 8, 252—258.

Hinton, D.E., Glaumann, H., Trump, B.F., 1978. Studies on the cellular toxicity of polychlorinated biphenyls (PCBs). I. Effect of PCBs on microsomal enzymes and on synthesis and turnover of microsomal and cytoplasmic lipids of rat liver — a morphological and biochemical study. Virchows Arch. B Cell Pathol. 27, 279—306.

Hoffman, E.C., Reyes, H., Chu, F.F., Sander, F., Conley, L.H., Brooks, B.A., Hankinson, O., 1991. Cloning of a factor required for activity of the Ah (dioxin) receptor. Science 252, 954—958.

Huang, P., Ceccatelli, S., Rannug, A., 2002. A study on diurnal mRNA expression of CYP1A1, AHR, ARNT, and PER2 in rat pituitary and liver. Environ. Toxicol. Pharmacol. 11, 119—126.

IARC working group on the evaluation of carcinogenic risks to humans: polychlorinated dibenzo-para-dioxins and polychlorinated dibenzofurans. Lyon, France, 4—11 February 1997. IARC Monogr. Eval. Carcinog Risks Hum. 69, 1997, 1—631.

James, O.F., Day, C.P., 1998. Non-alcoholic steatohepatitis (NASH): a disease of emerging identity and importance. J. Hepatol. 29, 495—501.

Jones, G., Greig, J.B., 1975. Pathological changes in the liver of mice given 2,3,7,8-tetrachlorodibenzo-p-dioxin. Experientia 31, 1315—1317.

Jones, S.A., Moore, L.B., Shenk, J.L., Wisely, G.B., Hamilton, G.A., McKee, D.D., Tomkinson, N.C., LeCluyse, E.L., Lambert, M.H., Willson, T.M., Kliewer, S.A., Moore, J.T., 2000. The pregnane X receptor: a promiscuous xenobiotic receptor that has diverged during evolution. Mol. Endocrinol. 14, 27—39.

Jou, J., Choi, S.S., Diehl, A.M., 2008. Mechanisms of disease progression in nonalcoholic fatty liver disease. Semin. Liver Dis. 28, 370—379.

Jung, H., Choe, Y., Kim, H., Park, N., Son, G.H., Khang, I., Kim, K., 2003. Involvement of CLOCK: BMAL1 heterodimer in serum-responsive mPer1 induction. Neuroreport 14, 15—19.

Kirpich, I.A., Gobejishvili, L.N., Bon Homme, M., Waigel, S., Cave, M., Arteel, G., Barve, S.S., McClain, C.J., Deaciuc, I.V., 2011. Integrated hepatic transcriptome and proteome analysis of mice with high-fat diet-induced nonalcoholic fatty liver disease. J. Nutr. Biochem. 22, 38—45.

Kodama, S., Koike, C., Negishi, M., Yamamoto, Y., 2004. Nuclear receptors CAR and PXR cross talk with FOXO1 to regulate genes that encode drug-metabolizing and gluconeogenic enzymes. Mol. Cell Biol. 24, 7931—7940.

Kawano, Y., Nishiumi, S., Tanaka, S., Nobutani, K., Miki, A., Yano, Y., Seo, Y., Kutsumi, H., Ashida, H., Azuma, T., Yoshida, M., 2010. Activation of the aryl hydrocarbon receptor induces hepatic steatosis via the upregulation of fatty acid transport. Arch. Biochem. Biophys. 504, 221—227.

Kern, P.A., Dicker-Brown, A., Said, S.T., Kennedy, R., Fonseca, V.A., 2002. The stimulation of tumor necrosis factor and inhibition of glucose transport and lipoprotein lipase in adipose cells by 2,3,7,8-tetrachlorodibenzo-p-dioxin. Metabolism 51, 65—68.

Kodama, S., Moore, R., Yamamoto, Y., Negishi, M., 2007. Human nuclear pregnane X receptor cross-talk with CREB to repress cAMP activation of the glucose-6-phosphatase gene. Biochem. J. 407, 373—381.

Kohli, K.K., Gupta, B.N., Albro, P.W., Mukhtar, H., McKinney, J.D., 1979. Biochemical effects of pure isomers of hexachlorobiphenyl: fatty livers and cell structure. Chem. Biol. Interact. 25, 139—156.

Koide, C.L., Collier, A.C., Berry, M.J., Panee, J., 2011. The effect of bamboo extract on hepatic biotransforming enzymes — findings from an obese-diabetic mouse model. J. Ethnopharmacol 133, 37—45.

Lahtela, J.T., Arranto, A.J., Sotaniemi, E.A., 1985. Enzyme inducers improve insulin sensitivity in non-insulin-dependent diabetic subjects. Diabetes 34, 911—916.

Lahvis, G.P., Lindell, S.L., Thomas, R.S., McCuskey, R.S., Murphy, C., Glover, E., Bentz, M., Southard, J., Bradfield, C.A., 2000. Portosystemic shunting and persistent fetal vascular structures in aryl hydrocarbon receptor-deficient mice. Proc. Natl. Acad. Sci. USA. 97, 10442—10447.

Lakshman, M.R., Campbell, B.S., Chirtel, S.J., Ekarohita, N., 1988. Effects of 2,3,7,8-tetrachlorodibenzo-p-dioxin (TCDD) on de novo fatty acid and cholesterol synthesis in the rat. Lipids 23, 904—906.

Lakshman, M.R., Ghosh, P., Chirtel, S.J., 1991. Mechanism of action of 2,3,7,8-tetrachlorodibenzo-p-dioxin on intermediary metabolism in the rat. J. Pharmacol. Exp. Ther. 258, 317—319.

Lammers, L.A., Achterbergh, R., de Vries, E.M., van Nierop, F.S., Klumpen, H.J., Soeters, M.R., Boelen, A., Romijn, J.A., Mathot, R.A., 2015. Short-term fasting alters cytochrome P450-mediated drug metabolism in humans. Drug Metab. Dispos. 43, 819—828.

Leclercq, I., Horsmans, Y., Desager, J.P., Delzenne, N., Geubel, A.P., 1998. Reduction in hepatic cytochrome P-450 is correlated to the degree of liver fat content in animal models of steatosis in the absence of inflammation. J. Hepatol. 28, 410—416.

Lee, C.C., Yao, Y.J., Chen, H.L., Guo, Y.L., Su, H.J., 2006. Fatty liver and hepatic function for residents with markedly high serum PCDD/Fs levels in Taiwan. J. Toxicol. Environ. Health A 69, 367—380.

Lee, J.H., Zhou, J., Xie, W., 2008. PXR and LXR in hepatic steatosis: a new dog and an old dog with new tricks. Mol. Pharm. 5, 60—66.

Lee, J.H., Wada, T., Febbraio, M., He, J., Matsubara, T., Lee, M.J., Gonzalez, F.J., Xie, W., 2010. A novel role for the dioxin receptor in fatty acid metabolism and hepatic steatosis. Gastroenterology 139, 653—663.

Li, C.C., Lii, C.K., Liu, K.L., Yang, J.J., Chen, H.W., 2007. DHA down-regulates phenobarbital-induced cytochrome P450 2B1 gene expression in rat primary hepatocytes by attenuating CAR translocation. Toxicol. Appl. Pharmacol. 225, 329—336.

Liu, P.C., Matsumura, F., 1995. Differential effects of 2,3,7,8-tetrachlorodibenzo-p-dioxin on the "adipose- type" and "brain-type" glucose transporters in mice. Mol. Pharmacol. 47, 65—73.

Longo, V., Ingelman-Sundberg, M., Amato, G., Salvetti, A., Gervasi, P.G., 2000. Effect of starvation and chlormethiazole on cytochrome P450s of rat nasal mucosa. Biochem. Pharmacol. 59, 1425—1432.

Lu, Y., Feskens, E.J., Boer, J.M., Muller, M., 2010. The potential influence of genetic variants in genes along bile acid and bile metabolic pathway on blood cholesterol levels in the population. Atherosclerosis 210, 14—27.

Lu, H., Cui, W., Klaassen, C.D., 2011. Nrf2 protects against 2,3,7,8-tetrachlorodibenzo-p-dioxin (TCDD)-induced oxidative injury and steatohepatitis. Toxicol. Appl. Pharmacol. 256, 122—135.

Lu, P., Yan, J., Liu, K., Garbacz, W.G., Wang, P., Xu, M., Ma, X., Xie, W., 2015. Activation of aryl hydrocarbon receptor dissociates fatty liver from insulin resistance by inducing fibroblast growth factor 21. Hepatology 61, 1908—1919.

Martin, J.V., 1984. Lipid abnormalities in workers exposed to dioxin. Br. J. Ind. Med. 41, 254—256.

Masson, D., Lagrost, L., Athias, A., Gambert, P., Brimer-Cline, C., Lan, L., Schuetz, J.D., Schuetz, E.G., Assem, M., 2005. Expression of the pregnane X receptor in mice antagonizes the cholic acid-mediated changes in plasma lipoprotein profile. Arterioscler Thromb. Vasc. Biol. 25, 2164−2169.

Masson, D., Qatanani, M., Sberna, A.L., Xiao, R., Pais de Barros, J.P., Grober, J., Deckert, V., Athias, A., Gambert, P., Lagrost, L., Moore, D.D., Assem, M., 2008. Activation of the constitutive androstane receptor decreases HDL in wild-type and human apoA-I transgenic mice. J. Lipid Res. 49, 1682−1691.

Matsumura, F., 1995. Mechanism of action of dioxin-type chemicals, pesticides, and other xenobiotics affecting nutritional indexes. Am. J. Clin. Nutr. 61, 695S−701S.

McCarver, D.G., Hines, R.N., 2002. The ontogeny of human drug-metabolizing enzymes: phase II conjugation enzymes and regulatory mechanisms. J. Pharmacol. Exp. Ther. 300, 361−366.

McMillan, B.J., Bradfield, C.A., 2007. The aryl hydrocarbon receptor is activated by modified low-density lipoprotein. Proc. Natl. Acad. Sci. USA. 104, 1412−1417.

Miao, J., Fang, S., Bae, Y., Kemper, J.K., 2006. Functional inhibitory cross-talk between constitutive androstane receptor and hepatic nuclear factor-4 in hepatic lipid/glucose metabolism is mediated by competition for binding to the DR1 motif and to the common coactivators, GRIP-1 and PGC-1α. J. Biol. Chem. 281, 14537−14546.

Miller, M., Burgan, R.G., Osterlund, L., Segrest, J.P., Garber, D.W., 1995. A prospective, randomized trial of phenytoin in nonepileptic subjects with reduced HDL cholesterol. Arterioscler Thromb. Vasc. Biol. 15, 2151−2156.

Minami, K., Nakajima, M., Fujiki, Y., Katoh, M., Gonzalez, F.J., Yokoi, T., 2008. Regulation of insulin-like growth factor binding protein-1 and lipoprotein lipase by the aryl hydrocarbon receptor. J. Toxicol. Sci. 33, 405−413.

Miyata, M., Nomoto, M., Sotodate, F., Mizuki, T., Hori, W., Nagayasu, M., Yokokawa, S., Ninomiya, S., Yamazoe, Y., 2010. Possible protective role of pregnenolone-16α-carbonitrile in lithocholic acid-induced hepatotoxicity through enhanced hepatic lipogenesis. Eur. J. Pharmacol. 636, 145−154.

Moore, L.B., Parks, D.J., Jones, S.A., Bledsoe, R.K., Consler, T.G., Stimmel, J.B., Goodwin, B., Liddle, C., Blanchard, S.G., Willson, T.M., Collins, J.L., Kliewer, S.A., 2000. Orphan nuclear receptors constitutive androstane receptor and pregnane X receptor share xenobiotic and steroid ligands. J. Biol. Chem. 275, 15122−15127.

Moreau, A., Teruel, C., Beylot, M., Albalea, V., Tamasi, V., Umbdenstock, T., Parmentier, Y., Sa-Cunha, A., Suc, B., Fabre, J.M., Navarro, F., Ramos, J., Meyer, U., Maurel, P., Vilarem, M.J., Pascussi, J.M., 2009. A novel pregnane X receptor and S14-mediated lipogenic pathway in human hepatocyte. Hepatology 49, 2068−2079.

Moya, M., Gomez-Lechon, M.J., Castell, J.V., Jover, R., 2010. Enhanced steatosis by nuclear receptor ligands: a study in cultured human hepatocytes and hepatoma cells with a characterized nuclear receptor expression profile. Chem. Biol. Interact. 184, 376−387.

Mukai, M., Tischkau, S.A., 2007. Effects of tryptophan photoproducts in the circadian timing system: searching for a physiological role for aryl hydrocarbon receptor. Toxicol. Sci. 95, 172−181.

Mukai, M., Lin, T.M., Peterson, R.E., Cooke, P.S., Tischkau, S.A., 2008. Behavioral rhythmicity of mice lacking AhR and attenuation of light-induced phase shift by 2,3,7,8-tetrachlorodibenzo-p-dioxin. J. Biol. Rhythms 23, 200−210.

Murray, M., 2006. Altered CYP expression and function in response to dietary factors: potential roles in disease pathogenesis. Curr. Drug Metab. 7, 67−81.

Nakamura, K., Moore, R., Negishi, M., Sueyoshi, T., 2007. Nuclear pregnane X receptor cross-talk with FoxA2 to mediate drug-induced regulation of lipid metabolism in fasting mouse liver. J. Biol. Chem. 282, 9768−9776.

Nebert, D.W., Gonzalez, F.J., 1987. P450 genes: structure, evolution, and regulation. Ann. Rev. Biochem. 56, 945−993.

Nebert, D.W., Roe, A.L., Dieter, M.Z., Solis, W.A., Yang, Y., Dalton, T.P., 2000. Role of the aromatic hydrocarbon receptor and [Ah] gene battery in the oxidative stress response, cell cycle control, and apoptosis. Biochem. Pharmacol. 59, 65−85.

Nguyen, P., Leray, V., Diez, M., Serisier, S., Le Bloc'h, J., Siliart, B., Dumon, H., 2008. Liver lipid metabolism. J. Anim. Physiol. Anim. Nutr. 92, 272−283.

Okey, A.B., 2007. An aryl hydrocarbon receptor odyssey to the shores of toxicology: the Deichmann Lecture, International Congress of Toxicology-XI. Toxicol. Sci. 98, 5−38.

Opitz, C.A., Litzenburger, U.M., Sahm, F., Ott, M., Tritschler, I., Trump, S., Schumacher, T., Jestaedt, L., Schrenk, D., Weller, M., Jugold, M., Guillemin, G.J., Miller, C.L., Lutz, C., Radlwimmer, B., Lehmann, I., von Deimling, A., Wick, W., Platten, M., 2011. An endogenous tumour-promoting ligand of the human aryl hydrocarbon receptor. Nature 478, 197−203.

Osabe, M., Sugatani, J., Fukuyama, T., Ikushiro, S., Ikari, A., Miwa, M., 2008. Expression of hepatic UDP-glucuronosyltransferase 1A1 and 1A6 correlated with increased expression of the nuclear constitutive androstane receptor and peroxisome proliferator-activated receptor α in male rats fed a high-fat and high-sucrose diet. Drug Metab. Dispos. 36, 294–302.

Partch, C.L., Green, C.B., Takahashi, J.S., 2014. Molecular architecture of the mammalian circadian clock. Trends Cell Biol. 24, 90–99.

Pelclova, D., Fenclova, Z., Preiss, J., Prochazka, B., Spacil, J., Dubska, Z., Okrouhlik, B., Lukas, E., Urban, P., 2002. Lipid metabolism and neuropsychological follow-up study of workers exposed to 2,3,7,8- tetrachlordibenzo- p-dioxin. Int. Arch. Occup. Environ. Health 75 (Suppl.), S60–S66.

Plee-Gautier, E., Antoun, J., Goulitquer, S., Le Jossic-Corcos, C., Simon, B., Amet, Y., Salaun, J.P., Corcos, L., 2012. Statins increase cytochrome P450 4F3-mediated eicosanoids production in human liver cells: a PXR dependent mechanism. Biochem. Pharmacol. 84, 571–579.

Poland, A., Glover, E., Kende, A.S., 1976. Stereospecific, high affinity binding of 2,3,7,8-tetrachlorodibenzo-p-dioxin by hepatic cytosol. Evidence that the binding species is receptor for induction of aryl hydrocarbon hydroxylase. J. Biol. Chem. 251, 4936–4946.

Potter, C.L., Menahan, L.A., Peterson, R.E., 1986. Relationship of alterations in energy metabolism to hypophagia in rats treated with 2,3,7,8-tetrachlorodibenzo-p-dioxin. Fundam. Appl. Toxicol. 6, 89–97.

Qu, W., Rippe, R.A., Ma, J., Scarborough, P., Biagini, C., Fiedorek, F.T., Travlos, G.S., Parker, C., Zeldin, D.C., 1998. Nutritional status modulates rat liver cytochrome P450 arachidonic acid metabolism. Mol. Pharmacol. 54, 504–513.

Qu, X., Metz, R.P., Porter, W.W., Neuendorff, N., Earnest, B.J., Earnest, D.J., 2010. The clock genes period 1 and period 2 mediate diurnal rhythms in dioxin-induced Cyp1A1 expression in the mouse mammary gland and liver. Toxicol. Lett. 196, 28–32.

Reisz-Porszasz, S., Probst, M.R., Fukunaga, B.N., Hankinson, O., 1994. Identification of functional domains of the aryl hydrocarbon receptor nuclear translocator protein (ARNT). Mol. Cell Biol. 14, 6075–6086.

Remillard, R.B., Bunce, N.J., 2002. Linking dioxins to diabetes: epidemiology and biologic plausibility. Environ. Health Perspect. 110, 853–858.

Ricketts, M.L., Boekschoten, M.V., Kreeft, A.J., Hooiveld, G.J., Moen, C.J., Muller, M., Frants, R.R., Kasanmoentalib, S., Post, S.M., Princen, H.M., Porter, J.G., Katan, M.B., Hofker, M.H., Moore, D.D., 2007. The cholesterol-raising factor from coffee beans, cafestol, as an agonist ligand for the farnesoid and pregnane X receptors. Mol. Endocrinol. 21, 1603–1616.

Richardson, V.M., Santostefano, M.J., Birnbaum, L.S., 1998. Daily cycle of bHLH-PAS proteins, Ah receptor and Arnt, in multiple tissues of female Sprague-Dawley rats. Biochem. Biophys. Res. Commun. 252, 225–231.

Riddler, S.A., Smit, E., Cole, S.R., Li, R., Chmiel, J.S., Dobs, A., Palella, F., Visscher, B., Evans, R., Kingsley, L.A., 2003. Impact of HIV infection and HAART on serum lipids in men. JAMA 289, 2978–2982.

Roth, A., Looser, R., Kaufmann, M., Meyer, U.A., 2008a. Sterol regulatory element binding protein 1 interacts with pregnane X receptor and constitutive androstane receptor and represses their target genes. Pharmacogenet Genomics 18, 325–337.

Roth, A., Looser, R., Kaufmann, M., Blattler, S.M., Rencurel, F., Huang, W., Moore, D.D., Meyer, U.A., 2008b. Regulatory cross-talk between drug metabolism and lipid homeostasis: constitutive androstane receptor and pregnane X receptor increase Insig-1 expression. Mol. Pharmacol. 73, 1282–1289.

Rysa, J., Buler, M., Savolainen, M.J., Ruskoaho, H., Hakkola, J., Hukkanen, J., 2013. Pregnane X receptor agonists impair postprandial glucose tolerance. Clin. Pharmacol. Ther. 93, 556–563.

Sakuma, T., Honma, R., Maguchi, S., Tamaki, H., Nemoto, N., 2001. Different expression of hepatic and renal cytochrome P450s between the streptozotocin-induced diabetic mouse and rat. Xenobiotica 31, 223–237.

Sberna, A.L., Assem, M., Gautier, T., Grober, J., Guiu, B., Jeannin, A., Pais de Barros, J.P., Athias, A., Lagrost, L., Masson, D., 2011. Constitutive androstane receptor activation stimulates faecal bile acid excretion and reverse cholesterol transport in mice. J. Hepatol. 55, 154–161.

Schmidt, J.V., Su, G.H., Reddy, J.K., Simon, M.C., Bradfield, C.A., 1996. Characterization of a murine Ahr null allele: involvement of the Ah receptor in hepatic growth and development. Proc. Natl. Acad. Sci. USA. 93, 6731–6736.

Shafran, S.D., Mashinter, L.D., Roberts, S.E., 2005. The effect of low-dose ritonavir monotherapy on fasting serum lipid concentrations. HIV Med. 6, 421–425.

Shi, X., Cheng, Q., Xu, L., Yan, J., Jiang, M., He, J., Xu, M., Stefanovic-Racic, M., Sipula, I., O'Doherty, R.M., Ren, S., Xie, W., 2014. Cholesterol sulfate and cholesterol sulfotransferase inhibit gluconeogenesis by targeting hepatocyte nuclear factor 4α. Mol. Cell Biol. 34, 485–497.

Shindo, S., Numazawa, S., Yoshida, T., 2007. A physiological role of AMP-activated protein kinase in phenobarbital-mediated constitutive androstane receptor activation and CYP2B induction. Biochem. J. 401, 735–741.

Shoelson, S.E., Lee, J., Goldfine, A.B., 2006. Inflammation and insulin resistance. J. Clin. Invest. 116, 1793–1801.

Sidhu, J.S., Omiecinski, C.J., 1999. Insulin-mediated modulation of cytochrome P450 gene induction profiles in primary rat hepatocyte cultures. J. Biochem. Mol. Toxicol. 13, 1–9.

Skett, P., Joels, L.A., 1985. Different effects of acute and chronic diabetes mellitus on hepatic drug metabolism in the rat. Biochem. Pharmacol. 34, 287–289.

Sookoian, S., Castano, G.O., Burgueno, A.L., Gianotti, T.F., Rosselli, M.S., Pirola, C.J., 2010. The nuclear receptor PXR gene variants are associated with liver injury in nonalcoholic fatty liver disease. Pharmacogenet Genomics 20, 1–8.

Sporstol, M., Tapia, G., Malerod, L., Mousavi, S.A., Berg, T., 2005. Pregnane X receptor-agonists down-regulate hepatic ATP-binding cassette transporter A1 and scavenger receptor class B type I. Biochem. Biophys. Res. Commun. 331, 1533–1541.

Staudinger, J.L., Goodwin, B., Jones, S.A., Hawkins-Brown, D., MacKenzie, K.I., LaTour, A., Liu, Y., Klaassen, C.D., Brown, K.K., Reinhard, J., Willson, T.M., Koller, B.H., Kliewer, S.A., 2001. The nuclear receptor PXR is a lithocholic acid sensor that protects against liver toxicity. Proc. Natl. Acad. Sci. USA. 98, 3369–3374.

Stedman, C.A., Liddle, C., Coulter, S.A., Sonoda, J., Alvarez, J.G., Moore, D.D., Evans, R.M., Downes, M., 2005. Nuclear receptors constitutive androstane receptor and pregnane X receptor ameliorate cholestatic liver injury. Proc. Natl. Acad. Sci. USA. 102, 2063–2068.

Stepanova, M., Hossain, N., Afendy, A., Perry, K., Goodman, Z.D., Baranova, A., Younossi, Z., 2010. Hepatic gene expression of Caucasian and African-American patients with obesity-related non-alcoholic fatty liver disease. Obes. Surg. 20, 640–650.

Su, G.M., Sefton, R.M., Murray, M., 1999. Down-regulation of rat hepatic microsomal cytochromes P-450 in microvesicular steatosis induced by orotic acid. J. Pharmacol. Exp. Ther. 291, 953–959.

Swift, L.L., Gasiewicz, T.A., Dunn, G.D., Soule, P.D., Neal, R.A., 1981. Characterization of the hyperlipidemia in guinea pigs induced by 2,3,7,8-tetrachlorodibenzo-p-dioxin. Toxicol. Appl. Pharmacol. 59, 489–499.

Tanimura, N., Kusunose, N., Matsunaga, N., Koyanagi, S., Ohdo, S., 2011. Aryl hydrocarbon receptor-mediated Cyp1a1 expression is modulated in a CLOCK-dependent circadian manner. Toxicology 290, 203–207.

Tanos, R., Murray, I.A., Smith, P.B., Patterson, A., Perdew, G.H., 2012. Role of the Ah receptor in homeostatic control of fatty acid synthesis in the liver. Toxicol. Sci. 129, 372–379.

Tarantino, G., Conca, P., Basile, V., Gentile, A., Capone, D., Polichetti, G., Leo, E., 2007. A prospective study of acute drug-induced liver injury in patients suffering from non-alcoholic fatty liver disease. Hepatol. Res. 37, 410–415.

Tarantino, G., Di Minno, M.N., Capone, D., 2009. Drug-induced liver injury: is it somehow foreseeable? World J. Gastroenterol. 15, 2817–2833.

Terashima, J., Habano, W., Gamou, T., Ozawa, S., 2011. Induction of CYP1 family members under low-glucose conditions requires AhR expression and occurs through the nuclear translocation of AhR. Drug Metab. Pharmacokinet. 26, 577–583.

Tilg, H., Moschen, A.R., 2010. Evolution of inflammation in nonalcoholic fatty liver disease: the multiple parallel hits hypothesis. Hepatology 52, 1836–1846.

Timsit, Y.E., Negishi, M., 2007. CAR and PXR: the xenobiotic-sensing receptors. Steroids 72, 231–246.

Venkatesh, M., Mukherjee, S., Wang, H., Li, H., Sun, K., Benechet, A.P., Qiu, Z., Maher, L., Redinbo, M.R., Phillips, R.S., Fleet, J.C., Kortagere, S., Mukherjee, P., Fasano, A., Le Ven, J., Nicholson, J.K., Dumas, M.E., Khanna, K.M., Mani, S., 2014. Symbiotic bacterial metabolites regulate gastrointestinal barrier function via the xenobiotic sensor PXR and Toll-like receptor 4. Immunity 41, 296–310.

Wada, T., Gao, J., Xie, W., 2009. PXR and CAR in energy metabolism. Trends Endocrinol. Metab. 20, 273–279.

Wang, X.L., Suzuki, R., Lee, K., Tran, T., Gunton, J.E., Saha, A.K., Patti, M.E., Goldfine, A., Ruderman, N.B., Gonzalez, F.J., Kahn, C.R., 2009. Ablation of ARNT/HIF1β in liver alters gluconeogenesis, lipogenic gene expression, and serum ketones. Cell Metab. 9, 428–439.

Waxman, D.J., Azaroff, L., 1992. Phenobarbital induction of cytochrome P-450 gene expression. Biochem. J. 281 (Pt 3), 577–592.

Weber, L.W., Lebofsky, M., Stahl, B.U., Gorski, J.R., Muzi, G., Rozman, K., 1991. Reduced activities of key enzymes of gluconeogenesis as possible cause of acute toxicity of 2,3,7,8-tetrachlorodibenzo-p-dioxin (TCDD) in rats. Toxicology 66, 133–144.

Wei, P., Zhang, J., Egan-Hafley, M., Liang, S., Moore, D.D., 2000. The nuclear receptor CAR mediates specific xenobiotic induction of drug metabolism. Nature 407, 920–923.

Wieneke, N., Hirsch-Ernst, K.I., Kuna, M., Kersten, S., Püschel, G.P., 2007. PPARα-dependent induction of the energy homeostasis-regulating nuclear receptor NR1i3 (CAR) in rat hepatocytes: potential role in starvation adaptation. FEBS Lett. 581, 5617–5626.

Xie, W., Barwick, J.L., Downes, M., Blumberg, B., Simon, C.M., Nelson, M.C., Neuschwander-Tetri, B.A., Brunt, E.M., Guzelian, P.S., Evans, R.M., 2000. Humanized xenobiotic response in mice expressing nuclear receptor SXR. Nature 406, 435–439.

Xie, W., Radominska-Pandya, A., Shi, Y., Simon, C.M., Nelson, M.C., Ong, E.S., Waxman, D.J., Evans, R.M., 2001. An essential role for nuclear receptors SXR/PXR in detoxification of cholestatic bile acids. Proc. Natl. Acad. Sci. USA. 98, 3375–3380.

Xie, W., Uppal, H., Saini, S.P., Mu, Y., Little, J.M., Radominska-Pandya, A., Zemaitis, M.A., 2004. Orphan nuclear receptor-mediated xenobiotic regulation in drug metabolism. Drug Discov. Today 9, 442–449.

Yang, X., Downes, M., Yu, R.T., Bookout, A.L., He, W., Straume, M., Mangelsdorf, D.J., Evans, R.M., 2006. Nuclear receptor expression links the circadian clock to metabolism. Cell 126, 801–810.

Yarushkin, A.A., Kachaylo, E.M., Pustylnyak, V.O., 2013. The constitutive androstane receptor activator 4-[(4R,6R)-4,6-diphenyl-1,3-dioxan-2-yl]-N,N-dimethylaniline inhibits the gluconeogenic genes PEPCK and G6Pase through the suppression of HNF4α and FOXO1 transcriptional activity. Br. J. Pharmacol. 168, 1923–1932.

Yoshinari, K., Takagi, S., Sugatani, J., Miwa, M., 2006. Changes in the expression of cytochromes P450 and nuclear receptors in the liver of genetically diabetic db/db mice. Biol. Pharm. Bull. 29, 1634–1638.

Younossi, Z.M., Baranova, A., Ziegler, K., Del Giacco, L., Schlauch, K., Born, T.L., Elariny, H., Gorreta, F., VanMeter, A., Younoszai, A., Ong, J.P., Goodman, Z., Chandhoke, V., 2005. A genomic and proteomic study of the spectrum of nonalcoholic fatty liver disease. Hepatology 42, 665–674.

Zhai, Y., Wada, T., Zhang, B., Khadem, S., Ren, S., Kuruba, R., Li, S., Xie, W., 2010. A functional cross-talk between liver X receptor-α and constitutive androstane receptor links lipogenesis and xenobiotic responses. Mol. Pharmacol. 78, 666–674.

Zhang, J., Huang, W., Chua, S.S., Wei, P., Moore, D.D., 2002. Modulation of acetaminophen-induced hepatotoxicity by the xenobiotic receptor CAR. Science 298, 422–424.

Zhang, Y.-K.J., Yeager, R.L., Klaassen, C.D., 2009. Circadian expression profiles of drug-processing genes and transcription factors in mouse liver. Drug Metab. Dispos. 37, 106–115.

Zhou, J., Zhai, Y., Mu, Y., Gong, H., Uppal, H., Toma, D., Ren, S., Evans, R.M., Xie, W., 2006. A novel pregnane X receptor-mediated and sterol regulatory element-binding protein-independent lipogenic pathway. J. Biol. Chem. 281, 15013–15020.

Zhou, C., Poulton, E.J., Grun, F., Bammler, T.K., Blumberg, B., Thummel, K.E., Eaton, D.L., 2007. The dietary isothiocyanate sulforaphane is an antagonist of the human steroid and xenobiotic nuclear receptor. Mol. Pharmacol. 71, 220–229.

Zhou, J., Febbraio, M., Wada, T., Zhai, Y., Kuruba, R., He, J., Lee, J.H., Khadem, S., Ren, S., Li, S., Silverstein, R.L., Xie, W., 2008. Hepatic fatty acid transporter Cd36 is a common target of LXR, PXR, and PPARγ in promoting steatosis. Gastroenterology 134, 556–567.

Zhou, C., King, N., Chen, K.Y., Breslow, J.L., 2009. Activation of PXR induces hypercholesterolemia in wild-type and accelerates atherosclerosis in apoE deficient mice. J. Lipid Res. 50, 2004–2013.

Zysset, T., Wietholtz, H., 1988. Differential effect of type I and type II diabetes on antipyrine disposition in man. Eur. J. Clin. Pharmacol. 34, 369–375.

Index

'*Note*: Page numbers followed by "f" indicate figures and "t" indicate tables.'

A

Absorption, distribution, metabolism, and
    elimination (ADME), 2–3
N-acetyltransferase (NAT)-mediated acetylation, 97
Alpha-1-glycoprotein (AGP), 195
Aryl hydrocarbon receptor, 258–259, 264–266
ATP-binding cassette B1, 150

B

Bacterial infections, 35
    helicobacter pylori, 35
    sepsis, 35
Bilateral renal ischemiaereperfusion, 97–98
Breast cancer resistance protein
    brain, 69–70
    intestine, 69
    liver, 69
    placenta, 70

C

Cardiorenal syndrome (CRS), 141–143, 142t, 144t
Cardiovascular (CV) disease
    cardiac arrest
        therapeutic hypothermia, 146–147
    cardiohepatic syndrome, 143–146
    CRS, 141–143, 142t, 144t
    cytochrome P450, 147
    defined, 140–147
    heart failure, 140
    overview, 139–140
    pharmacogenomics, 148–153
        acute coronary syndrome and percutaneous
          coronary intervention, 150–151
        angiotensin receptor blockers and
          CYP2C9, 149
        β-blockers and CYP2D6, 148–149
        carboxylesterase-1, 152
        clopidogrel and CYP2C19, 150–151
        CYP2C9, 151–152
        dabigatran, 152
        digoxin and ATP-binding cassette B1, 150

drug metabolism variation, 148
dyslipidemia, 152–153
heart failure and hypertension, 148–150
HMG-CoA reductase inhibitors, 152–153
SLCO1B1, 152–153
thromboembolism, 151–152
VKORC1, 151–152
warfarin, 151–152
Cerebral blood flow (CBF), 118–119
Cerebral hypoperfusion, 118–119
Chlorzoxazone metabolism, 126–127
Chronic heart failure (CHF), 10–11
Chronic inflammation, 75
    cholestasis, 79–80
    chronic renal failure, 79
    inflammatory bowel disease, 77–78
    rheumatoid arthritis, 75–77
Chronic kidney disease (CKD), 141
    altered drug metabolism mechanism, 105–107
        modified gene/protein expression, 105–106
        posttranslational modifications, 106–107
    conventional drug-dosing paradigm, 92–93, 93f
    drug metabolism, 94–98, 94t
    experimental models, metabolism in, 95–97, 95t
        acute kidney injury, 97–98, 98t
    human drug metabolism, 99–104
        altered nonrenal clearance, 99–102, 100t
        phenotypic assessments metabolic pathways,
          102–104
    nonrenal clearance, 93
Chronic obstructive pulmonary disease (COPD), 9
Chronic renal failure (CRF), 94
Constitutive androstane receptor, 259–260, 266–270
Crigler–Najjar syndrome, 8
CRS. *See* Cardiorenal syndrome (CRS)
Cytochrome P450 enzymes, 147, 184–190
    bacterial infections, 35
    cardiac arrest, 127–132, 129t–130t
    critical care medicine, 115–116
    epoxyeicosatrienoic acids (EETs), 116–117,
        117f

Cytochrome P450 enzymes (*Continued*)
20-hydroxyeicosatetraenoic acid (20-HETE), 116–117, 117f, 121–123
liver disease, 32–33
metabolism, 117, 118f
parasitic infections, 35–37
sterile inflammation, 37–43
stroke, 118–123, 120t–121t
traumatic brain injury, 123–127, 124t–125t
viral infections, 33–35

D
Dapsone metabolisms, 126–127
Digoxin, 150
Dihydroxyeicosatetraenoic acids (DHETs), 116–117
Direct competitive inhibition, 106–107
Doxorubicin, 101
Drug metabolism
absorption parameters, 8–10
gastric emptying time changes, 9–10
gut and lung surface area changes, 9
permeability changes, 8–9
blood flow to organs, 10–11
disease effects on, 5–8
chronic kidney disease, 7
genetic disorders, 8
infection and inflammation, influence of, 6–7
liver disease, 6
overview, 4f, 5–8
protein binding changes, 11–13
protein therapeutics, 12–13
small molecules, 12
transporter expression, disease effects on, 13–14
Drug-metabolizing enzymes (DMEs)
disease-dependent drug–drug interactions, 43–44
inflammatory mediators
proinflammatory cytokines, 29–31
TLR ligands, 28–29
inflammatory response, 23–27
acute phase proteins, 25–27
APP genes, 25
cytokines, 25–27
initiation, 23–24, 24f
interleukin-1, 26–27
interleukin-6, 25–26, 26f
liver innate immune response, 27
propagation, 24–25
tumor necrosis factor α, 27
P450 enzymes
bacterial infections, 35
liver disease, 32–33
parasitic infections, 35–37
sterile inflammation, 37–43
viral infections, 33–35

regulation mechanisms, 44–47
posttranscriptional mechanisms, 46–47
transcriptional mechanisms, 44–46
Drug transporters
ABC efflux transporters, 62–75, 63f–65f
bile salt export pump, 72–73
breast cancer resistance protein
brain, 69–70
intestine, 69
liver, 69
placenta, 70
chronic inflammation, 75
cholestasis, 79–80
chronic renal failure, 79
inflammatory bowel disease, 77–78
rheumatoid arthritis, 75–77
multidrug resistance-associated proteins, 70–72
liver, 71–72
other tissues, 72
P-glycoprotein, 63–68
brain, 67–68
intestine, 66–67
kidney, 67
liver, 65–66
placenta, 68
solute carrier uptake transporting family, 73–75
kidney, 74
liver, 74
placenta, 74–75
Dyslipidemia, 152–153

E
Enzyme-linked immunosorbent assay (ELISA) analysis, 124–126
Epoxyeicosatrienoic acids (EETs), 116–117, 117f
Erythromycin breath tests (EBTs), 95–96
EST. *See* Estrogen sulfotransferase (EST)
Estrogen
steroid sulfatase (STS), 241–243, 242f
chronic liver disease, 248–251, 250f
homeostasis, 248–251, 250f
Estrogen sulfotransferase (EST), 241–243, 242f
homeostasis, 241–243, 242f
liver ischemia and reperfusion response, 245–247, 247f
sepsis response regulation, 243–245, 244f

F
Fasting plasma glucose (FPG), 162
Flavin-containing monooxygenase-5 (FMO5), 168–169
Flurbiprofen metabolisms, 126–127
Food and Drug Administration (FDA), 103

G

Gastrointestinal tract (GIT), 4
Gene Expression Omnibus database (GSE32504), 248—249
Glucose metabolism, 268—269

H

Hemorrhagic strokes, 118
Hepatic drug metabolism
    hepatic blood flow, 194—195
    hepatic drug transporters, 196
    intrinsic hepatic clearance, 184—194
        CYP1A2, 184—186
        CYP2A, 186—187
        CYP3A, 189—190
        CYP2C, 187—188
        CYP2D, 188
        CYP2E, 188—189
        hepatic CYP enzymes, 182f, 184—190, 185t
        hepatic UGT enzymes, 190—194, 191t—192t, 193f
    ontogeny, 181—183
    plasma protein binding, 195
Hepatic metabolism, 103—104
HMG-CoA reductase inhibitors, 152—153
Hormonal regulation, pregnancy, 221—230
    cortisol, 227—230, 229t
    estrogen, 221—225, 223t—224t
    growth hormone, 227t—228t, 226—227
    placental lactogen, 226—227, 227t—228t
    progesterone, 225—226
    prolactin, 226—227, 227t—228t
20-hydroxyeicosatetraenoic acid (20-HETE), 116—117, 117f, 121—123
Hypoalbuminemia, 12

I

Immunotherapy, 7
Inflammation
    acute inflammation, 60—61
        drug transporters, 62—75
        models, 61—62
        overview, 59—60
Insulin resistance, 261—262, 263f, 268—269
Intensive care units (ICUs), 115—116
Intracerebral hemorrhage (ICH), 118
Isoform-specific probe drugs, 102

K

Ketoconazole, 10

L

Lipid metabolism, 266—268
Lipopolysacharide (LPS), 243

L (continued)

Lipoprotein homeostasis, 269—270
Lipoprotein lipase (LPL), 171

M

Meglitinides
    drug-metabolizing enzyme coding gene mutations, 164
    drug transporter coding gene mutations, 164—165
    mechanism, 163—164
    other gene mutations, 165—166
R-mephenytoin (R-MP), 103
S-mephenytoin (S-MP), 103
Mephenytoin metabolism, 126—127
Metformin
    drug transporter coding gene mutations, 166—168
    mechanism, 166
    other gene mutations, 168—169
Model-based approach, 193
Morphine, 194
Multidrug resistanceeassociated protein 2 (MRP2), 196

N

Neurogenic differentiation 1 (NEUROD1), 165
Nonalcoholic fatty liver disease, 260—261
Nonalcoholic steatohepatitis, 260—261
Nuclear receptor subfamily 1 group I member 2 (NR1I2), 165

O

Oral antidiabetic drugs (OADs)
    DPP-4 inhibitors, 173
    α-glucosidase inhibitors, 172
    meglitinides
        drug-metabolizing enzyme coding gene mutations, 164
        drug transporter coding gene mutations, 164—165
        mechanism, 163—164
        other gene mutations, 165—166
    metformin
        drug transporter coding gene mutations, 166—168
        mechanism, 166
        other gene mutations, 168—169
    overview, 158, 159t—161t
    sulfonylureas
        drug-metabolizing enzyme coding gene mutations, 161—162
        mechanism, 158
        other gene mutations, 162—163
    thiazolidinediones, 169—172
        drug-metabolizing enzyme coding gene mutations, 169—170
        drug transporter coding gene mutations, 170

Oral antidiabetic drugs (OADs) (*Continued*)
    mechanism, 169
    other gene mutations, 170−172
Organic anionetransporting polypeptide 1B1
    (OATP1B1), 164
Organic anion transporter proteins (OATPs), 12
Organic anion transporting polypeptide (OATP), 195

P
Paired box gene 4 (PAX4), 165
Parasitic infections
    amebiasis, 37
    leishmaniasis, 37
    liver flukes, 37
    malaria, 35−36
    schistosomiasis, 36−37
P-glycoprotein, 63−68
    brain, 67−68
    intestine, 66−67
    kidney, 67
    liver, 65−66
    placenta, 68
Pharmacokinetics (PK), 92
Physiological adaptations, pregnancy, 208−210
    filtration, 210
    gastrointestinal function, 210
    hematology, 209
    hemodilution, 209
    hemodynamics, 209
    renal blood flow, 210
    respiratory, 209
Posttranscriptional mechanisms
    microRNAs, 47
    nitric oxide, 46−47
Pregnancy
    bile acid metabolism and transport, 230−234, 231f
        phase I, 231
        phase II, 231
        transcription factors, 232−233
        translational implications, 233−234
        transport, 232
    extrahepatic regulation, 230
    hepatic phase I enzymes, 210−215
        carboxylesterase, 214−215
        cytochrome P450, 210−214, 211t−213t
        paraoxanase enzymes, 214−215
    hepatic phase II enzymes, 215−218
        GST, 217
        sults, 217−218
        uridine 50-diphosphoglucuronosyltransferases
           (UGT), 215−217, 216t
    hepatic transporters, 218−220
        ATP-binding cassette (ABC) transporters, 218−220

        solute carrier (SLC) transporters, 218
    hormonal regulation, 221−230
        cortisol, 227−230, 229t
        estrogen, 221−225, 223t−224t
        growth hormone, 226−227, 227t−228t
        placental lactogen, 226−227, 227t−228t
        progesterone, 225−226
        prolactin, 226−227, 227t−228t
    nuclear receptors, 220−221
    overview, 208
    physiological adaptations, 208−210
        filtration, 210
        gastrointestinal function, 210
        hematology, 209
        hemodilution, 209
        hemodynamics, 209
        renal blood flow, 210
        respiratory, 209
Pregnane X receptor, 259−260, 266−270
Proinflammatory cytokines, 105
    cytokines, 31
    cytokines participation, 30−31
    hepatocytes, 29−30
    interleukin-6, 30−31
    interleukin-1β, 31
    tumor necrosis factor α, 27
Propofol, 194−195
Pyrrolidine dithiocarbamate (PDTC), 243−244

R
Reboxetine, 100−101
Rosiglitazone, 169−170

S
SAH. *See* Subarachnoid hemorrhage (SAH)
SLCO1B1, 152−153
Solute carrier organic anion transporter family
    member 1B1 (SLCO1B1), 164
Solute carrier uptake transporting family, 73−75
    kidney, 74
    liver, 74
    placenta, 74−75
Sparteine, 103
Specificity protein 1 (SP1), 168
Sterile inflammation
    arthritis, 38
    behçet disease, 42
    bone marrow transplantation, 43
    cancer, 39−42, 40t−41t
    congestive heart failure (CHF), 43
    critical illness, 43
    lupus erythematosus, 42
    vaccination, 37−38

Steroid sulfatase (STS), 241–243, 242f
Subarachnoid hemorrhage (SAH), 118–121
Sulfonylureas
    drug-metabolizing enzyme coding gene mutations, 161–162
    mechanism, 158
    other gene mutations, 162–163
Sulfotransferases (SULT), 242

T
Therapeutic hypothermia
    cardiac arrest, 146–147
Thiazolidinediones, 169–172
    drug-metabolizing enzyme coding gene mutations, 169–170
    drug transporter coding gene mutations, 170
    mechanism, 169
    other gene mutations, 170–172
Thromboembolism, 151–152
TLR ligands
    toll-like receptor 2, 28
    toll-like receptor 3, 28–29
    toll-like receptor 4, 28
Transcriptional mechanisms
    direct repression, 24f, 26f, 44
    epigenetic mechanisms, 46
    induction mechanisms, 45–46
    positive transcription factors
        downregulation, 45
        inhibitory binding, 45
Tumor necrosis factor alpha (TNF), 6

U
Uremic toxins, 105
Uridine diphosphate-glucuronosyltransferase (UGT)-mediated glucuronidation, 97

V
Viral infections
    hepatitis A virus, 35
    hepatitis B virus, 34
    hepatitis C virus, 33–34
    human immunodeficiency virus, 33
    influenza, 33

W
Warfarin, 151–152

X
Xenobiotic receptors
    drug metabolism, 258–260
        aryl hydrocarbon receptor, 258–259
        Circadian CLOCK and Feeding–Fasting switch, 263–264
        diabetes effect and insulin resistance, 261–262, 263f
        energy metabolism, 260–264
        nonalcoholic fatty liver disease, 260–261
        nonalcoholic steatohepatitis, 260–261
        pregnane X receptor and constitutive androstane receptor, 259–260
    energy metabolism
        aryl hydrocarbon receptor, 264–266
        drug metabolism, 264–270
        glucose metabolism, 268–269
        insulin resistance, 268–269
        lipid metabolism, 266–268
        lipoprotein homeostasis, 269–270
        pregnane X receptor and constitutive androstane receptor, 266–270
    overview, 258

Z
Zidovudine, 194